D0268114

Unexplained somatic complaints c

A. Have you been bothered by continuing aches or pains or other physical complaints for which a cause has not been found (eg nausea, vomiting, diarrhoea, shortness of breath, chest pain, headaches, abdominal pain)? . . . . ❏

If YES to any of the above, continue below

1. Have you seen more than one doctor for these problems? . . . . ❏

2. Have you seen any specialists about these problems? . . . . ❏

3. Have you experienced these pains or different physical problems for longer than six months? . . . . ❏

4. Low mood or loss of interest or pleasure? . . . . ❏

5. Worried, anxious or tense? . . . . ❏

6. How much alcohol do you drink in a typical week (number of standard drinks/week)? . . ❏

Summing up

Positive to A and also to at least one from 1 to 3, and negative to 4, 5 and 6: consider **unexplained somatic complaints**. . . . . ❏

B. Because of these problems during the past month:

- how many days were you unable fully to carry out your usual daily activities? . . . . ❏
- how many days did you spend in bed in order to rest? . . . . ❏

Anxiety checklist

A. **Feeling tense or anxious?** . . . . ❑

B. **Worrying a lot about things?** . . . . ❑

If YES to any of the above, continue below

1. Symptoms of arousal and anxiety? . . . . ❑   1.

2. Experienced intense or sudden fear unexpectedly or for no apparent reason? . . . . ❑   2.
   - Fear of dying . . . . ❑
   - Fear of losing control . . . . ❑
   - Pounding heart . . . . ❑
   - Sweating . . . . ❑
   - Trembling or shaking . . . . ❑
   - Chest pains or difficulty breathing . . . . ❑
   - Feeling dizzy, light-headed or faint . . . . ❑
   - Numbness or tingling sensations . . . . ❑
   - Feelings of unreality . . . . ❑
   - Nausea . . . . ❑

3. Experienced fear/anxiety in specific situations? . . . . ❑
   - Leaving familiar places . . . . ❑
   - Travelling alone, eg train, car, plane . . . . ❑
   - Crowds/confined places/public places . . . . ❑

4. Experienced fear/anxiety in social situations? . . . . ❑
   - Speaking in front of others . . . . ❑
   - Social events . . . . ❑
   - Eating in front of others . . . . ❑
   - Worry a lot about what others think, or self-conscious? . . . . ❑

Summing up

ive to A, B and 1, recurring regularly, negative to 2, 3 and 4:

   n of **generalized anxiety** . . . . ❑

   1 and 2: indication of **panic disorder** . . . . ❑

   2 and 3: indication of **agoraphobia** . . . . ❑

   3 and 4: indication of **social phobia** . . . . ❑

ng housework or household tasks? . . . . ❑

cial activities, seeing friends? . . . . ❑

emembering things? . . . . ❑

WHO Guide to Mental and Neurological Health in Primary Care

A Guide to Mental and Neurological Ill Health in Adults, Adolescents and Children

Adapted for the UK, with permission, from *Diagnostic and Management Guidelines for Mental Disorders in Primary Care: ICD-10 Chapter V Primary Care Version*

Editorial Board:
Rachel Jenkins, Charles Warlow, Barry Lewis, Albert Persaud, Debbie Sharp, Eric Taylor, Jim Thompson, André Tylee, Nigel Wellman and Edzard Ernst

Overall direction of the project by Rachel Jenkins

The WHO Collaborating Centre for Research and Training for Mental Health gratefully acknowledges financial support towards the development costs of the second edition of the Guide from the Department of Health

The Royal Society of Medicine Press gratefully acknowledges financial support for printing costs from an unrestricted educational grant from Janssen-Cilag Ltd.

UK Edition

World Health Organization Collaborating Centre
for Research and Training for Mental Health

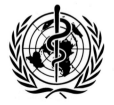

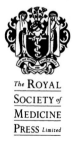

The ROYAL
SOCIETY *of*
MEDICINE
PRESS *Limited*

Adapted with permission from *Diagnostic and Management Guidelines for Mental Disorders in Primary Care: ICD-10 Chapter V Primary Care Version*, published on behalf of the World Health Organization by Hogrefe & Huber Publishers, Rohnsweg 25, D-37085 Goettingen, Germany. ISBN 0 88937 148 2.
© 1996 World Health Organization

Published by the Royal Society of Medicine Press Ltd., 1 Wimpole Street, London W1G 0AE, UK
Tel: +44 (0)20 7290 2921
Fax: +44 (0)20 7290 2929
E-mail: publishing@rsm.ac.uk
Website: http://www.rsmpress.co.uk

First edition 2000
Reprinted 2001 (three times)
Second edition 2004
Reprinted 2005

The authors have worked to ensure that all information in this book containing drug dosages, schedules and routes of administration is accurate at time of publication and consistent with standards set by the World Health Organization (WHO) and the general medical community. As medical research and practice advance, however, therapeutic standards may change. For this reason, and because human and mechanical errors sometimes occur, we recommend that readers follow the advice of a physician who is directly involved in their care or in the care of a member of their family.

Reference this book as: Jenkins, R ed. *WHO Guide to Mental and Neurological Health in Primary Care*. London: Royal Society of Medicine Press, 2004.

British Library Cataloguing in Publication Data
A catalogue record is available for this book from the British Library

ISBN 1 85315 560 8

The clinical terms (the Read Terms) is Crown Copyright data reproduced by permission of the Controller of Her Majesty's Stationery Office.

Phototypeset by Phoenix Photosetting, Chatham, Kent, UK
Printed in India by Replika Press Pvt. Ltd

Foreword to second edition

We are very pleased to support this second edition of the WHO Guide to Mental and Neurological Health in Primary Care.

The first edition was a UK adaptation of the *'Diagnostic and Management Guidelines for Mental Disorders in Primary Care: ICD-10 Chapter V'*. Published in 2000, it has proved invaluable as an easily and speedily accessible guide for primary-care professionals to help in the immediate care of their patients, as a resource for more detailed reference, and as a source of practical information and resources for patients and their families. It is also commonly found on the desks of staff in specialist teams, although it was primarily written for the needs of general practice. The first edition was signposted in the National Service Framework for Mental Health as a resource to help primary-care teams in delivering Standard Two and contributing to Standard Four. It has sold out several times, going into a number of reprints, and has now sold over 30 000 copies. In addition it is in the National Electronic Library and receives around 200 hits a day.

Last year, the Department of Health commissioned a second edition. Like the first edition, it has been produced by an extensive process of review and consensus, involving primary-care professionals, specialists, academics and user organizations. The result is an expanded guide which reflects not only recent developments in the evidence base and clinical practice, but also includes whole new sections on the disorders of childhood and adolescence, personality disorder, self harm, domestic violence and sexual abuse. The issues of differential diagnosis and/or comorbidity with mental disorders and a number of common neurological disorders including stroke are also included altogether making this a truly comprehensive resource for generalist staff.

We hope that use of this guide continues to support good practice, communication and collaboration among all who have a stake in the provision of good primary mental and neurological health care.

Lesley Southgate
President, The Royal College of General Practitioners

Sylvia Denton
President, The Royal College of Nursing

Charles Warlow
Chair, Royal College of Physicians Joint Specialty Committee for Neurology

Mike Shooter
President, The Royal College of Psychiatrists

André Tylee
Professor of Primary Care Mental Health, Institute of Psychiatry and Chairman, Primary Care Board, National Institute for Mental Health in England

Foreword to first edition

In a general-practice surgery, every third or fourth patient seen has some form of mental disorder. Levels of disability among primary care patients with such disorders are high; greater on average than disability among primary care patients with common chronic diseases such as hypertension, diabetes, arthritis and back pain. Simple effective treatments are available for many mental disorders and some can be treated more effectively than hypertension or coronary heart disease.

Changes in the way services are provided also emphasize the importance of primary care as a setting for mental healthcare. Over the past 30 years, the number of hospital beds available for people with mental illness has fallen, while the number of GPs and psychiatrists has risen. A direct result is that people in primary care need to work more closely with those in mental health services. Good mental healthcare is a collaborative effort. The Primary Care Team includes practice nurses, district nurses, health visitors, counsellors, clinical psychologists and school nurses, as well as GPs, all of whom may have a role in mental healthcare. The Community Mental Health Team may include nurses, occupational therapists, clinical psychologists, social workers and support workers, as well as psychiatrists. Families and friends, self-help and community groups also provide crucial support to people with a whole range of mental disorders: from transient distress to enduring psychotic illness. They need to talk to one another, respect each other's contribution and jointly agree who will provide which service to whom.

Despite this, mental health provision has been dogged, perhaps more than any other area of healthcare, by differences in how we think about mental health and the words we use. This makes it hard for different professional groups and non-professionals to talk to each other. This handbook aims to ameliorate this problem. The diagnostic and management summaries it contains are based on the *WHO International Diagnostic and Management Guidelines for Mental Disorders in Primary Care* and are wholly compatible with ICD-10 Chapter V — which is the diagnostic framework used by psychiatric professionals. However, they have been simplified and extensively piloted to ensure that they are relevant to primary care. They also include management strategies based on a multiaxial approach — emphasizing the information needs of patients and their families, and simple social and psychological management strategies, in addition to medication.

This handbook is a resource that can be used in a number of ways. It can be used by an individual practitioner in the care of his or her patients; it can also be used by a primary care team or a primary care organization (or local health group) to review, jointly with mental health teams, the service they provide, identifying gaps and training needs or developing locally appropriate, shared criteria for referral to specialist services. We support this handbook and hope that its use improves communication and collaboration between all who have a stake in the provision of good primary mental healthcare.

Dr John Cox
President, Royal College of Psychiatrists

Claire Rayner
President, Patient's Association

Professor André Tylee
Director, Royal College of General Practitioners Unit for Mental Health Education in Primary Care

Christine Hancock
President, Royal College of Nursing

Contents

Child & adolescent disorders

Learning disability   199

A guide to Mental Health Act assessments

The Children Act 1989   217

Template chart for local resources: statutory services   218

Template chart for local resources: voluntary agencies   219

Resource directory   220

Mental health in your practice: what does your practice offer?   243

Suggested issues for practice and PCT audit   245

Psychological therapies: what are they?   247

Complementary and alternative treatment   249

Training for primary care teams in mental health skills   250

Interactive summary cards: for discussion by professional and patient together

Contents of CD-ROM

Self-help leaflets for patients

Management strategies useful for a large number of disorders
01-1 Solving problems and achieving goals
01-2 Learning to relax
01-3 Coping with side-effects of medication

Acute stress reaction
02   Psychological responses to traumatic stress: what to expect

Alcohol misuse
03-1 Responsible drinking guidelines
03-2 How to cut down on your drinking

Anxiety disorders
04-1 Anxiety
04-2 Dealing with anxious thinking
04-3 Overcoming particular fears (phobias)
04-4 Helping someone else overcome a phobia
04-5 Distinguishing between a panic attack and a heart attack

Bipolar disorder
05-1 What is bipolar disorder?
05-2 Lithium toxicity

Depression
06-1 Depression
06-2 Activity planning
06-3 Dealing with depressive thinking
06-4 Ideas for enjoyable things to do

Drug misuse
07-1 Harm minimization: advice about safer drug use
07-2 Sample drug-use diary

Psychosis
08-1 What you may expect after an acute episode of psychosis
08-2 What is schizophrenia?
08-3 Coping with difficult behaviour
08-4 Early warning signs form

Sleep problems
09   Sleep problems

Unexplained physical complaints
10   Unexplained physical problems

Checklists for professionals
11-1 CAGE questionnaire: screen for alcohol misuse
11-2 AUDIT questionnaire: screen for alcohol misuse

Connections between ICD-10 PHC and ICD-10 Chapter V

To load CD-Rom, place CD in CD-drive, double click on the 'My Computer' icon, double click on the relevant CD-drive (often but not always the 'D' drive).

Introduction

Mental and neurological disorders are common and affect all of us at some time; if not ourselves directly, then friends, family or work colleagues. Most people who suffer from mental and neurological disorders and who receive care from the health service do so in primary care. Mental health problems alone are now implicated in one in four primary care consultations, making mental health consultations second only to those for respiratory infections.[1,2] Depression is the third most common reason for consultation in UK general practice.[3] While most people suffer from mild conditions and recover quickly, a significant proportion suffer from chronic conditions[4] that cause moderate or high disability.[5]

Standard two of the *National Service Framework for Mental Health*[6] emphasizes the importance of primary care in addressing mental health problems:
'Any service user who contacts their primary healthcare team with a common mental health problem should:

- have their mental health needs identified and assessed
- be offered effective treatments, including referral to specialist services for further assessment, treatment and care, if they require it.

To achieve this standard, each primary care group will need to work with the support of specialized mental health services to:

- develop the resources within each practice to assess mental health needs
- develop the resources to work with diverse groups in the population
- develop the skills and competencies to manage common mental health problems
- agree the arrangements for referral for assessment, advice or treatment and care
- have the skills and necessary organizational systems to provide the physical healthcare and other primary care support needed, as agreed in their care plan, for people with severe mental illness.

This *Guide* has been written to support primary care professionals, primary care organizations and local user groups in their delivery of primary care mental and neurological health services. It deals with conditions frequently seen in primary care, or those that have a high profile, and which can be managed effectively by general practitioners (GPs) and their teams, supported as appropriate by secondary care.

In response to feedback from the first edition and the sister publication *Mental Health in Primary Care in Prison*,[7] this second edition now includes guidelines on the following:

- Child and adolescent mental health disorders and related problems, such as bullying and abuse. For a few conditions, for example, Obsessive-compulsive disorder, Psychosis and Sleep problems, the special considerations particular to children and adolescents have been described at the end of the relevant adult guideline.
- Common neurological disorders for example, Epilepsy, Headache and Stroke. We received a number of requests to include common neurological conditions, and so have included several relatively common ones, which can all be severe and disabling.
- Domestic violence, Personality disorder, Postnatal disorders, Obsessive-compulsive disorder, Self-harm and Smoking cessation.

Most of the conditions in the *Guide* are classified in ICD-10; however, a few are behavioural problems that do not have an ICD-10 code. These, for example domestic violence, are included here at the request of the Department of Health (DoH). The current ICD-10 classification does not distinguish between adults and children and adolescents for disorders such as depression.

Personality disorder is encoded under ICD-10 but was omitted from the first edition

1

because it was not included in the original World Health Organization (WHO) version. It is included in this second edition at the request of the DoH.

A brief summary of how to diagnose and manage each condition is given. The management summaries include information for the patient, advice and support, descriptions of treatment methods and indications for liaison and specialist referrals. They are supported by a linked set of resources to help the GP or other members of the primary care team to carry out the management strategies recommended, as well as contact details of relevant voluntary sector organizations.

Resources provided

- **A mental disorder assessment guide.** This is to help the assessment of depression, anxiety, alcohol, sleep, chronic tiredness and unexplained somatic complaint disorders. To use it, start with the screening questions (in top boxes) to explore the presence of disorders and, if the disorder exists, you can continue below.
- **Interactive summary cards.** For the six disorders most common in primary care (depression, anxiety, alcohol problems, chronic fatigue, unexplained somatic complaints and sleep problems) two-page summaries have been produced. One page contains information for the practitioner, the other for the patient. With less information than the main summaries, but easier to see at a glance, they are meant to be used interactively. These are found on pages 283–295. They may be printed out and mounted on either side of a piece of A4 card and used to facilitate discussion between practitioner and patient within a consultation.
- **A linked set of patient information and self-help leaflets** giving more information about the treatment and self-help strategies recommended. These can be found on the CD-ROM and can be printed out and given to patients to help reinforce the information that has been provided and also to encourage active participation in treatment. These vary in length and complexity. Some (eg the one-page problem-solving sheet) are suitable for use by GPs in a consultation. Others are more likely to be used by another member of the team, such as a counsellor, nurse or physiotherapist. The notation 'R: x–x' appears in the text of a summary to indicate the existence of a linked resource leaflet. Leaflets from the first edition have been retained because they have been found to be useful, but leaflets have not been provided for those guidelines new to the second edition, owing to the plethora of information now available on the Internet.

Why were these disorders chosen?

The book contains categories of mental disorders from the ICD-10 classification, together with some common neurological disorders from the ICD-10 classification and several common behavioural issues, such as domestic violence and bullying, which are not all classified in ICD-10.

The choice of disorder is the result of a selection process that reflects the following:

- The public health importance of disorders (ie prevalence, morbidity or mortality, disability resulting from the condition, burdens imposed on the family or community, healthcare resources needed). A few rarer disorders (eg Attention-deficit/hyperactivity disorder and Autism spectrum disorders) are included because of their high profile.
- Availability of effective and acceptable management (ie interventions with a high probability of benefit to the patient or their family are readily available within primary care and are acceptable to the patient and the community).
- A reasonable consensus exists among primary care practitioners and mental and neurological health professionals regarding the diagnosis and management of the condition.
- Cross-cultural applicability (ie suggestions for identification and management are applicable in different cultural settings and healthcare systems).
- Consistency with the main ICD-10 classification scheme (ie each diagnosis and

diagnostic category corresponds to those in ICD-10) (with the exception of those problems included at the request of the DoH — domestic violence and bullying, which do not have ICD-10 codes).

We have also set out the clinical terms equivalents for the ICD-10 codes, because these are more widely used in UK primary care practice than are the ICD-10 codes.

All disorders included in this *Guide* are fairly common in primary care settings and a management plan can be written for each of them.

The section for people with a learning disability has been identified separately because recognition and treatment of mental disorders present particular difficulties in this group and because mainstream adult mental health services might not be appropriate for them. Learning disability is, of course, not itself a mental disorder.

How the diagnostic and management summaries were developed

WHO developed a state-of-the-art classification of mental disorders for use in clinical practice and research. The *Tenth Revision of the International Classification of Diseases* (ICD-10) has many features that improve the diagnosis of mental disorders. To extend this development to primary care settings, where most patients with mental disorders are seen, diagnostic and management guidelines were combined into the WHO book *Diagnostic and Management Guidelines for Mental Disorders in Primary Care (ICD-10 Chapter V, Primary Care Version)*. The guidelines were developed by an international group of GPs, family physicians, mental health workers, public health experts, social workers, psychiatrists and psychologists with a special interest in mental health problems in primary care, using a consensus approach. The WHO guidelines were field-tested extensively in over 40 countries by 500 primary care physicians to assess their relevance, ease of use and reliability. This work has been published.[8,9] Field trials using the WHO guidelines continue in various centres in the UK.

The diagnostic and management summaries in this handbook consist of the WHO's *International Diagnostic and Management Guidelines for Mental Disorders in Primary Care*, specially adapted (and updated) for use in the UK. They have been adapted in two stages. The first stage of adaptation to the UK setting was carried out in south Bristol by a panel of GPs and multidisciplinary representatives from community mental health teams, using a consensus methodology. A randomized controlled trial of the handbook in 30 general practices in Bristol, measuring a range of mental health outcomes, was then carried out.

The second stage of adaptation was carried out by a national editorial team coordinated by the WHO Collaborating Centre of the Institute of Psychiatry, London. The evidence base was reviewed (see below), information on psychological therapies was added, and information (on the Mental Health Act of England and Wales 1983, community resources and referral) was made appropriate to the whole of the UK. Representatives of primary care nurses, counsellors and patient groups have made valuable suggestions to ensure that the information is accessible to these important groups. Several rounds of consensus, including a conference, were held to debate the amendments and agree the final text. Names of those involved in this stage can be found in the Acknowledgements section.

For this second edition, guidelines from the first edition and new guidelines have been produced and reviewed by specialists, GPs and the voluntary sector, intensively discussed at a consensus meeting, and piloted by a number of general practices.

The interactive handy cards, the diagnostic checklist and most of the patient information leaflets were produced by the WHO's Division of Mental Health and Prevention of Substance Abuse, and endorsed by The Collegium Internationale Neuro-Psychopharmacologicum, the World Organization of National Colleges, Academies and Associations of General Practitioners and Family Physicians, and the World Psychiatric Association. Some of the leaflets were developed by the WHO Collaborating Centre for Mental Health and Substance Abuse, as part of the Treatment Protocol Project.

The evidence on which the summaries are based

Where applicable, the diagnosis sections are based on the ICD-10 classification of disorders. ICD-10 is itself a consensus document and has been tested for reliability. The ICD-10 PHC diagnostic criteria presented here have been tested among primary care professionals to check for validity and usefulness.

References supporting evidence have been given in line with the principles set out below.

Treatments (medication and psychotherapies)

The recommendations about medication are all in line with the *British National Formulary* (BNF). Where recommendations about medication are unexceptional and in line with both the BNF and established practice for many years, references have not been given.

References have been reserved for key statements about medication and about particular psychotherapies or for statements about which evidence and opinion are divided. It should be noted that most studies have been carried out in a secondary care setting. The mixed presentations of disorders found in primary care means that, generally speaking, both drugs and psychotherapies prove less efficacious (compared with placebo) in that setting than they do in more selected groups in secondary care. We have therefore included some discussion about what the evidence says, along with the references to the studies themselves. A grading of the quality of the evidence is also provided in the reference/notes section. Where possible, evidence has been given from Cochrane reviews, high-quality published reviews and meta-analyses or randomized controlled trials (RCTs). Discussions have been held with experts and authors of key areas of research.

The evidence has been graded as follows:

Strength of the evidence supporting the recommendation

A = Good evidence to support
B = Fair evidence to support
C = Preliminary evidence to support.

Quality of the evidence supporting the statement

I = Evidence obtained from a meta-analysis of trials, including one or more well-designed RCTs
II = Evidence obtained from one well-designed RCT
III = Evidence obtained from one or more controlled trials, without randomization
IV = Evidence obtained from one or more uncontrolled studies
V = Opinions of respected authorities, based on clinical experience, descriptive studies or reports of expert committees. Occasionally, the 'respected authorities' comprise collective patient experience. Where this is the case, it is clearly stated.

Where a qualitative review of previously published literature without a quantitative synthesis of the data is referenced, it has been graded in accordance with the type of studies the review includes.

Information and advice

The sections on 'Essential information for patient and family' and 'General management and advice to patient and family' are primarily the result of consensus. There are no trials comparing the outcome of patients given different sorts of advice by their GP. The advice itself is based on a mixture of evidence and consensus of professionals and/or patients. A small number of references to supporting evidence have been given.

Referrals

The referral recommendations are based on consensus and will vary from place to place, depending on services available in all care sectors.

Connections to ICD-10 and NHS Clinical terms

The first edition of this guide was based on the disorders included in *the ICD-10 PC Chapter V Mental Disorders Classification, Primary Care Version,* is a 'user-friendly' version of the Tenth revision of the *International Classification of Diseases (ICD-10) Chapter V.* For practical reasons, the ICD-10 PC is a condensed version of *ICD-10 Chapter V* for easy application in busy primary care settings. It has 23 categories instead of 457. It intends to cover the universe of mental disorders seen in primary care settings in adults. As a classification, it is 'jointly exhaustive and mutually exclusive'. It may seem simplistic; however, it corresponds to the ICD-10 main volume. A chart that shows the grouping of the detailed specialty-adaptation categories into ICD-10 PC categories can be found on the CD-ROM. This second edition now includes a number of additional neurological, behavioural and childhood disorders. Where possible, relevant ICD-10 codes and NHS clinical terms have been given. A table of these codes can be seen below.

Adult mental and neurological disorders

Disorder	ICD-10 codes	Clinical terms codes
Acute psychotic disorders	F23.9	Eu23
Adjust disorder (including acute stress reaction)	F43.2	Eu43.2
Alcohol misuse	F10	Eu10
Bereavement and loss	Z63.4	E2900
Bipolar disorder	F31	Eu31
Chronic fatigue syndrome/ME	G93.3	
Chronic mixed anxiety and depression	F41.2	Eu41.2
Chronic psychotic disorders	F29	Eu20
Delirium	F05	EU05
Dementia	F03	Eu00.
Depressive disorders	F32	Eu32
Dissociative (conversion) disorder	F44	Eu44
Domestic violence (new)		
Drug use disorders	F10–19 Mental and behavioural disorders due to use of: F11 opioids F12 cannabinoids F13 sedatives or hypnotics F14 cocaine F15 other stimulants, including caffeine F16 hallucinogens F17 tobacco F18 volatile solvents F19 multiple drug use and use of other psychoactive substances	Eu11
Eating disorders	F50	Eu50
Epilepsy	G40.9	F25
Fatigue states, including Chronic fatigue	F48.0	Eu46.0
Generalized anxiety	F41.1	Eu41.1
Headache (including migraine)	R51 headache G43.9 migraine G44.2 tension G44.0 cluster	R040

5

Adult mental and neurological disorders – *continued*

Disorder	ICD-10 codes	Clinical terms codes
Motor Neurone disease	G12.2	F152
Multiple Sclerosis	G35	F20
Panic disorder	F41.0	Eu41.0
Parkinson's disease	G20	F12
Perinatal disorders		Eu204
Personality disorder (new)	F60	Eu6
Phobic disorders	F40	Eu40
PTSD	F43.1	Eu43.1
OCD (new)	F42	Eu42
Sexual disorders (female)	F52	Eu52
Sexual disorders (male)	F52	Eu52
Sleep problems (insomnia)	F51	Eu51
Smoking (new)	F17.1	(no letter 137) i.e. it's a symptom not a disorder
Stroke	I64	G66
Suicide/deliberate self-harm (new)	X60–X84	U2...
Unexplained somatic complaints	F45	Eu45
Learning disabilities	F81.9	Eu70

Children and adolescents mental and neurological disorders

Disorders of childhood and adolescence F90–F98. Where there is no appropriate code within F90–F98, we have used the relevant adult codes.

Disorder	ICD-10 codes	Clinical terms codes
Abuse	Z61.4	ZV612
Autism	F84.0	Eu840
Asperger	F84.5	Eu845
Anxiety (including phobia, OCD)	F93	Eu93
Conduct disorder	F91	Eu91
Bullying at school		13ZF.
Bereavement and loss	Z63.4	Eu2900
Adolescent psychosis	No ICD code of adolescence	No clinical term for adolescent
Substance misuse	No ICD code for adolescence	No clinical term for adolescent
Depression in adolescence	No ICD code for adolescence	
ADHD	F90.0	Eu97
CFS and somatoform	G93.3	Eu460
Deliberate self-harm/suicide	X60-X84	Eu2
Eating disorders	F98.2 This code is for infants and early childhood only	Eu50
Mental health needs of refugee and asylum seeking children	No ICD code	No clinical term

How an individual practitioner might use the handbook

In the field trials, some practitioners used the summaries as a resource between consultations, to look something up. Others used the summaries interactively with the patient, to help explain the disorder and determine a treatment plan. The appropriate information and/or self-help leaflet can be printed out and given to the patient to reinforce what is said in the consultation. The interactive summary cards can be used to facilitate discussion between clinician and patient.

The leaflets have been placed on the CD-ROM as Word.doc files. GPs or other team members, with regular access to a computer, could install the handbook on their computer, for ease of searching. The *Guide* is also available on the web (see www.http://www.mentalneurologicalprimarycare.org).

The handbook will also be a useful resource for educators of all generalist doctors and nurses.

Patients as partners

It is important that patients and practitioners can negotiate a shared understanding of the problems before a management plan can be agreed. A successful dialogue during which patient and professional communicate well with each other can have a positive effect on clinical outcome[10,11] and will help to reduce the well-documented high level of 'non-adherence', where people do not take the medication prescribed for them. However, medication is not the only answer, particularly for mild to moderate conditions. A partnership approach will help patients to understand ways in which they might be able to help themselves, and to make informed decisions about what is likely to work for them. Many patients want to take part in making decisions about their treatment and care, and they can get better faster or cope better with chronic illness if they are actively involved in understanding what is happening to them and making changes to their lifestyle. This approach applies to all patients, but shared understanding is particularly important where the cultural background of the professional is different from that of the patient.

Beyond diagnosis: a multi-axial approach

Patients presenting in primary care with mental and neurological health problems often have a mixture of social, psychological, physical, medical and emotional difficulties, and primary care mental and neurological health services are being encouraged to develop a multi-axial approach, rather than a purely medical perspective.

A short diagnostic summary cannot capture the full clinical and social picture. The summaries focus on the diagnosis, severity and duration of the disorder, as an essential prerequisite of a specific management plan. The practitioner needs to add to this as appropriate, assessing other factors such as social stresses linked to the symptoms, physical health, past and family history and the level of social support available from family and friends. Some of the management strategies outlined in the summaries and patient leaflets are easier for a patient who has good support from family or friends. Increased professional support could perhaps then be focused on those people who are more isolated.

Care programme approach

Where a patient is receiving care from mental health services, they should have a care programme (comprising a written care plan reviewed regularly, and a named key worker who coordinates their care). There needs to be clear agreement about which elements of care are provided by the GP and which by the community team. Both team and patient need to know what the plan is in case of relapse, and have names and telephone numbers of the key people (eg the care manager, identified on the front page of the notes) to contact easily to hand. The summaries assume that these discussions will take place.

Medication

Wherever possible, medication recommendations refer to a class of drug or a generic form. Where it is considered particularly useful or important, however, examples of particular named drugs are given. *These are examples only and should not be taken as a WHO recommendation to prescribe that particular brand.* The summaries should be read in conjunction with the BNF, which contains information on every individual drug.

Self-help

Self-help materials are mostly available as books or computer programs and are designed to teach patients how to self-manage and overcome their symptoms and related difficulties. It is becoming increasingly relevant in the management of chronic mental illness, not least because of the shortage in some areas of staff trained in providing psychotherapy both in primary and secondary care. Self-help has a number of advantages:[12]

- Patients like the idea of working on their own to deal with their problems and reducing their reliance on professional help.
- Taking responsibility for self-management may be empowering, which could be particularly important in dealing with feelings of hopelessness and despair. It also gives the patient a sense of control over their illness.
- Self-help can be returned to as often as the patient wants and whenever they want.
- Self-help is more accessible and may be able to provide some psychological and social support without delay.

Self-help material is included in the resource section of the guidelines although there is still limited evidence for the effectiveness of individual publications. For some people and some conditions, self-help could be an effective option.[12]

Contact details of voluntary organizations, many of which run local groups, are also given at the end of each guideline.

How a practice team, primary care organization or local health group might use the handbook

Team working and training within primary care

The diagnostic and management summaries assume that the resources available to primary care teams will vary widely. The 'advice to patient and family' can be offered by any member of the primary care team who has suitable training and skills. GP, nurse, health visitor, school nurse, practice counsellor and psychologist may all contribute, and discussion to clarify the roles of each is essential. It will be helpful to carry out an assessment of the mental health skills available within the team (see page 243), in order to make best use of the skills of all members and inform practice training plans, as well as referral to external resources. This assessment could be done by an individual practice, group of practices or whole primary care organization. A list of sources of training in primary mental healthcare and a checklist of ways a practice can respond to the mental health needs of its patients is provided on pages 250–253.

Team working between primary, secondary and social care

Primary care organizations could use the diagnostic and management summaries as a basis to discuss and agree locally appropriate referral criteria with specialist mental health services. It would be possible to work on a small number of disorders or to work through all of them. This process might reveal gaps in local services, for example in the availability of structured psychological therapies for affective disorders. Primary care organizations might wish to consider ways of addressing these gaps in their service development plans or in the commissioning plans of training consortia.

Some primary care organizations or health groups might wish to go further and address systems for communication between primary and secondary care. Effective communication is a crucial element of effective care, and misunderstandings between primary care and mental health services are very common. Primary care teams and community mental health teams may wish to meet to agree the roles, responsibilities and expectations of each member of both teams. Various different models have been tried, to improve communication as a whole and to improve the care of patients who are 'shared' between primary and secondary care in particular. Joint case registers of people with chronic mental illness is one of these. Suggested issues for practice and PCT audit are on pages 245–246.

Information about resources in the community

The primary care organization or local health group might also produce a locally appropriate directory of services and community resources (see pp. 220–242) and distribute this to its constituent practices. The information could be made available on computer or in a wall-chart format. Consideration will need to be given to regular updating of this information. Within each practice, the practice manager or other team member will need to consider how best to make the patient information leaflets available, how to obtain and insert the information about local services into the template wall charts and how best to make that information readily accessible to patients and all members of the practice team.

Localization

The diagnostic and management summaries are meant as a resource to local agencies. They will only be useful if they are actively disseminated at practice, primary care organization and Health Authority levels. Local adaptation of the summaries to suit particular situations is welcomed and encouraged. To make it possible, we have included the text of the summaries in electronic format on a CD-ROM. Locally adapted pages can be inserted easily, where required. A template, to be filled in with information about local services, is provided on page 250. Although the diagnostic information is standard and used internationally, the management plan, particularly the referral criteria, will vary according to the availability of services locally and the training of healthcare workers.

The copyright for the diagnostic and management summaries rests with the WHO. Where a primary care organization or local health group is producing locally adapted guidelines using the WHO summaries as a basis, we ask that you contact Professor Rachel Jenkins at the WHO Collaborating Centre Office, Institute of Psychiatry, De Crespigny Park, Denmark Hill, London SE5 8AF, UK. Tel: +44 20 7848 0383; E-mail: r.jenkins@iop.kcl.ac.uk.

Special considerations

Needs of carers

The term 'carer' is taken to mean informal caregivers, rather than those providing care in the statutory sector on an organized and paid basis. Three in five people in the UK will become carers at some point in their lives.[13] The strain on these informal carers, particularly those living with the ill person or young carers who may feel burdened by the responsibility, can be severe, resulting in an increased risk of both physical and mental ill health. Many carers have to give up work in order to look after their relative or friend, and become economically disadvantaged and socially isolated. Carers often have no respite from their role, and may find themselves experiencing feelings such as frustration, resentment, guilt, anger, fear, depression and loneliness.

Those caring for people with a mental or even neurological illness often have the additional burden of stigma to cope with. About half of those with severe mental illness live with family or friends, and many others receive considerable support from them. It is important to review how the carer is managing and to encourage them to find ways of reducing the stress on them. Self-help groups, day care and respite care can all help. The assessment and care planning process should take the mental and physical health of carers, and their ability to continue coping, into account. Standard Six of the Mental Health National Service Framework lays down guidance to ensure that health and social services assess the needs of carers who provide regular and

9

substantial care for those with severe mental illness, and provide care to meet their needs.

Checklist for GPs and primary care teams:[6]

- Have you identified those patients who are carers, and patients who have a carer?
- Do you check carer's physical and emotional health whenever a suitable opportunity arises?
- Do you routinely tell carers that they can ask social services for an assessment of their own needs?
- Do you always ask patients who have carers whether they are happy for health information about them to be told to a carer?
- Do you know whether there is a carers' support group or carers' centre in your area, and do you tell carers about them?

Carers are entitled to an assessment of the needs of the carer (under the Carer's Recognition and Services Act 1995) and this can be requested from the local Social Services department. This advice is relevant to all chronic disorders; it is not repeated on each individual summary.

Gender[14]

Service delivery should be sensitive to gender issues. Mental and neurological ill health is common in both men and women, but important differences in the family and social context of their lives, and the presentation and type of their mental illness, will influence their care and treatment needs:

- Anxiety, depression (particularly during pregnancy and in the post-partum period) and eating disorders are more common in women; substance misuse and antisocial personality disorder are more common in men.[15]
- Women often present with a combination of physical complaints and mental ill health, and the former can obscure the recognition of the latter.
- Women must often juggle many roles; the competing demands of work and major responsibility for the home and care of children and other dependent family members can place them under considerable stress and have an adverse effect on their mental health.
- Women are more vulnerable to poverty and social isolation, which are strongly associated with mental ill health. They generally outlive their partners, are less likely to work, and if they do, earn less; they are less likely to own a car. Lone mothers are three times more likely to be depressed than any other group of women.
- Women are more likely to experience abuse and violence, both in childhood and adulthood.
- Women who have children under 5, particularly if lone parents, are vulnerable to mental ill health.
- A woman's mental ill health may have wide repercussions for children and other dependent relatives.
- Although psychological therapies should be considered routinely for mental health problems, women are more likely to be prescribed psychotropic drugs, particularly antidepressants, anxiolytics and hypnotics, than men. This practice will also have consequences for fetal development or breast-feeding, or the effectiveness of contraception.

Specific issues identified for general practice in *Women's Mental Health: Into the Mainstream* are as follows:

- Recognition and appropriate treatment of depression (including postnatal depression), anxiety and eating disorders, such as increased availability of psychological treatments and appropriate use of antidepressants/anxiolytics.
- Review of long-term prescribing, particularly of benzodiazepines.

- Detection and management of issues/conditions that often remain hidden — self-harm, substance misuse, and experience of violence and abuse.
- Access to support services, such as benefits or housing advice.

Among the key components of assessment and care planning should be experience of violence and abuse, caring responsibilities, social and economic support, physical health, ethnicity and culture (see below), dual diagnosis with substance misuse, and risk assessment and management.

Ethnicity and culture[16,17]
Service delivery must also be sensitive to different cultural needs.

- Minority ethnic communities are over-represented among the lower social classes, with higher unemployment rates and poorer housing and employment status, all of which are associated with poor mental health. In addition, in some cases racism might contribute to increased levels of stress and distress.
- If the practitioner and patient are from different ethnic groups, there is a higher likelihood that misunderstanding may occur, particularly if they hold different explanatory models of illness. It is important to ensure that adequate time is set aside for these consultations.
- There may be a language barrier between doctor and patient:
  — The use of skilled professional interpreters wherever possible is essential. Family and friends fulfilling this role is not adequate — accurate interpretation cannot be relied upon, confidentiality cannot be maintained, a patient may not reveal details of their problem, and issues such as domestic violence might remain hidden.
  — Access to fully trained medical translators is often limited, and the practitioner must be extra vigilant, using clear terminology and giving precise instructions and guidance both to the translator and the patient.
  — Simple language and open questions should be used as much as possible to enhance understanding; for example, 'What do you think caused your problem?' 'Why do you think it started when it did?' 'What does your illness do to you?'
  — Two-way checking (ie that the practitioner has understood the patient's concerns and the patient has understood and agreed to the management plan) is important to avoid misunderstanding.
  — Written information prepared with the translator can be invaluable for patients to take home with them.
- Cultural differences:
  — Different beliefs about causes, interventions and outcomes of illness will affect when and how people present, and how they understand messages about treatment. Exploring these issues will maximize the ability to address a patient's concerns and ensure as collaborative a relationship as possible.
  — How symptoms are displayed may be different; for example, depression might manifest as severe headaches. It is helpful to consider this possibility, while never assuming the case.
  — Patients might not share a Western view of the difficulties they experience. Psychological problems are often described by terms — for example, nervous breakdown, broken hearted — that might not be understood by non-Western cultures or *vice versa*.
  — Familiarity with Western methods of treatment should never be assumed; for example, the concept of 'talking as a cure' might not be accepted. Clear explanations and rationales for these should be given.
  — Families might make use of other health resources within their communities (eg a herbal Chinese practitioner) before consulting their GP.
- Children:
  — Most children from ethnic minority communities will have been born in the UK, but many might need to negotiate two different cultures. It can be very complex

for a child to manage two possibly conflicting belief systems (ie the family and the peer group). Worries and stresses arising from this are unlikely to be volunteered and thought needs to be given to asking about these, if appropriate.

— These children may be at higher risk of experiencing bullying and racism.

Refugees and asylum seekers

In addition to the points listed above under Ethnicity and culture, those working in primary healthcare need to be aware of the following:

- the range of experiences that asylum seekers and refugees may have suffered in their home country
- the likelihood that they will experience ongoing difficulties of poverty and isolation in the host country
- asylum cases may take years to be resolved, a process that can have psychological implications.

It is estimated that over 50% of refugees suffer from a mental health disorder.[18] Common symptoms in refugees and asylum seekers include depression, anxiety, panic attacks, agoraphobia, sleep difficulties, loss of memory and poor concentration, and there are high levels of Post-traumatic stress disorder.[19] Patients may also be suffering bereavement following the loss of, or the loss of contact with, friends and relatives.

They have often been exposed to traumatic events (eg torture, imprisonment, rape and war), and separation from family and friends. They then face further stress and anxiety from relocation to a country where they may have no contacts, common language or knowledge of social and legal systems. They might have a lingering distrust of authority. They could suffer racial discrimination and abuse, as well as poverty and social isolation. Experiences en route to and within the host country should not be overlooked as factors that could undermine mental health. Problems can stem predominantly from the dislocating experience of seeking refuge, rather than from experiences in the home country. Often facilitation of support groups and even just the opportunity for social meeting can be of benefit by reducing feelings of social isolation.

Asylum cases can take a long time to be resolved fully, and until refugee status is granted the asylum process can have an impact on the progress and maintenance of mental health problems.

Further support to primary-care teams

1. The NHS Plan 2000 contained two targets specifically focused on supporting primary care — first, new graduate primary-care workers and second, gateway workers. Information about both of these is on the Department of Health website (www.doh.gov.uk/mentalhealth).
2. The National Institute of Mental Health for England established a primary care mental health programme in Spring 2003, see NIMHE for further details. The aim is capacity-building in primary care around service modernization to improve access, choice and responsiveness of services.
3. There is a Doctors' Support Network (www.dsn.org.uk) and Doctors' Support Line (www.doctorssupport.org) for doctors who need anonymous and confidential support and/or information. The Doctors' Support Line (0870 7650001) is staffed Monday–Friday from 6pm to 10pm; in addition it is staffed on Tuesdays from 9am to 2pm and 6pm to 11pm, and Sundays from 10am to 10pm. The Doctors' Support Network can be contacted on 07071 223372.

References

1 McCormick A, Fleming D, Charlton J. *Morbidity Statistics from General Practice: Fourth National Study 1991–1992*. London: HMSO, series MB5 no 3, 1995.

2 Ustun TB, Sartorius N. *Mental Illness in General Healthcare: An International Study*. Chichester: John Wiley & Sons, 1995.

3 NHS Centre for Reviews and Dissemination. Improving the recognition and management of depression in primary care. *Effect Healthcare Bull* 2002, 7(5): 1–12.

4 Mann A, Jenkins R, Besley E. The twelve-month outcome of patients with neurotic illness in general practice. *Psychol Med* 1981, 11: 535–550.

5 Meltzer H, Gill B, Petticrew M, Hinds K. *OPCS Survey of Psychiatric Morbidity in Great Britain Report 3: Economic Activity and Social Functioning of Adults With Psychiatric Disorders*. London: HMSO, 1995.

6 Department of Health. *National Service Framework Mental Health*. London: HMSO, 1999.

7 *Mental Health in Primary Care in Prison*. London: Royal Society of Medicine Press Ltd, 2002.

8 Goldberg D, Sharp D, Nanayakkara K. The field trial of the mental disorders section of ICD-10 designed for primary care (ICD10-PHC) in England. *Family Practice* 1995, 12(4): 466–473.

9 Ustun B, Goldberg D, Cooper J *et al*: A new classification of mental disorders based on management for use in primary care (ICD10-PHC). *B J Gen Pract* 1995, 45: 211–215.

10 Kai J, Crosland A. Perspective of people with enduring mental ill health from a community-based qualitative study. *Br J Gen Pract* 1995 2001, 51: 730–737.

11 Peck E, Gulliver P, Towel D. Information, consultation or control: user involvement in mental health services in England at the turn of the century. *J Mental Health* 2002, 11(4): 441–451.

12 Lewis G, Anderson L, Araya R *et al*. Self-help interventions for mental health problems. www.nimhe.org.uk.

13 Carers UK. *It Could Be You*. London: Carers UK, 2001.

14 Department of Health. *Women's Mental Health: Into the Mainstream*. London: Department of Health, 2002.

15 Gold J. Gender differences in psychiatric illness and treatments: a critical review. *J Nervous Mental Dis* 1998, 186(12): 769–775.

16 Bhugra D (ed). *Mental Health Practice in Multicultural Britain*. London: Royal College of Psychiatry, 1999.

17 Malek M, Joughin C. *Mental Health Services for Minority Ethnic Children and Adolescents*. London: Jessica Kingsley, 2003.

18 Bruntland GH. Mental health of refugees, internally displaced persons and other populations affected by conflict. *Acta Psychiatrica Scand* 2000, 102(3): 159–161.

19 Burnett A, Peel M. Health needs of asylum seekers and refugees. *BMJ* 2001, 322: 544–547.

Prevalence of mental disorders

Prevalence of mental disorders in men and women (rates per 1000)[1]

	Men	Women	Total
All neurosis	135	194	164
Mixed anxiety and depression	68	108	88
Generalized anxiety	43	46	44
Depression	23	28	26
Phobias	13	22	18
Obsessive-compulsive disorder	9	13	11
Panic	7	7	7
Personality disorder	54	34	44
Obsessive-compulsive	26	13	19
Avoidant	10	7	8
Schizoid	9	8	8
Paranoid	12	3	7
Borderline	10	4	7
Antisocial	10	2	6
Dependant	2	0	1
Schizotypal	0	1	1
Histrionic	–	–	–
Narcissistic	–	–	–
Probable psychosis	6	5	5

Adults with a neurotic disorder are more likely to be:
- women
- aged between 35 and 54
- separated or divorced
- living as a one-person family unit or as a lone parent
- have no formal educational qualifications
- have a predicted IQ of <90
- come from social class V
- economically inactive
- tenants of Local Authorities and Housing Associations
- have moved two to three times in past two years
- living in an urban area
- also suffering from a physical complaint.

Prevalence of substance abuse in men and women[1]

Alcohol abuse	Men	Women	Total
Hazardous drinking (score 8 and over on audit) in the past year	38%	15%	26%
Mean audit score	7	4	5
Illicit substance use in past year of any drug – All ages – 20–24-year-olds	8% 37%	13% 29%	11% 33%

Prevalence of mental disorders in children and adolescents by gender (rates per 1000)[2]

	Boys aged 5–10	Girls aged 5–10	Boys aged 11–15	Girls aged 11–15	All children and adolescents
Anxiety	3.2	3.1	3.9	5.3	3.8
Depression	0.2	0.3	1.7	1.9	0.9
Conduct disorder	6.5	2.7	8.6	3.8	5.3
Hyperkinetic disorder	2.6	0.4	2.3	0.5	1.4
Less common disorders, eg Obsessive-compulsive disorder, phobia	0.8	0.2	0.5	0.7	0.5
Any disorder	10.4	5.9	12.8	9.6	9.5

Children with a mental disorder are more likely to:
- live in social-sector housing
- live with a lone parent
- have problems with the police
- have bereavement
- have poor physical health
- have a parent with no educational qualifications
- have both parents unemployed
- have mentally-ill parents.

Prevalence of mental disorders by ethnic group (rates per 1000 adult population)[3]

	White	Irish	Black Caribbean	Bangladeshi*	Indian	Pakistani
All neurosis	158	185	173	126	181	196
Mixed anxiety and depression	109	116	120	90	119	123
Generalized anxiety	14	30	13	6	12	14
Depression	29	28	24	19	38	45
Phobias	18	·21	15	7	8	21
Obsessive-compulsive disorder	9	10	10	10	12	17
Panic	5	17	13	13	21	12

*After adjusting for differences in age structure between the different ethnic groups, only the lower prevalence of all neuroses in Bangladeshi women compared with white women remained statistically significant.

References

1 Singleton N, Bumpstead R, O'Brien M *et al. Psychiatric Morbidity Among Adults Living in Private Households, 2000*. Office of National Statistics. London: The Stationery Office, 2001. URL http://www.statistics.gov.uk/downloads/theme_health/psychmorb.pdf.

2 Meltzer H, Gatward R, Goodman R, Ford T. *Mental Health of Children and Adolescents in Great Britain*. London: The Stationery Office, 2000. URL http://www.statistics.gov.uk/downloads/theme_health/KidsMentalHealth.pdf.

3 Sproston K, Nazroo J. *The Ethnic Minority Psychiatric Morbidity Survey*. London: The Stationery Office, 2002.

Incidence and prevalence of some neurological conditions

Condition	Incidence: number of new cases per 100,000 that develop each year	Prevalence: total number of people per 100,000	Source
Alzheimer's disease/dementia	25,000 per 100,000 in over 65 year olds	1,000	Alzheimer's Society based on ONS population estimate 1996
CJD	per 100,000		Alzheimer's Society
vCJD	27 new cases in year 2000	101 cases since 1995	Alzheimer's Society
Epilepsy	80 per 100,000	500	Clinical Standards Advisory Group *Services for people with epilepsy* 2000 and *Lancet;* 336: 1267–71
Headache	Migraine 400 per 100,000[1]	15,000 (8,000,000)	1. Steiner TJ et al Epidemiology of migraine in England **Cephalalgia**
	Cluster Headache 4 per 100,000[2]	100	2. Olesen J, Goadsby PJ, Cluster Headache and related conditions in Olesen J (Ed) *Frontiers in Headache Research* Vol 9, OUP 1999
	Paroxysmal Hemicrania[3]	10	3. Goadsby PJ, Lipton RB. A review of paroxysmal hemicranias *Brain* 1997; 120: 193–209
	Chronic Migraine[4] Chronic tension-type headache[4]	3,000	4. Silberstein SD et al, *Headaches in Primary Care* Oxford/Isis Medical Media 1999
Motor neurone disease	4 per 100,000	7 per 100,000	Motor Neurone Disease Association
Multiple Sclerosis		144 (85,000)	MS Society and MS Research Trust — estimates based on UK area studies and international data
Myalgic Encephalomyelitis (ME)		300–500	Dowsett E G, Richardson J The *Epiemiology of Myalgic Encephalomyelitis (ME) in the UK 1919–1999* Evidence submitted to the All Party Parliamentary Group of MPs on ME 23.11.1999
Parkinson's disease		200	Parkinson's Disease Society — advice from medical adviser

General referral criteria for adults with mental health problems

A main objective of the *WHO Guide to Mental Health in Primary Care* is to extend the expertise of the primary-care clinician and improve the cooperation and communication between primary care and secondary mental health services. With this understanding, the following guidelines have been prepared.
Referral to secondary mental health services should be considered in the following circumstances:

- where the patient is displaying signs of suicidal intent or if there seems to be a risk of harm to others
- where the patient is so disabled by their mental disorder that he/she is unable to leave his/her home, look after his/her children or fulfil other activities of daily living
- where the GP requires the expertise of secondary care to confirm a diagnosis or implement specialist treatment
- where the GP feels that the therapeutic relationship with the patient has broken down
- where primary care interventions and voluntary/non-statutory options have been exhausted
- where there is severe physical deterioration of the patient
- where particular psychotropic medication is required (eg clozapine, lithium or donezepil)
- if the patient requests a referral.

When making a referral to secondary mental health services, Social Services or voluntary/non-statutory organizations, the GP should:

- have access to a local resource directory
- consider coordination issues around the referral (eg Care Programme approach, care manager)
- consider implications for the continuing care of the physical health of the patient.

All referral criteria constitute part of the guideline for that particular disorder and assume that, as far as possible, the guideline for diagnosis and management has been followed.

Referral letters
It is helpful if referral letters include as many as possible of the following:

- patient's name, hospital number (if known), date of birth, address and telephone number
- presenting complaint
- reason for referral, including whether for advice only for GP to manage, or for psychiatrist to manage
- past psychiatric history
- background
- current mental state
- current medication, details of any medication tried in the past few weeks
- drugs and alcohol history
- details of carers and significant others.

General referral criteria for children and adolescents with mental health problems

Referral to Child and Adolescent Mental Health Services (CAMHS) should be considered in the following circumstances:

- where the young person is displaying signs of suicidal intent
- where assessment of the young person is not suitable for primary care (eg psychotic symptoms, attention-deficit/hyperactivity disorder [ADHD])
- where the young person is likely to require medication, and treatment is not suitable for primary care (eg depressive disorder in a child, severe obsessive-compulsive disorder)
- where the young person is so disabled that they cannot go to school or see friends
- if the young person or parent requests a referral
- where primary care or other options have failed.

Referral to other agencies may be necessary. Criteria include the following:

- any form of suspected abuse (Social Services)
- young person who is no longer in the care of their parents and is at risk of harming themselves or others (Social Services)
- young person who is at risk of harming other children or adults (Police)
- young person with school attendance problems (Educational Welfare Service)
- young person with suspected specific learning disability (school special needs department)
- young person with a substance misuse problem (local young person's drug and alcohol services).

Voluntary organizations can often help children and adolescents with emotional or behavioural problems — for example, the NSPCC, local parental support groups (eg ADHD groups) and parenting groups run through programmes such as Sure Start. When making a referral to other service providers, the GP should have access to a local resource directory.

Referral letters

It is helpful if referral letters include as many as possible of the following:

- patient's name, hospital number (if known), date of birth, address and telephone number
- presenting complaint
- reason for referral, including who wants what from whom
- past medical and psychiatric history or contact, including whether this child or a sibling has been seen by CAMHS before
- family and social background
- developmental history
- current medication
- any drug and alcohol history
- details of carers and significant others.

General recommendations for prescribing in children and adolescents

In child and adolescent psychiatry, medication usually forms only part of the treatment, although it is finding a larger place.[1] Most youngsters who have mental disease severe enough to require medication will generally be referred to a specialist. However, much of the repeat prescribing will be done by GPs. In order to take over the prescribing, the GP will want to know:

- the diagnosis
- what the medicine is being used for
- the form of the medicine
- the dose and frequency
- anticipated side-effects, special precautions and possible interactions
- who will be responsible for any monitoring required and for changing or stopping the medication.

The informed use of unlicensed medications or licensed medicines for unlicensed applications is deemed to be necessary in paediatric practice. The checking of doses can be problematic but formularies such as *Medicines for Children* should be consulted.[2] As youngsters can be very sensitive to psychotropic medicines, a cautious approach is recommended. Some monitoring may be necessary, such as blood pressure, liver function tests or ECG, depending on the choice of drug. Start with a low dose and increase it slowly, monitoring for beneficial and adverse effects. Avoid rapid withdrawal.

Another problem area concerns the taking of drugs with abuse potential, eg methylphenidate and dexamphetamine, to school. The use of controlled-release preparations will avoid the need for lunchtime doses. If a midday dose is necessary, arrangements with the local community should be made so that a separately labelled dose can be taken at school.[3]

References

1 Bramble D. The use of psychotrophic medications in children: a British view. *J Child Psychol Psychiatry* 2003, 44: 169–179.

2 Royal College of Paediatrics and Child Health. *Medicines for Children*. London: RCPCH Publications, 1999.

3 Bellingham C. Starting out right: the children's NSF. *The Pharmaceutical Journal* 2003, 270: 539–540.

Key to signs used in the main text

R: 1–1	A resource relevant to the point in the text may be found on the CD-ROM — usually a patient information and self-help leaflet or a diagnostic questionnaire. (R = resource. The number refers to the number of the leaflet or questionnaire.)
F23	This is the code in *ICD-10 PC Chapter V* (ie the International Classification of Diseases, primary care version, mental health chapter. A full list of how the primary care codes relate to the codes from the main ICD-10 volume can be found on the CD-ROM.
G30	This is the code in ICD-10 VI, neurology chapter.
Eu23	This is the clinical term (or closest equivalent).

The '#' code is used in *ICD-10 PC Chapter V* only. It refers to 'condensed' codes. For example, 'F00# — Dementia' refers to all different types of dementia listed in F00–F03 and their related fourth and fifth character codes.

Reference numbers: A grading of the evidence can be found in the reference section. The evidence has been graded as described in the Introduction.

Eu – mental health clinical terms

F – neurological clinical terms

G – cardiovascular clinical terms

ADULT DISORDERS

Acute psychotic disorders — F23.9

Includes first-episode psychosis, acute schizophrenia-like psychosis, acute delusional psychosis and other acute and transient psychotic disorders
(Clinical term: Acute and transient psychotic disorders Eu23)

Presenting complaints
Patients might experience:

- hallucinations, eg hearing voices when no one is around, seeing visions
- strange beliefs or fears
- apprehension, confusion
- perceptual disturbances.

Families and other agencies (eg schools, social workers, probation and housing services) might ask for help with behaviour changes that cannot be explained, including strange or frightening behaviour (eg withdrawal, suspiciousness, self-neglect and threats).

Young adults, particularly when experiencing their first episode of psychosis, may present with persistent changes in functioning, behaviour or personality (eg multiple physical complaints, withdrawal or deterioration in social, academic or occupational performance), but without florid psychotic symptoms.

Diagnostic features
Recent onset of:

- hallucinations (false or imagined sensations, eg hearing voices when no one is around, seeing visions)
- delusions (firmly held ideas that are often false and not shared by others in the patient's social, cultural or ethnic group, eg patient believes they are being poisoned by neighbours, receiving messages from the television, or being looked at by others in some special way)
- disorganized or strange speech
- agitation or bizarre behaviour
- extreme and labile emotional states.

These symptoms could be preceded by a period of deteriorating social, occupational and academic functioning.

Differential diagnosis
- Physical disorders that can cause psychotic symptoms include:
  — drug-induced psychosis (especially stimulants such as amphetamines or cocaine)
  — alcoholic hallucinosis
  — infectious or febrile illness
  — **'Epilepsy — G40, G41'** (or other organic intracranial pathology).
- Refer to **'Delirium — F05'** for other potential causes.

To exclude organic conditions, it might be useful to perform urine and blood investigations.

Essential information for patient and family
- Agitation and strange behaviour can be symptoms of a mental disorder.
- Acute episodes often have a good prognosis,[1] and it is important to remain positive in view of the proven benefits of treatments and support from various agencies.

- The long-term course of the illness can be difficult to predict from an acute episode.
- The sooner psychotic symptoms are identified and treated, the better the outcome.
- Advise patient and family about the importance of medication, how it works and possible side-effects (R: 1–3).
- Continued treatment may be needed for several months after symptoms resolve.
- Psychotic illness is no one's fault and has nothing to do with parenting.

If the patient requires treatment under the Mental Health Act, advise family about related legal issues (see guide to the Mental Health Acts, pages 204–216).

General management and advice to patient and family (R: 8–1)

- Ensure the safety of the patient and those caring for them:
  — family or friends should be available for the patient if possible
  — ensure that the patient's basic needs (eg food, drink and accommodation) are met.
- Minimize stress and stimulation: do not argue with psychotic thinking (you may disagree with the patient's beliefs but do not try to argue they are wrong).
- Avoid confrontation or criticism, unless it is necessary to prevent harmful or disruptive behaviour.[2]
- If there is a significant risk of suicide, violence or neglect, admission to hospital or close observation in a secure place might be required. If the patient refuses treatment, legal measures might be needed.
- The DVLA must be notified in all cases. Advise patient to inform DVLA: driving should cease during the acute illness (cars and motorbikes) and until patient has been stable and well for at least three years with insight into their condition (LGV/PSV driver).[3]
- Encourage resumption of normal activities as soon as possible.
- It is important to offer psychological and social support to both patient and family/carer. This may include advice about benefits and housing. Specific referral for family intervention may also be appropriate.

Medication

- Antipsychotic medication can reduce psychotic symptoms over 10–14 days. Where access to a specialist is speedy and symptoms relatively mild, especially for a first referral, the specialist may prefer to see the patient unmedicated.
- If you decide to treat prior to the patient seeing a specialist, then the first-line treatment should be an atypical antipsychotic.[4] Examples include olanzapine (5–10 mg a day) if sedation is required, or risperidone (4–6 mg per day), which is relatively non-sedating (*BNF* section 4.2.1). The use of a typical drug (eg haloperidol) as first-line treatment is no longer recommended. Patients experiencing a first episode of psychosis require lower doses of medication and should be prescribed an atypical drug.[5] In a case of relapse where the patient has previously responded to a drug, restart that drug. The dose should be the lowest possible for the relief of symptoms.[6]
- Anti-anxiety medication can also be used for the short term in conjuction with neuroleptics to control acute agitation (*BNF* section 4.1.2). Examples include diazepam (5–10 mg up to four times a day) or lorazepam (1–2 mg up to four times a day). If required, diazepam can be given rectally or lorazepam IM (although this must be kept refrigerated).
- In a first episode, continue antipsychotic medication for at least six months after symptoms resolve.[7] Close supervision is usually needed in order to encourage patient agreement.
- Be alert to the risk of co-morbid use of street drugs (eg amphetamines) and alcohol.
- Monitor for side-effects of medication:
  — Acute dystonias or spasms may be managed with oral or injectable antiparkinsonian drugs (*BNF* section 4.9.2), for example procyclidine (5 mg three times a day) or orphenadrine (50 mg three times a day).

— Parkinsonian symptoms (eg tremor, akinesia) may be managed with oral antiparkinsonian drugs (*BNF* section 4.9.2), for example procyclidine (5 mg three times a day) or orphenadrine (50 mg three times a day). Withdrawal of antiparkinsonian drugs should be attempted after two to three months without symptoms, because these drugs are liable to misuse and might impair memory.

— Akathisia (severe motor restlessness) may be managed with dosage reduction or beta-blockers (eg with propranolol [30–80 mg a day]) (*BNF* section 2.4). Switching to a low-potency antipsychotic (eg olanzapine or quetiapine) may help.

— Tardive dyskinesia is a particularly important side-effect to monitor for. It is associated with longer term use of traditional antipsychotic medication, is severely disabling and can be irreversible.

— Other side-effects (eg weight gain and sexual dysfuction) are under-reported and are important reasons for poor adherence. Quetiapine (an atypical antipsychotic) is least likely to elevate serum prolactin and lead to weight gain and should be considered when these side-effects become troublesome.

More detail on antipsychotic drugs and their differing side-effect profiles can be found in the *Maudsley Prescribing Guidelines* and the UKPPG.[8,9]

Referral

Referral should be made under the following conditions:

- As an emergency, if the risk of suicide, violence or neglect is considered significant.
- Urgently for ALL first episodes to the Early Intervention Service, to confirm the diagnosis and arrange care planning and appointment of key worker. A home visit may be required. Specific interventions for people experiencing their first episode of psychosis, including specific psychoeducation of the patient and family,[10] is one of the requirements of the *National Service Framework for Mental Health*.[11]
- For ALL relapses, to review the effectiveness of the care plan, unless there is an established previous response to treatment and it is safe to manage the patient at home.
- If there is non-adherence with treatment, treatment resistance, problematic side-effects, failure of community treatment, or concerns about co-morbid drug and alcohol misuse.

Particularly on relapse, referral may be to the Community Mental Health Team or to a member of it, such as a community mental health nurse (community psychiatric nurse [CPN]), as well as to a psychiatrist.

If there is fever, rigidity and/or labile blood pressure, stop antipsychotic medication and refer immediately to the on-call physician for investigation of Neuroleptic malignant syndrome.

Special considerations in children and adolescents

Acute disturbance in children and teenagers is usually due to causes other than psychosis, and anxiety symptoms may masquerade as hallucinations or delusions. The diagnosis of psychosis should be made by a specialist and the appropriate specialist referral will usually be to the Child and Adolescent Mental Health Service.

Resources for patients and families
Resource leaflets: 1–3 *Coping with the side-effects of medication* and 8–1 *What to expect after an acute episode of psychosis*

Rethink (formerly the National Schizophrenia Fellowship)
England: 020 8974 6814 (Advice line: 10am–3pm, Monday–Friday)
Email: advice@rethink.org; website: http://www.rethink.org
Scotland: 0131 557 8969
Northern Ireland: 02890 402 323
Monthly social groups for clients with schizophrenia living in the community and support for relatives.

Schizophrenia Association of Great Britain 01248 354 048
Email: info@sagb.co.uk; website: http://www.sagb.co.uk
Offers information and support to sufferers, relatives, friends, carers and medical workers.

MINDinfoLINE 08457 660 163 (Helpline 9.15am–5.15pm, Monday–Friday)
Email: info@mind.org.uk; website: http://www.mind.org.uk
Information service for matters relating to mental health.

SANELine 08457 678000 (Helpline 12noon–2.00am)
Website: http://www.sane.org.uk
A helpline offering information and advice on all aspects of mental health for those experiencing illness, or for their families or friends.

Hearing Voices Network 0161 228 3896 (10.30am–3pm, Monday–Wednesday, Friday)
Website: http://www.hearing-voices.org.uk
Self-help groups to allow people to explore their voice-hearing experiences.

The UK NHS Portal for Schizophrenia
Website: http://www.nhs.uk/schizophrenia
A web-based information resource for people with schizophrenia and their carers. The site contains a number of user-friendly sections: Evidence-based treatment summaries; What is schizophrenia? How is schizophrenia diagnosed? Managing schizophrenia; Living with schizophrenia; Support for carers; and Legal issues.

Mental Health Care
Website: http://www.mentalhealthcare.org.uk
This site provides mental health information and research news from the Institute of Psychiatry and the South London and Maudsley NHS Trust in partnership with Rethink.

The Mental Health Foundation produces the information booklet *Understanding Schizophrenia*. Publications, The Mental Health Foundation, 7th Floor, 83 Victoria Street, London SW1H 0HW, UK. Tel: 020 7802 0304. website: http://www.mentalhealth.org.uk

Living With Schizophrenia: a Holistic Approach to Understanding, Preventing and Recovering from Negative Symptoms by John Watkins. South Yarra, Australia: Hill of Content Publishing (now Michelle Anderson Publishing), 1996.

Working with Voices by R Coleman and M Smith. Handsell Publishing, Gloucester, UK, 1997
Workbook to help voice-hearers manage their voices.

Hearing Voices: A Common Human Experience by John Watkins. South Yarra, Australia: Hill of Content Publishing (now Michelle Anderson Publishing), 1998.

Adjustment disorder — F43.2 (including acute stress reaction)

(Clinical term: Adjustment disorders Eu43.2)

Presenting complaints
- Patients feel overwhelmed or unable to cope.
- There may be stress-related physical symptoms, such as insomnia, headache, abdominal pain, chest pain and palpitations.
- Patients may report symptoms of acute anxiety or depression.
- Use of alcohol or other substances may increase.

Diagnostic features
- Acute reaction to a recent stressful or traumatic event.
- Extreme distress resulting from a recent event, or preoccupation with the event.
- Symptoms may be primarily somatic.
- Other symptoms may include the following:
  — low or sad mood
  — anxiety
  — worry
  — feeling unable to cope.

Acute reaction usually lasts from a few days to several weeks.

Differential diagnosis and co-existing conditions
Acute symptoms may persist or evolve over time. Patients should be followed up after 1–2 weeks. If significant symptoms persist, consider an alternative diagnosis.

- If significant symptoms of depression persist, see **'Depression — F32#'**.
- If significant symptoms of anxiety persist, see **'Generalized anxiety — F41.1'** or **'Panic disorder — F41.0'**.
- If significant symptoms of both depression and anxiety persist, see **'Chronic mixed anxiety and depression — F41.2'**.
- If stress-related somatic symptoms persist, see **'Unexplained somatic complaints — F45'**.
- If symptoms are due to a loss, see **'Bereavement and loss — Z63'**.
- If anxiety is long-lasting and focused on memories of a previous traumatic event, see **'Post-traumatic stress disorder — F43.1'**.
- If dissociative symptoms (sudden onset of unusual or dramatic somatic symptoms) are present, see **'Dissociative (conversion) disorder — F44'**.

Essential information for patient and family
- Stressful events often have mental and physical effects. The acute state is a natural reaction to events (R: 2).
- Stress-related symptoms usually last only a few days or weeks.

General management and advice to patient and family[12]
- Elicit and explain patient's concerns (this is important for preventing somatic symptoms from continuing).
- Review and reinforce positive steps the patient has taken to deal with the stress.
- Identify steps the patient can take to modify the situation that produced the stress. If the situation cannot be changed, discuss coping strategies (R: 1–1).
- Identify relatives, friends and community resources able to offer support.

- Encourage a return to usual activities within a few weeks.
- Short-term rest and relief from stress may help the patient. Consider short-term sickness certification.
- Encourage the patient to acknowledge the personal significance of the stressful event.
- Offering a further consultation with a member of the primary-care team, to see how the situation develops, can be valuable in helping the patient through the episode.

Medication

Most acute stress reactions will resolve without the use of medication. Skilled GP advice and reassurance is as effective as benzodiazepines.[13] However, if severe anxiety symptoms occur, consider using anti-anxiety drugs for up to three days. If the patient has severe insomnia, use hypnotic drugs for up to three days. Doses should be as low as possible (*BNF* sections 4.1.1 and 4.1.2).

Referral

See 'General referral criteria'. Usually self-limiting.
Routine referral to secondary mental health services is advised if:

- symptoms persist and general referral criteria are met
- unsure of the diagnosis.

Consider recommending a practice counsellor or voluntary/non-statutory counselling[14] services in all other cases where symptoms persist.

Resources for patients and families

Resources leaflets: 1–1 *Problem-solving sheet* and 2 *What to expect after traumatic stress.*

BACP (British Association for Counselling and Psychotherapy) 0870 443 5252
Website: http://www.counselling.co.uk
Provides advice on sources of individual counselling and family therapy in the UK.

The Samaritans National phone number 08457 909 090 (24-hour helpline)
Email: jo@samaritans.org; website: http://www.samaritans.org.uk
Offers confidential emotional support to any person who is despairing or suicidal.

Victim Support 0845 3030 900 (Support line 9am–9pm, Monday–Friday; 9am–7pm, Saturday/Sunday; 9am–5pm, bank holidays)
Email: contact@victimsupport.org.uk; website: http://www.victimsupport.com
Provides emotional support and practical information for anyone who has suffered the effects of crime, regardless of whether the crime has been reported.

Citizens Advice Bureau (see local telephone directory)
Main website: http://www.citizensadvice.org.uk (gives directory of all offices and advice by email); Advice Guide website: http://www.adviceguide.org.uk
Provides a wide range of free and confidential advice and help. Subjects include social security benefits, housing, family and personal matters, money advice and consumer complaints.

Relate 01788 573 241/0845 456 1310
Email: enquiries@relate.org.uk; website: http://www.relate.org.uk
Counselling for adults with relationship difficulties, whether married or not.

International Stress Management Association (ISMA) UK 0700 780 430 (helpline)
Email: stress@isma.org.uk; website: http://www.isma.org.uk
Promotes knowledge and best practice in the prevention and reduction of acute stress.

Coping with stress at work. Talking Life, 1A Grosvenor Road, Hoylake, Wirral CH47 3BS, UK. Tel: 0151 632 0662; website: http://www.talkinglife.co.uk
This is a tape teaching you to recognize stress symptoms. It includes a relaxation exercise.

Alcohol misuse — F10
(Clinical term: Mental and behavioural disorders due to use of alcohol Eu10)

Presenting complaints
Patients may present with:

- depressed mood
- nervousness
- insomnia
- physical complications of alcohol use (eg ulcer, gastritis, liver disease or hypertension)
- accidents or injuries due to alcohol use
- poor memory or concentration
- evidence of self-neglect (eg poor hygiene)
- failed treatment for depression.

There may also be:

- legal and social problems due to alcohol use (eg marital problems, domestic violence, child abuse or neglect, missed work)
- signs of alcohol withdrawal (eg sweating, tremors, sickness, hallucinations [usually visual], seizures).

Patients might sometimes deny or be unaware of alcohol problems. Family members may request help before patient does (eg because patient is irritable at home or missing work). Problems may also be identified during routine health promotion screening.

Diagnostic features
- Harmful alcohol use:
  — heavy alcohol use (eg >28 units a week for men and >21 units a week for women)
  — overuse of alcohol has caused physical harm (eg liver disease, gastrointestinal bleeding), psychological harm (eg depression or anxiety), or has led to harmful social consequences (eg loss of job or breakdown of a relationship).
- Alcohol dependence is present when three of the following are present:
  — a strong desire or compulsion to use alcohol
  — difficulty controlling alcohol use
  — withdrawal symptoms (eg anxiety, tremors, sweating) when drinking is ceased
  — tolerance (eg drinks large amounts of alcohol without appearing intoxicated)
  — continued alcohol use despite harmful consequences
  — neglect of other activities due to alcohol.

Blood tests such as gamma-glutamyl transferase (GGT) and mean corpuscular volume (MCV) can help identify heavy drinkers. Administering the CAGE (R: 11–1) or AUDIT (R: 11–2) questionnaire may also help diagnosis.

Differential diagnosis and co-existing conditions
Symptoms of anxiety or depression may occur with heavy alcohol use. Alcohol use can also mask other disorders, eg agoraphobia, social phobia and generalized anxiety. Assess and manage symptoms of depression or anxiety if symptoms continue after a period of abstinence. See 'Depression — F32#' or 'Generalized anxiety — F41.1'.

Drug misuse may also co-exist with this condition. Presentation of other psychiatric disorders should trigger inquiry about alcohol and drug misuse history.

Essential information for patient and family

- Alcohol dependence is an illness with serious consequences.
- Ceasing or reducing alcohol use will bring mental and physical benefits.
- Drinking during pregnancy may harm the baby.
- Goal-setting needs to be negotiated and matched to individual needs and assessment, as well as to overall pattern of drinking and dependence.
- For most patients with alcohol dependence, physical complications of alcohol abuse or psychiatric disorder, abstinence from alcohol is the preferred goal.[15] Sometimes, abstinence is also necessary for social crises, to regain control over drinking or because of failed attempts at reducing drinking. Because abrupt abstinence can cause withdrawal symptoms, medical supervision is necessary.
- In some cases of harmful alcohol use, controlled or reduced drinking is a reasonable goal, or a reasonable *starting* goal where the alcohol-dependent patient is unwilling or unable to quit.
- As in many chronic behavioural disorders, relapse is common. Controlling or ceasing drinking often requires several attempts. Outcome depends on the motivation and confidence of the patient.

General management and advice to patient and family[16,17]

- In assessing patients with alcohol or other type of addictive behaviour, the framework of cycles of change can be helpful in assessing the patient's readiness for change. A patient may be:
  — pre-contemplative (ie not considering any change)
  — contemplative (ie considering change or prepared to change behaviour), or
  — in an action phase, where they are actually in the process of change.
  Of course, because of the relapsing nature of these disorders, patients might shift from an action phase back to a pre-contemplative phase and then move through the phases of change. Assessment can be a prompt for some to move into a contemplative or action phase.
- For all patients:
  — discuss costs and benefits of drinking from the patient's perspective
  — feedback information about health risks, including the results of GGT and MCV
  — emphasize personal responsibility for change
  — give clear advice to change and discuss alternative strategies to alter drinking pattern
  — assess and manage physical health problems and nutritional deficiencies (eg vitamin B)
  — consider options for problem-solving or targeted counselling to deal with life problems related to alcohol use
  — brief interventions in primary-care settings are effective in cases of hazardous drinking.[18]
- If there is no evidence of physical or psychological harm due to drinking and the patient is not dependent, a controlled drinking programme is a reasonable goal:
  — negotiate a clear goal for decreased use (eg no more than two drinks per day, with two alcohol-free days per week).
  — discuss strategies to avoid or cope with high-risk situations (eg social situations and stressful events)
  — introduce self-monitoring procedures (eg a drinking diary) and safer drinking behaviour (eg time restrictions, drinking more slowly, interspersing with non-alcoholic drinks) (R: 3–2).
- For patients with physical or mental illness and/or dependency, or failed attempts at controlled drinking, an abstinence programme is indicated.
- For patients willing to stop now:
  — set a definite day to quit
  — discuss symptoms and management of alcohol withdrawal

— discuss strategies to avoid or cope with high-risk situations (eg social situations and stressful events)

— make specific plans to avoid drinking (eg ways to face stressful events without alcohol, ways to respond to friends who still drink)

— help patients to identify family members or friends who will support ceasing alcohol use

— consider options for support after withdrawal.

- For patients not willing to stop or reduce now, a harm-reduction programme is indicated:

— do not reject or blame

— clearly point out medical and social problems caused by alcohol

— consider thiamine preparations

— make a future appointment to re-assess health and alcohol use.

- For patients who do not succeed, or who relapse:

— identify and give credit for any success

— discuss the situations that led to relapse

— return to earlier steps above

— avoid blame or criticism

— be aware of the patient's sense of failure or self-criticism and give support if needed.

Self-help organizations (see below), voluntary and non-statutory agencies are often helpful for patients, families and other people involved.[19]

Doctors have a responsibility to inform patients that they are obligated to inform the DVLA if they have been given a diagnosis of alcohol misuse or dependency; licence restoration only occurs after a period free from alcohol problems and satisfactory medical reports.[3] This advice should be documented in the medical records.

Medication[17]

Detoxification

- For patients with mild withdrawal symptoms, frequent monitoring, support, reassurance, adequate hydration and nutrition are sufficient treatment without medication.[20]

- Patients with a moderate withdrawal syndrome may also require benzodiazepines and vitamins. Most can be detoxified, with a good outcome, as outpatients or at home.[21] Community detoxification should only be undertaken by practitioners with appropriate training and supervision.

- Patients at risk of a complicated withdrawal syndrome (eg with a history of fits or delirium tremens, very heavy use and high tolerance, significant polydrug use, benzodiazepine dependence, severe co-morbid medical or psychiatric disorder) who lack social support or are a significant suicide risk may require specialist input and probably inpatient detoxification, which should be carried out in liaison with specialist alcohol services.

- Chlordiazepoxide (Librium; 10 mg) is recommended. The initial dose should be titrated against withdrawal symptoms, within a range of 5–40 mg four times a day (*BNF* section 4.10). This requires close, skilled supervision.

- The following regimen is commonly used, although the dose level and length of treatment will depend on the severity of alcohol dependence and individual patient factors (eg weight, sex and liver function):

Days 1 and 2:	20–30 mg qds
Days 3 and 4:	15 mg qds
Day 5:	10 mg qds
Day 6:	10 mg bd
Day 7:	10 mg nocte

- Naltrexone may decrease alcohol consumption in people with alcohol dependency but their compliance with treatment appears problematic.[22]

- Chlomethiazole is not recommended for outpatient detoxification under any circumstances.[23]
- Dispensing should be daily or involve the support of family members to prevent the risk of misuse or overdose. Confirm abstinence by checking the breath for alcohol, or using a saliva test or breathalyser for the first three to five days.
- Thiamine (150 mg a day in divided doses) should be given orally for one month.[24] As oral thiamine is poorly absorbed, transfer patient immediately to a general hospital or clinic with appropriate resuscitation facilities for parenteral supplementation if any *one* of the following is present: ataxia, confusion, memory disturbance, delirium tremens, hypothermia and hypotension, ophthalmoplegia or unconsciousness.
- Daily supervision is essential in the first few days, then advisable thereafter, to adjust dose of medication, assess whether the patient has returned to drinking, check for serious withdrawal symptoms and maintain support.

Supporting abstinence

- Anxiety and depression often co-occur with alcohol misuse. The patient may have been using alcohol to self-medicate. If symptoms of anxiety or depression increase or remain after a period of abstinence of >2–3 weeks, see **'Depression — F32#'** or **'Generalized anxiety — F41.1'**. Selective serotonin re-uptake inhibitor (SSRI) antidepressants are preferred to tricyclics because of the risk of tricyclic–alcohol interactions (fluoxetine, paroxetine and citalopram do not interact with alcohol). Other newer drugs, such as venlafaxine and mirtazepine, can also be considered (*BNF* section 4.3.3). For anxiety, benzodiazepines should be avoided because of their high potential for abuse[25] (*BNF* section 4.1.2).
- Disulfiram (Anatabuse) produces an aversive reaction including flushing, headaches, palpitations and nausea if combined with alcohol. Extreme reactions can produce hypotension, cardiac arrythmias and collapse, resulting in several contraindications and limiting its use. It is more effective if supervised (*BNF* section 4.10).[26]
- Acamprosate may help to maintain abstinence from alcohol as an adjunct to psychosocial treatment in some cases.
- Naltrexone has a similar profile to Acamprosate, but is not currently licensed for this indication in the UK.

For information on brief interventions for people whose drinking behaviour puts them at risk of becoming dependent, see Alcohol Concern's *Brief Intervention Guidelines*.[27]

Referral

Consider referral:

- to non-statutory Alcohol Advice and Counselling Agency, if available, and if no psychiatric illness is present
- to a specialist NHS alcohol service if the patient has alcohol dependence and requires an abstinence-based group programme or has an associated psychiatric disorder, or if there are no appropriately trained practitioners available in primary care
- for general or specialist hospital inpatient detoxification if the patient does not meet the criteria for community detoxification (see above)
- to targeted counselling, if available, to deal with the social consequences of drinking (eg relationship counselling)
- non-urgently to secondary mental health services if there is a severe mental illness (see relevant disorder), or if symptoms of mental illness persist after detoxification and abstinence.

If available, both specific social skills training[28] and community-based treatment packages[29] may be effective in reducing drinking.

Resources for patients and families

Resource leaflet: 1–1 *Problem solving*, 3–1 *Responsible drinking guidelines* and 3–2 *How to cut down on your drinking*

Al-Anon Family Groups UK and Eire 020 7403 0888 (24-hour helpline)
Website: http://www.al-anonuk.org.uk
Understanding and support for families and friends of alcoholics whether still drinking or not.

Alcoholics Anonymous 0845 769 7555 (24-hour helpline)
Website: http://www.alcoholics-anonymous.org.uk
Helpline and support groups for men and women trying to achieve and maintain sobriety and help other alcoholics to get sober.

National Association for Children of Alcoholics 0117 924 8005
Email: help@nacoa.org.uk Website: www.nacoa.org.uk

Drinkline National Alcohol Helpline 0800 917 8282 (11am–7pm, Monday–Friday)
Secular Organisations for Sobriety (SOS) 020 8698 9332/020 8291 5572 (helpline)
A non-religious self-help group.

Northern Ireland Community Addiction Service 02890 664 434
Alcohol Focus Scotland 0141 572 6700
Email:jacklaw@alcohol-focus-scotland.org.uk; website: http://www.alcohol-focus-scotland.org.uk
Formerly the Scottish Council on Alcohol, initiates and supports actions to promote a healthy approach to the use of alcohol.

Health Education Authority 020 7430 0850
Health Development Agency (HDA) 020 7430 0850
Recorded alcohol information is also available on freephone 0500 801802
Email: communications@hda-online.org.uk; website: http://www.hda-online.org.uk
Produces leaflets on sensible drinking.

Health Education Board for Scotland 0131 536 5500
Website: http://www.hebs.scot.nhs.uk
Provides leaflets to support brief interventions for people at risk of becoming dependent on alcohol.
Leaflets are available from the Royal College of Psychiatrists
(http://www.rcpsych.ac.uk): *Alcohol, Alcohol and Depression, Alcohol and Other Drug Misuse*

Bereavement and loss — Z63.4

(Clinical term: Grief reaction E2900)

Presenting complaints

An acute grief reaction is a normal, understandable reaction to loss. Patients present in different ways, but typically they:

- feel overwhelmed by loss
- are preoccupied with the loss
- may present with somatic symptoms following loss.

Individual grief experiences vary enormously; they depend on:

- the type of loss (eg a loved one, health, social status and lifestyle through the loss of a job, or the breakdown of a relationship)
- the nature of the loss (expected versus unexpected, traumatic loss, concurrent multiple stressful events, multiple losses)
- the individual suffering the loss (eg coping strategies, age, spiritual health, previous experience of loss) and their social context (eg family systems, access to support, cultural context).

Grief may precipitate or exacerbate other psychiatric conditions. It can also become pathological, eg it can be absent, delayed (grief reaction triggered some time after loss) or chronic (intrusive and fixed emotions of grief). Broadly speaking, difficulties arise when the response becomes unusually dysfunctional to the individual and those around them.

Diagnostic features

Besides the emotional response to loss, symptoms resembling depression can occur:

- low or sad mood
- disturbed sleep
- loss of appetite
- loss of interest
- restlessness
- guilt or self-criticism about actions not taken by the person before the death of the loved one
- transient hallucinations of the deceased person, such as hearing their voice
- thoughts of joining the deceased.

The patient may:

- withdraw from usual activities and social contacts
- find it difficult to think of the future
- increase his/her use of drugs or alcohol.

Patient presentation can be obvious, but it can also be hidden. Adverse reactions to loss may only be revealed after careful questioning. It might be possible to identify certain individuals who are at particular risk (eg social isolation, history of mental illness, previous unresolved grief). Assessing the impact of the loss and the coping strategies available is important in guiding management. Taking time, perhaps over a couple of appointments, may be necessary.

Differential diagnosis

- **'Depression — F32#'.** Knowing when to use the medical model for depression can be difficult and it is important not to medicalize the problem. That said, disabling depressive symptoms that become protracted (about 4–6 months) or severe (eg retardation, overwhelming guilt, hopelessness, suicidal ideation) may be helped by treatment for depression.

- **'Generalized anxiety — F41.1'.**
- **'Sleep problems — F51'.**

Essential information for patient and family

- Everybody grieves differently.
- Important losses are often followed by intense sadness, crying, anger, disbelief, anxiety, guilt or irritability.
- Bereavement typically includes preoccupation with the deceased (including hearing or seeing the person).
- A desire to discuss the loss is normal and beneficial.
- Inform patients, especially those at greater risk of developing an abnormal grief reaction, of local agencies, which offer bereavement counselling and aim to help guide people through their normal grief.[30]

General management and advice to patient and family[31]

- If a loss can be predicted, lead the patient and their family through the challenges facing them with appropriately paced and guided discussion, shared understanding based on the patient's world view and optimal physical care.
- Enable the bereaved person to talk about the deceased and the circumstances of the death. This can provide them with a useful narrative about their loss, which will help them in the future.
- Answer questions to enable the bereaved to understand what happened at the time of death.
- Encourage free expression of feelings about the loss (including feelings of sadness, guilt or anger). In bereavement, be prepared to hear and acknowledge any expressions of anger directed at health professionals, including you. Sensitive management of this anger can be crucial.
- Offer reassurance that recovery will take time (grief has to run its course). Some reduction in burdens (eg work or social commitments) may be necessary.
- Explain that intense grieving will fade slowly and that reminders of the loss might continue to provoke feelings of loss and sadness.
- Social structures (eg families) are vulnerable at times of bereavement. Group coping strategies can increase or decrease subsequent individual morbidity and group functioning.
- Take into account the cultural context of the loss.
- Listening and giving a sense of 'being there' for the patient may be all that is needed.

There is no 'catch-all' advice for the patient and family, but the following might be helpful:

- Do cry if the need is there, and don't be surprised if you cry more than normal, even if it is in unusual places.
- Do accept help from others, but don't let people pressure you to do things that don't feel right or before you are ready.
- Don't feel guilty if you do not always feel upset. There will be many occasions when you need to carry on with everyday things.
- Do remember that children and young people need to grieve as well. Let the teachers and school know.
- Do remember that people react to grief in different ways; within a family, this can be difficult.
- Do take care of yourself and try to eat sensibly and rest.
- Do try to keep life as normal as possible, with some sort of routine. Do, if you can, avoid any major changes in the first year, such as moving house.

- Do take things a day at a time when you are feeling low, but be ready, as time passes, to try new things and meet people.

Medication

Avoid medication if possible. If the grief reaction becomes abnormal, see **'Depression — F32#'** for advice on the use of antidepressants.

Disturbed sleep is to be expected. If severe insomnia occurs, short-term use of hypnotic drugs may be helpful but use should be limited to two weeks.

Referral

If the patient is failing to respond to the measures outlined above, or symptoms are severe and persistent, or if the patient is particularly at risk, then more formal grief counselling may help and can be arranged via:

- a practice counsellor
- Cruse Bereavement Care (adult bereaved)
- Compassionate Friends (for those bereaved through the loss of a child)
- hospice bereavement services (for those bereaved of hospice patients)
- Relate (for those who are suffering through the loss of a relationship).

Referral to secondary mental health services is advised:

- if the patient is severely depressed, threatening suicide (never be afraid to ask), or showing psychotic features
- non-urgently, if symptoms have not subsided by one year despite bereavement counselling.

Refer bereaved people with a learning disability to a specialist disability team or specialist learning disability counsellor.

Resources for patients and families

Cruse Bereavement Care 0870 167 1677 (Helpline 9.30am–5.00pm, Monday–Friday)
Email: info@crusebereavementcare.org.uk; website:
http://www.crusebereavementcare.org.uk
Offers support, information, training and direct telephone help to anyone who has been affected by a death. Over 150 branches throughout the UK.

The Compassionate Friends 0117 953 9639 (Helpline 10am–4pm, 6.30pm–10.30pm)
Email: info@tcf.org.uk; website: http://www.tcf.org.uk
Organization of bereaved parents offering friendship and understanding to others after the death of a child.

Stillbirth and Neonatal Death Society (SANDS) 020 7436 5881 (Helpline 10am–3pm)
Email: support@uk-sands.org; website: http://www.uk-sands.org
Provides support for parents and families whose baby is stillborn, or dies shortly after birth.

Foundation for the Study of Infant Deaths (FSID) 0870 787 0554 (helpline)
Email: fsid@sids.org.uk; website: http://www.sids.org.uk
National helpline, local parent groups and befrienders to bereaved families who have suffered a cot death.

Papyrus 01706 214 449
Website: http://www.papyrus-uk.org
Self-help for parents of young people who have committed suicide.

Relate 01788 573 241
Website: http://www.relate.org.uk
Counselling for adults with relationship difficulties, whether married or not.

Growthhouse.org http://www.growthhouse.org
This is an award-winning website for those facing the end of life and bereavement.

Coping with Bereavement. The Royal College of Psychiatrists. Talking Life, 1A Grosvenor Rd, Hoylake, Wirral CH47 3BS. Tel: 0151 632 0662. website: http://www.talkinglife.co.uk

A programme on tape of practical advice and support to people of all ages who have been bereaved.

Leaflets are available from the Royal College of Psychiatrists (http://www.rcpsych.ac.uk): *Bereavement, Sleeping Well, Bereavement Information Pack: for those bereaved by suicide or other sudden death*.

Bipolar disorder — F31
(Clinical term: Bipolar affective disorder Eu31)

Presenting complaints
Patients may have a period of depression, mania, mixed manic and depressive symptoms, or unusual or abnormal behaviour, with the pattern described below.
  Referral may be made by others, owing to the patient's lack of insight.

Diagnostic features
- Periods of mania with:
  — increased energy and activity
  — elevated mood or irritability
  — rapid speech
  — loss of inhibitions, including financial and sexual inhibitions
  — decreased need for sleep
  — increased importance of self
  — delusions, hallucinations, disturbed or illogical thinking.
- The patient may be easily distracted.
- The patient may also have periods of depression with:
  — low or sad mood
  — loss of interest or pleasure
  — disturbed sleep
  — poor concentration or irritability
  — guilt or low self-worth
  — disturbed appetite
  — fatigue or loss of energy
  — suicidal thoughts or acts
  — delusions, hallucinations, disturbed or illogical thinking.

Either type of episode may predominate. Episodes may alternate frequently or may be separated by periods of normal mood. Psychotic phases include strange or illogical beliefs, or disturbed or illogical thinking.
  Mixed states are very common; even if criteria for mixed states are not met, depressive symptoms are very common in manic episodes and associated manic symptoms can occur in bipolar depression.
  Lesser degrees of mania and hypomania can be missed on a brief interview and collateral information from relatives is vital.

Differential diagnosis
- 'Alcohol misuse — F10' or 'Drug use disorder — F11#' can cause similar symptoms.
- 'Chronic psychotic disorders — F20#' (psychotic subtype, schizoaffective disorder or schizophrenia) or major 'Depression — F32#', especially where psychotic symptoms are present.

Essential information for patient and family
- Unexplained changes in mood and behaviour can be symptoms of an illness.
- Effective treatments are available. Long-term treatment can help prevent future episodes.
- If left untreated, manic episodes may become disruptive or dangerous. Manic episodes often lead to loss of job, legal problems, financial problems or high-risk sexual behaviour. When the first, milder symptoms of mania or hypomania occur, referral is often indicated and the patient should be encouraged to see their GP straight away.

- Inform patients who are on lithium of the signs of lithium toxicity (see Medication below) (R: 5–2).
- Manic symptoms can be followed by depressive symptoms; the patient's GP should be informed of major changes in the patient's mood and the occurrence of suicidal ideas.

General management and advice to patient and family (R: 5–1)

- Remain optimistic and emphasize the patient's strengths and abilities, rather than his/her deficits.
- In acute manic or depressive episodes, refer urgently to secondary care.
- During depression, assess risk of suicide. (Has the patient frequently thought of death or dying? Does the patient have a specific suicide plan? Have they made serious suicide attempts in the past? Can the patient be sure not to act on suicidal ideas?) Ask about risk of harm to others (see **'Depression — F32#'** and **Self-harm**).
- During manic periods:
  — avoid confrontation unless necessary, to prevent harmful or dangerous acts
  — advise caution about impulsive or dangerous behaviour
  — close observation by family members is often needed
  — if agitation or disruptive behaviour are severe, hospitalization may be required
  — suicide is not unknown, especially in mixed states. Identify early warning signs with the patient and family.
- During depressed periods, consult management guidelines for depression (see **'Depression — F32#'**).
- Describe illness and possible future treatments.
- Encourage the family to consult, even if the patient is reluctant.
- Women with bipolar disorder who are planning pregnancy or become pregnant should seek early advice about control and prevention of the illness and use of medication ante- and postnatally. The risk of relapse is high postnatally. Specialist advice is indicated.
- Work with patient and family to identify early warning symptoms of mood swings, in order to avoid major relapse.
- The treatment plan should include recognition of early warning signs and the agreed management of crises should be clearly recorded in the medical records; a copy of the plan should be given to the patient, and with the patient's permission, to the family/carers.
- For patients able to identify early symptoms of a forthcoming 'high' (sleep disturbance is the most important warning sign for mania), advise:
  — planning for a good night's sleep
  — avoid taking major decisions
  — taking steps to limit capacity to spend money (eg give credit cards to a friend)
  — avoiding stimulating or stressful situations (eg parties).[32]
- Therapeutic alliances build on respect and feeling valued; encourage the patient to build relationships with key members of the practice team, eg by seeing the same doctor or nurse at each appointment. Use the relationship to discuss the treatment plan, including medication.
- The DVLA must be notified in all cases. Advise patient to inform DVLA. Driving should cease during the acute illness (cars and motorbikes) and until patient has been stable and well for at least three years with insight into their condition (LGV/PSV driver).[3]
- Cognitive behavioural therapy may be of benefit in relapse prevention of mania and the treatment of depressive episodes.

Medication

- If the patient displays psychotic symptoms, increasing agitation, excitement or disruptive behaviour, antipsychotic medication might be needed initially[33] (BNF section 4.2). Antipsychotic medication has a specific anti-manic action. The doses should be the lowest possible for the relief of symptoms.[34] If antipsychotic medication causes acute dystonic reactions (eg muscle spasms) or marked extrapyramidal symptoms (eg stiffness or tremors), antiparkinsonian medication (*BNF* section 4.9) — eg procliclidine, 5 mg orally up to three times a day — may be helpful. Routine use is not necessary. Atypical antipsychotics (eg olanzapine) are now widely used and usually obviate the need for antiparkinsonian medication.

- Benzodiazepines may also be used in the short term with or without antipsychotic medication and mood stabilizers to control acute agitation[35] (*BNF* section 4.1.2) and re-establish a normal sleep pattern. Examples include diazepam (5–10 mg up to four times a day) or lorazepam (1–2 mg up to four times a day). If required, diazepam can be given rectally, or lorazepam IM (although it must be kept refrigerated).
- Lithium can help relieve mania[36] and depression[37] and can prevent episodes from recurring.[38,39] One usually commences or stops taking lithium only with specialist advice. Some GPs are confident about restarting lithium treatment after a relapse. Alternative mood-stabilizing medications include carbamazepine and sodium valproate.[40]

If lithium is prescribed:
— It takes several days to show effects and is probably slower to act than the antipsychotics.
— There should be a clear agreement between the referring GP and the specialist as to who is monitoring lithium treatment. Lithium monitoring is ideally carried out using an agreed protocol. If carried out in primary care, monitoring should be done by a suitably trained person.
— Levels of lithium in the blood should be measured frequently, when adjusting the dose, and every three months in stable patients, 10–14 hours post-dose (desired blood level is 0.4–1.0 mmol/L [*BNF* section 4.2.3]; locally recommended levels may vary slightly). **If blood levels are >1.5 mmol/L or there is diarrhoea and vomiting, stop the lithium immediately**. If there are other signs of lithium toxicity (eg tremors, diarrhoea, vomiting, nausea or confusion), stop lithium and check blood level. Renal and thyroid function should be checked every two to three months when adjusting the dose, and every 12 months in stable patients.[41]
— Never stop lithium abruptly (except in the presence of toxicity) — relapse rates are twice as high under these conditions.[39,42] Lithium should be continued for at least six months after symptoms resolve (longer-term use is usually necessary to prevent recurrences). Lithium should be tapered off over at least four weeks, and rebound mania is substantially reduced if the patient is co-prescribed an atypical antipsychotic.

- Antidepressant medication is often needed during phases of depression but can precipitate mania when used alone (see '**Depression — F32#**'). If the patient becomes hypomanic, stop the antidepressant.

Liaison and referral

Referral to secondary mental health services is advised:

- as an emergency if very vulnerable (eg if there is significant risk of suicide or disruptive behaviour)
- urgently if significant symptoms continue or escalate despite treatment.

Non-urgent referral or advice from specialist worker is recommended:

- for assessment, care planning and allocation of key worker under the Care Programme Approach
- before starting lithium
- for medication review and for other treatment strategies, eg cognitive behavioural therapy

- because of lithium's teratogenicity, for preconceptual counselling or contraception advice; for all women with a history of bipolar disorder to plan prevention and management of high risk (up to 50%) of puerperal psychosis.

Resources for patients and families

Resource leaflets: 5–1 *Living with bipolar disorder* and 5–2 *Lithium toxicity*

The Manic Depression Fellowship (MDF)
England: 020 7793 2600
Email: mdf@mdf.org.uk; website: http://www.mdf.org.uk
Scotland: 0141 560 2050; Email: manic@globalnet.co.uk
Wales: 01633 244 244; Email: mdf.wales@btclick.com; website:
http://www.manicdepressionwales.org.uk
    Advice, support, local self-help groups and publications list for people with a manic depressive illness.
    A leaflet is available from the Royal College of Psychiatrists
(http://www.rcpsych.ac.uk): *Manic Depressive Illness*

Overcoming Mood Swings by Jan Scott. Constable & Robinson, 2001
Self-help manual.

Inside Out: A Guide to Self-Management of Manic Depression. Available from the Manic Depression Fellowship, Castle Works, 21 St George's Road, London SE1 6ES. Tel: 020 7793 2600

Living Without Depression and Manic Depression: a Workbook for Maintaining Mood Stability by Mary Ellen Copeland. New Harbinger Press, USA

New Hope for People with Bipolar Disorder by Jan Fawcett. Crown Publications 2000, Victoria, Canada

Chronic fatigue syndrome (CFS or CFS/ME — G93.3)

CFS is commonly referred to as (benign) myalgic encephalomyelitis (encephalopathy) or ME.

A range or spectrum of disorders exists, characterized by abnormal levels and unusual types of fatigue, along with other features and symptoms. Whether these represent distinct entities or variations on a common theme is uncertain. Aetiology and pathogenesis are not always known. Terminology is therefore problematic.

Terminology and concepts

International terminological differences exist. The terminology used may reflect incidental factors such as specialty of clinician, historical or social factors — all of which can influence different recording practices both nationally and internationally. The terms used derive from the following:

- The apparent trigger (eg Post-viral fatigue syndrome).
- The research/surveillance definition (Chronic fatigue syndrome).
- A clinically characterized entity falling short of CFS criteria ([idiopathic] chronic fatigue). All terms focus on fatigue, even though the patient experience may go well beyond this single symptom.
- An historical term implying a particular locus and process of disease (ME, [benign] myalgic encephalomyelitis/encephalopathy). This term has also been incorporated emblematically into lay parlance; it is used by many as synonymous with CFS but is also used by some to designate a discrete entity.
- A different historical term derived from an earlier model of disorders of nervous system dysfunction (neurasthenia), which is now rarely used clinically in the UK but remains popular in many countries.

The terms 'Post-viral fatigue syndrome' and '(benign) myalgic encephalomyelitis' (classified under G93.3 'neurological disorders') have been used where there is excessive fatigue following a specific trigger such as a viral disease and/or where the symptoms do not fulfil the criteria for F48.0. 'Fatigue syndrome', both chronic and not, with or without an established physical precursor, has been classified under 'neurasthenia', F48.0. In practice, there is extensive overlap in symptoms (up to 96%).

In the absence of a simple biological marker or test, the diagnosis of CFS and other fatigue states requires the fulfilment of clinical criteria.

The research/surveillance definition for CFS has enabled better characterization of this disorder; however, it implies a distinction from other fatigue states that may be artefactual, since research has shown considerable overlap in the symptoms of many chronic fatigue states. The approach to clinical management is similar for these fatigue states, although differences in severity and type influence the level and model of management used.

Fatigue states associated with other medical conditions, such as inflammatory, autoimmune or malignant disorders, may have clinical similarities, and may respond similarly to treatment, usually aimed at perpetuating factors such as poor sleep, depression and lack of exercise. Likewise, fatigue and other symptoms can characterize certain mental health disorders.

Common presenting complaints and main symptoms
- intrusive fatigue and lack of energy — physical and mental
- post-exertional malaise
- musculoskeletal aches and pains
- sleep disturbances, especially hypersomnia and non-refreshing sleep quality
- headaches of a new type or pattern
- other somatic symptoms.

CFS may additionally be characterized by the following:[43]

- increased symptoms after physical or mental activity, often delayed
- prolonged recovery times, despite rest
- subjectively tender cervical lymph nodes
- a wide variety of other somatic symptoms
- onset after infection or other physical or psychological stressors
- insidious onset in a minority of cases.

All definitions state that CFS in adults can be diagnosed when substantial physical and mental fatigue of new onset lasts for more than six months, is substantial and impairs daily activities, and there are no relevant findings on physical examinations or laboratory investigations. Early diagnosis might help with treatment and improve prognosis (see Box 1).[44]

Severity
The severity of the illness among some, its prevalence among children, and its impact on people of all ethnic backgrounds and class are often misunderstood and were highlighted in the Chief Medical Officer Working Group on CFS/ME.[43] This working group set out a helpful categorization of severity in CFS/ME, although care must be taken not to diminish inadvertently the experience of any patient by descriptors of severity.

- **Mild**: Patients are mobile and can care for themselves and can do light domestic tasks with difficulty. Most will still be working; however, in order to remain in work, they will have stopped all leisure and social pursuits, often taking days off. Most will use the weekend to rest in order to cope with the week.
- **Moderate**: Patients have reduced mobility and are restricted in all activities of daily living, often having peaks and troughs of ability, dependent on the degree of symptoms. They have usually stopped work and require rest periods, often sleeping in the afternoon for one or two hours. Sleep quality at night is generally poor and disturbed.
- **Severe**: Patients are able to carry out minimal daily tasks only — for example, face washing and teeth cleaning; they have severe cognitive difficulties and are wheelchair-dependent for mobility. They are often unable to leave the house except on rare occasions, leading to a severe and prolonged after-effect from the effort.
- **Very severe**: Patients are unable to mobilize or carry out any daily tasks for themselves and are in bed most of the time. They are often unable to tolerate any noise, and are generally extremely sensitive to light.

Differential diagnosis and co-existing conditions
Patients with many medical conditions may exhibit fatigue as a symptom, but do not meet the case definition of CFS or lack other characteristic features.
Other diagnoses to consider include:

- 'Depression — F32#' (if low or sad mood is prominent)
- 'Chronic mixed anxiety and depression — F41.2'
- 'Panic disorder — F41.1' (if anxiety attacks are prominent)
- Somatization disorders.

Co-morbidity of CFS and mood disorder is common.[45] Patients may have both; and both will need management. In clinical practice, the two are not mutually exclusive, although the research definitions necessarily try to avoid co-morbidity.

Assessment

Clinical history is crucial. A well-taken history might also help the patient in validating their problem, and encourage a good clinician–patient relationship.[46,47]

Physical examination is obligatory, usually normal, and largely serves to exclude other conditions. Assessment must also include examination of the patient's mental state and a psychosocial assessment.

Investigations should include a full blood count, C-reactive protein (CRP) (or erythrocyte sedimentation rate [ESR]), thyroid function tests, urea and electrolytes, blood sugar and liver function tests. If clinically indicated, screening for gluten-sensitive enteropathy or autoimmune disease might be helpful.

Alternative diagnoses should be considered in particular circumstances, for example where there is:

- significant weight loss
- a history of foreign travel
- any documented fever
- extremes of life (very young or very old)
- any physical sign
- myalgic symptoms only after exertion and not associated with any symptoms of mental fatigability (suggests possible myopathy).

Essential information for patient and family

- Fatigue as a symptom is extremely common and could relate to a diversity of underlying physical and/or psychological pathologies.
- Chronic fatigue often improves spontaneously.
- Management of chronic fatigue is possible with good results.
- No single management approach to CFS has been found to be universally successful, but effective treatment does exist. The patient's belief about their condition may guide the choice of treatment.
- Symptoms are genuinely disabling and are not 'all in the mind'. Symptoms following exertion are not synonymous with physical damage and long-term disability.

General management and advice to patient and family

- Management of the fatigue state should focus on maximizing useful and sustainable functional activity, while avoiding levels and types of activity that cause setbacks. It should also focus on recognizing individual perpetuating factors.
- Approaches that have been shown to be successful include[48] cautiously implemented graded exercise programmes,[49,50] cognitive behavioural therapy.[51] 'Pacing' and/or 'living within limits' is considered by some to be useful.
- Gather information from the patient's previous experience to identify level of functioning, types of triggers for setbacks and factors leading to improvements. A diary might be useful.
- The patient may be able to build endurance by gradually increasing activity. Start with a manageable level and increase a little each week, if tolerable and sustainable without increased symptoms or disability.
- Emphasize pleasant or enjoyable activities to balance necessary tasks. Consider mixing the types of activity.
- Assess sleep patterns and normalize as much as possible. Encourage a regular sleep routine and, where appropriate, avoid daytime sleep. Consider medication (see below).
- Avoid excessive rest and/or sudden changes in activity.
- Recognize and treat psychological or physical co-morbidities.

- Explore what the patient thinks their symptoms mean. Offer appropriate explanations and reassurance.
- Involving families could be important, and is essential when the patient is a child (see **'Unexplained medical symptoms including chronic fatigue'**).

Medication

- Pain and poor sleep might respond to low-dose tricyclic 'antidepressants'. (Their rationale should be explained.)
- Anxiety and depression might respond to the less sedating antidepressants in full doses.
- Antidepressants have not been shown to be effective, but are widely used in the management of CFS in the absence of mood disorder.
- Consider analgesics for headache or muscle pain.
- Severe or neuropathic pain might require management by a specialist pain service or neurologist.
- Be aware that some patients are sensitive to a wide variety of drugs, and doses may need to be reduced accordingly.

Referral

- Consider referral to an appropriate specialist physician if there is uncertainty about diagnosis.
- Referral to secondary services for assessment and management of CFS depends on local provision. Services might be provided by liaison psychiatrists, infectious diseases consultants, pain clinics or rheumatologists.
- Referral to Community Mental Health Teams may be indicated in special circumstances:
  — where there is a risk of suicide
  — in cases of bipolar disorder
  — in patients with eating disorders.
- Complex and bed- or house-bound patients might need domiciliary medical and social care; a small percentage may require admission for specialized rehabilitation programmes.[52,53]
- Misunderstanding about the purpose and nature of referrals is common. Explanation and shared decision-making, which may include carers, are important.

Resources for patients and families
Action for ME (AfME) 01749 670799
Email: admin@afme.org.uk; website: http://www.afme.org.uk
This is a national charity campaigning for patients and a useful source of information.

M.E. A Guide to Symptoms, Causes and Treatments. Available from: Action for ME, PO Box 1302, Wells, Somerset BA5 1YE, UK. Tel: 01749 670799, Email: admin@afme.org.uk. Price: £2.

Coping with Chronic Fatigue by Trudie Chalder, Sheldon Press, 1995
A book with self-help advice.

Facing and Fighting Fatigue: A Practical Approach by B Natelson, Yale University Press, 1998.

Chronic Fatigue Syndrome: The Facts by M Sharpe and F Campling, Oxford University Press, 2000
Self-help advice for more severe symptoms.

The King's College London website: Chronic Fatigue and Chronic Fatigue Syndrome: A Practical Self Help Guide, http://www.kcl.ac.uk/cfs
This site includes a full patient-management package for more severe symptoms of chronic fatigue syndrome. It provides information on the disorder and suggestions to aid self-management, as well as special material for families and children.

Box 1: Criteria for CFS (as defined by Fukuda *et al.*, 1994)[44]

These have become the most internationally accepted criteria for the diagnosis of CFS for research and surveillance purposes and have proved remarkably robust in various settings. However, clinicians must recognize that there are no agreed or validated clinical criteria for use in clinical practice. The constraints of the existing definitions designed for research or surveillance need modification in this setting, especially in respect of allowing for co-morbid conditions, for example.
Fukuda criteria:

1. Clinically evaluated, unexplained, persistent or relapsing chronic fatigue that:
   - is of new or definite onset (ie has not been life-long)
   - is not the result of ongoing exertion
   - is not substantially alleviated by rest
   - results in substantial reduction in occupational, educational, social or personal activities.

2. The concurrent occurrence of four or more of the following symptoms, all of which must have persisted or recurred during six or more consecutive months of illness and must not have pre-dated the fatigue:
   - self-reported impairment in short-term memory or concentration, severe enough to cause substantial reduction in previous levels of activities
   - sore throat
   - tender cervical or axillary lymph nodes
   - muscle pain
   - multi-joint pain without joint swelling or redness
   - headaches of a new type, pattern or severity
   - unrefreshing sleep
   - post-exertional malaise lasting more than 24 hours.

3. The following conditions exclude a patient from the diagnosis of unexplained chronic fatigue:
   - Any active medical condition that may explain the presence of chronic fatigue, such as untreated hypothyroidism, sleep apnoea, narcolepsy and the side-effects of medication.
   - Any previously diagnosed medical condition whose continued activity might explain the chronic fatiguing illness, such as previously treated malignancies and unresolved cases of Hepatitis B or C infection.
   - Any past or current diagnosis of a major depressive disorder, with psychotic or melancholic features, bipolar affective disorders, schizophrenia of any subtype, delusional disorders of any subtype, dementias of any subtype, anorexia nervosa or bulimia nervosa.
   - Alcohol or other substance abuse within two years before the onset of the chronic fatigue and at any time afterward.
   - Severe obesity, as defined by a body mass index of ≥ 45.

Chronic mixed anxiety and depression — F41.2
(Clinical term: Mixed anxiety and depressive disorder Eu41.2)

Many people in the community report significant levels of depression and/or anxiety that do not meet the diagnostic criteria for either depressive episode or the anxiety disorders. There are a variety of ways of classifying this group within ICD-10, including dysthymia, mixed anxiety, and depression.

Presenting complaints
One or more physical symptoms (eg pains, poor sleep, fatigue), and various anxiety and depressive symptoms, present for more than six months.

Diagnostic features
• Low or sad mood
• Loss of interest or pleasure
• Prominent anxiety or worry
• Multiple associated symptoms, for example:
  — disturbed sleep   — disturbed appetite
  — tremor   — suicidal thoughts or self-harm
  — fatigue or loss of energy   — dry mouth
  — palpitations   — tension and restlessness
  — poor concentration   — irritability
  — dizziness   — sexual dysfunction.

Differential diagnosis and co-existing conditions
• If more severe depression or anxiety are present, see **'Depression — F32#'** or **'Generalized anxiety — F41.1'**.
• If marked fear/anxiety in particular situations (eg crowds, enclosed spaces, travel), see **'Phobic disorders — F40'**.
• If history of manic episodes (eg excitement, elevated mood, rapid speech), see **'Bipolar disorder — F31'**.
• If somatic symptoms predominate without an adequate physical explanation, see **'Unexplained somatic complaints — F45'**.
• If drinking heavily or using drugs, see **'Alcohol misuse — F10'** and **'Drug use disorders — F11'**.

Essential information for patient and family
• Anxiety and depression have many physical and mental effects that are likely to be worse at times of personal stress. Aim to help the patient reduce symptoms.
• The problems are not due to weakness or laziness.
• Regular structured visits can be helpful — state their frequency and include arranged visits to other professionals if necessary.

General management and advice to patient and family
• If physical symptoms are present, discuss their link to mental distress (see **'Unexplained somatic complaints — F45'**).
• Advise relaxation methods to relieve physical symptoms (R: 1–2).
• Cut down caffeine intake (coffee, tea, stimulant drinks).
• Discuss ways to challenge negative thoughts or exaggerated worries (R: 4–2 and 6–3).
• Encourage simple cognitive strategies and structured problem-solving between appointments:
  — identify events that trigger undue worry (eg a young woman presents with worry, tension, nausea and insomnia, which began after her son was diagnosed with asthma: her anxiety worsens when he has asthma episodes)

— list as many solutions as possible (eg meet the nurse to learn about asthma management; discuss concerns with parents of other asthmatic children; write down a management plan for asthma episodes)
— list the pros and cons of each possible solution.
- At appointments, help the patient to:
— choose their preferred approach
— work out the steps necessary to achieve the plan
— set a date to review the plan; identify and encourage whatever seems to be working.
- Assess risk of suicide — see **'Self-harm'**.
- Encourage use of self-help books, tapes and/or leaflets, and voluntary organizations (see below)[54] (R: 6–1 and 4–1).
- These patients risk developing more severe disorders and should be monitored regularly.

Medication
- Medication is a secondary treatment of uncertain value.
- If prescribed, medication should be simple, reviewed regularly, and only continued if definitely helping.
- Avoid multiple psychotropics.
- Can try a tricyclic or SSRI antidepressant if depression or anxiety are marked[55] (*BNF* section 4.3). See **'Depression — F32#'** for severity threshold for initiating medication and specific guidance about it.

Referral
See general referral criteria.

Stress/anxiety management,[56] problem-solving,[57] cognitive behaviour therapy or counselling[58] might help and be given in primary care or the voluntary sector. It is unusual to refer for psychological treatment unless the disorder becomes severe. Refer to secondary mental healthcare as an emergency if suicide risk is significant — see **'Self-harm'**.

Consider recommending voluntary/non-statutory/self-help organizations.

Resources for patients and families (see also 'Depression — F32#' for more resources)
Resource leaflets: 1–1 *Problem-solving*, 1–2 *Learning to relax*, 4–1 *Anxiety and how to reduce it*, 6–1 *Depression and how to cope with it*, 4–2 *Dealing with anxious thoughts*, and 6–3 *Dealing with depressive thinking*

Depression Alliance
England: 020 8768 0123
Wales: 029 2069 2891 (10am–4pm, Monday–Friday)
Scotland: 0131 467 3050
Website: http://www.depressionalliance.org
Provides information and support groups.

Aware Defeat Depression Ltd. (local groups) 02871 260 602
Email: info@aware-ni.org; website: http://www.aware-ni.org
Provides information leaflets, lectures and runs support groups for sufferers and relatives.

The Samaritans 08457 909090 (24-hour helpline; see telephone directory for local branches)
Website: http://www.samaritans.org.uk

The Samaritans offer confidential emotional support to any person who is despairing or suicidal.

SANEline 0845 767 8000 (12pm–2am)
Website: http://www.sane.org.uk
This is a helpline offering information and advice on all aspects of mental health for those experiencing illness or their families or friends.

First Steps to Freedom 01926 851 608 (24-hour helpline)
Email: info@firststeps.demon.co.uk; website: http://www.first-steps.org

CITA (Council for Involuntary Tranquilliser Addiction) 0151 949 0102 (helpline 10am–1pm, Monday–Friday; emergency weekend number available)
Offers advice on withdrawing from tranquilisers and help with anxiety and depression.
Leaflets are available from the Royal College of Psychiatrists (http://www.rcpsych.ac.uk): *Worries and Anxieties, Anxiety & Phobias, Anxiety*

Helping You Cope: A Guide To Starting And Stopping Tranquillisers and Sleeping Tablets by the Mental Health Foundation: now out of print, but available online: http://www.mentalhealth.org.uk/page.cfm?pagecode=PBBF

Anxiety, Phobias and Panic Attacks: Your Questions Answered by Elaine Sheehan, Vega Books, 2002
Information and advice on types of anxiety and the treatments available, including self-help strategies and what to expect.

Living With Fear, 2nd edition, by Isaac M Marks. McGraw Hill, 2001. Tel: 01628 252 700; Email: orders@mcgraw-hill.co.uk.
This is a self-help manual.

Managing Anxiety and Depression by Nicholas Holdsworth and Roger Paxton. London: The Mental Health Foundation, 1999. Publications, The Mental Health Foundation, 7th Floor, 83 Victoria Street, London SW1H 0HW. Tel: 7802 0304. www.mentalhealth.org.uk

Restoring the Balance: A Self-Help Program for Managing Anxiety and Depression by Fred Yates. London: The Mental Health Foundation, 2000. Publications, The Mental Health Foundation, 7th Floor, 83 Victoria Street, London SW1H 0HW, UK. Tel: 020 7802 0304; website: http://www.mentalhealth.org.uk.
This is a self-help CD-ROM for people with mild to moderate anxiety and depression.

Chronic (persistent) psychotic disorders* — F29

(Clinical term: Schizophrenia Eu20)

Includes schizophrenia, schizoaffective disorders, schizotypal disorder, persistent delusional disorders, induced delusional disorder, other non-organic psychotic disorders

Presenting complaints

Many patients will have an established history of psychosis; others, however, may be unknown to specialized services, particularly those with more insidious presentations or those who have disengaged or are homeless.

Patients may present with the following:

- difficulties with thinking or concentrating (eg they think that the television is talking to them, or that their thoughts are being read)
- reports of hearing voices or seeing visions
- strange beliefs (eg having supernatural powers or being persecuted)
- extraordinary physical complaints (eg strange sensations or having unusual objects inside their body)
- problems or questions related to antipsychotic medication
- problems in managing work, studies or relationships
- physical healthcare problems (eg weight, respiratory or cardiac problems)
- lack of energy or motivation and an inability to feel emotion
- depression or suicidal thinking.

Families might seek help because of apathy, withdrawal, poor hygiene, or strange behaviour.

Diagnostic features

- Persistent problems with the following features:
  - social withdrawal and/or poor social integration
  - low motivation, interest or self-neglect
  - disordered thinking (exhibited by strange or disjointed speech).
- Periodic episodes of:
  - depression (co-existing depression is common, and is sometimes a serious consequence of persistent psychosis; there is a serious risk of suicide)
  - agitation or restlessness
  - bizarre behaviour
  - hallucinations (false or imagined perceptions, eg hearing voices)
  - delusions (firm beliefs that are often false, eg patient is related to royalty, receiving messages from their television, being followed or persecuted)
  - intense fear, anxiety and distress.

It can be difficult to ask patients about strange thoughts and hallucinations. Useful questions include, 'Have you had the feeling lately that people are talking or plotting about you, or trying to hurt you?' 'Is there anything special about you that would make anyone want to do that?' 'Have there been times lately when you have heard noises or voices or seen strange things when no one else was about and there was nothing else to explain it?'

*Chronic psychosis has become a pejorative term: persistent psychosis embraces the possibility of recovery.

Differential diagnosis and co-existing conditions

- 'Depression — F32#' (if low or sad mood, pessimism and/or feelings of guilt; co-morbid depression is common).
- 'Bipolar disorder — F31' (if symptoms of mania excitement, elevated mood, exaggerated self-worth is prominent).
- 'Alcohol misuse — F10' or 'Drug use disorders — F11#'. Chronic intoxication or withdrawal from alcohol or other substances (stimulants, hallucinogens) can cause psychotic symptoms.

Patients with persistent psychosis might misuse drugs and/or alcohol.

Essential information for patient and family

- Agitation and strange behaviour can be symptoms of a mental disorder.
- Symptoms may come and go over time.
- Medication should be part of an overall holistic and multi-axial approach to care and can help by reducing current difficulties and the risk of relapse.
- Stable living conditions (eg stable accommodation, adequate income, daily work or activities) are a pre-requisite for effective rehabilitation and recovery.
- It is important for family/carers to work with the doctors to learn to recognize early warning signs of relapse and for an advance agreement to be established with the patient and family/carers on how crises should be managed (R: 8-4).
- Voluntary organizations can provide valuable information, support and self-management courses to the patient and carers.

General management and advice to patient and family

- Remain optimistic and emphasize the patient's strengths and abilities, rather than deficits.
- Recovery often takes place in small steps and, for the patient, being engaged in an activity that is meaningful to them might be as important as symptom control.
- Discuss a treatment plan with the patient, in line with NICE good practice;[5] provide information on the condition, treatment choices and informed discussion. The treatment plan should include recognition of early warning signs and the agreed management of crises should be clearly recorded in the medical records. A copy of the plan should be given to the patient and, with their permission, to the family/carers (R: 8-3).
- Explain that drugs help prevent relapse, and discuss information on effects and side-effects with the patient (R: 1–3).
- The DVLA must be notified in all cases. Advise patient to inform DVLA: driving should cease until patient has been stable and well for at least three years and has insight into his/her condition (LGV/PSV driver).[3]
- Support patient to function in the areas that are important to him/her (eg work, recreation, relationships).
- It is important proactively to offer patients the same health promotion and prevention measures as the general population (eg smoking cessation, weight control, screening for diabetes and sexual health).
- Substance misuse (seen in over 30% of cases) will increase the chance of relapse.
- Psychological therapies for both the patient and family/carers might help prevent relapse, promote recovery, and are increasingly available in local services. Encourage the patient to engage with psychological therapies where available (eg cognitive behavioural therapy, family therapy, problem-solving interventions).
- Family interventions or problem-solving work might help improve patient and carer health.
- Therapeutic alliances build on respect and feeling valued. Encourage the patient to build relationships with key members of the practice team, for example by seeing the same doctor or nurse at each appointment. Use the relationship to discuss the

treatment plan, including advantages of medication and to review the effectiveness of the care plan (R: 11–4).

- Refer to 'Acute psychotic disorder — F23' for advice on the management of agitated or excited states.
- If care is shared with the Community Mental Health Team, agree who is to do what.
- Support of the carer is essential for effective treatment and rehabilitation. An assessment of the patient's needs and those of the carer (under the Carer's Recognition and Services Act) can be requested from the local Social Services department.

Medication

- Antipsychotic medication may reduce psychotic symptoms (*BNF* section 4.2.1).
- Some patients remain stable on the older medications (eg trifluoperazine, chlorpromazine). If effective and well tolerated, NICE guidance suggests the drug should be continued.[5] If ineffective or poorly tolerated, NICE guidance suggests an atypical medication should be considered.[5]
- Atypical antipsychotics, for example olanzapine (5–10 mg a day) or risperidone (2–4 mg per day), should be considered as a first-line treatment.[5]
- Inform the patient that continued medication helps reduce risk of relapse. In general, antipsychotic medication should be continued for at least one year.
- The dose should be the lowest possible for relief of symptoms and effective daily functioning.
- If, after team support, the patient is reluctant or erratic in taking medication, injectable long-acting antipsychotic medication could be considered in order to ensure continuity of treatment and reduce risk of relapse.[59] It should be reviewed at 4–6-monthly intervals, and a weight gain and physical annual heath check is essential to decrease the risk of cardiac and respiratory effects of medication and a sedentary lifestyle. Doctors and nurses who give depot injections in primary care need training to do so.[60] If available, specific counselling about medication is also helpful.[61] As part of the 'shared care plan', decide who is to contact the patient, should he/she fail to attend an appointment.
- Discuss the potential side-effects with the patient. Common motor side-effects, particularly with older antipsychotics, include the following:
  — Acute dystonias or spasms and parkinsonian symptoms (eg tremor and akinesia), which can be managed with antiparkinsonian drugs (eg orphenadrine [50 mg three times a day]; *BNF* section 4.9).
  — Withdrawal of antiparkinsonian drugs should be attempted after two to three months without symptoms, as these drugs are liable to misuse and might impair memory.
  — Akathisia (severe motor restlessness) can be managed with dosage reduction, or beta-blockers (eg propranolol at 30–80 mg a day; *BNF* section 2.4). A change in medication might be necessary.
  — Tardive dyskinesia is a particularly important side-effect for which to monitor. It is associated with longer-term use of traditional antipsychotic medication, is severely disabling and can be irreversible.
- Other side-effects can include glucose intolerance, weight gain, galactorrhoea and photosensitivity. Patients suffering from drug-induced photosensitivity are eligible for sunscreen on prescription.
- Avoid poly-pharmacy, particularly concurrent prescribing of typical and atypical antipsychotics, and prescribing in excess of *BNF* guidelines.

Liaison and referral

Referral to secondary mental health services is advised:

- Urgently:
  — if there are signs of relapse (unless there is an established previous response to treatment and it is safe to manage the patient at home)

55

— if there is a risk to self or others.
- Non-urgently:
  — if there is a poor response to treatment
  — to clarify diagnosis and ensure most appropriate treatment, including family interventions and cognitive behavioural therapy for psychosis
  — if there is non-compliance with treatment, problematic side-effects, failure of community treatment or breakdown of living arrangements (eg threat of loss of home).

Patients with complex mental-health, occupational, social and financial needs are normally managed by specialist services, under the Care Programme Approach and shared care with primary healthcare teams once stable.

Community Mental Health Services can be able to provide concordance therapy,[61] family interventions,[62] cognitive behaviour therapy[63] and rehabilitative facilities.

Special considerations in children and adolescents

- In younger teenagers, psychosis is less common than in adults, and in pre-pubertal children it is decidedly rare. When it does occur, however, it often takes a particularly severe and persistent form.
- For children and teenagers, family-based management and specialist education are particularly important.
- Only atypical antipsychotics should be used and depot preparations are seldom necessary or appropriate.

Child and Adolescent Mental Health Services should usually be the specialist advisors for children and teenagers.

Resources for patients and families

Resource leaflets: 1–3 *Coping with the side-effects of medication*, 8–2 *About schizophrenia*, 8–3 *Coping with difficult behaviours*, and 8–4 *Early warning signs* form

Rethink (*formerly* the National Schizophrenia Fellowship)
England: 020 8974 6814 (Advice line: 10am–3pm, Monday–Friday)
Email: advice@rethink.org; website: http://www.rethink.org
Scotland: 0131 557 8969
Northern Ireland: 02890 402 323
Monthly social groups for clients with schizophrenia living in the community and relatives support.

Schizophrenia Association of Great Britain 01248 354 048
Email: info@sagb.co.uk; website: http://www.sagb.co.uk
Offers information and support to sufferers, relatives, friends, carers and medical workers.

MINDinfoLINE 08457 660 163 (9.15am–5.15pm, Monday–Friday).
Email: info@mind.org.uk; website: http://www.mind.org.uk
Information service for matters relating to mental health.

SANELine 08457 678 000 (helpline 12noon–2.00am)
Website: http://www.sane.org.uk
Helpline offering information and advice on all aspects of mental health for those experiencing illness or their families or friends.

Hearing Voices Network 0161 228 3896 (10.30am–3pm, Monday–Wednesday, Friday)
Self-help groups to allow people to explore their voice-hearing experiences.

The UK NHS Portal for Schizophrenia
Website: http://www.nhs.uk/schizophrenia
This is a web-based information resource for people with schizophrenia and their carers. The site contains a number of user-friendly sections: Evidence-based treatment summaries; What is schizophrenia? How is schizophrenia diagnosed? Managing schizophrenia; Living with schizophrenia; Support for carers; and Legal issues.

IRIS (Initiative to Reduce the Impact of Schizophrenia) 01922 858 044
Website: http://www.iris-initiative.org.uk
In conjunction with Rethink, IRIS has developed clinical guidelines for practitioners and consumers.

Mental Health Care http://www.mentalhealthcare.org.uk
This site provides mental health information and research news from the Institute of Psychiatry and the South London and Maudsley NHS Trust in partnership with Rethink.
The Mental Health Foundation produces the information booklet *Understanding Schizophrenia*. Publications, The Mental Health Foundation, 7th Floor, 83 Victoria Street, London SW1H 0HW, UK. Tel: 020 7802 0304; website: http://www.mentalhealth.org.uk.

Living With Schizophrenia: A Holistic Approach to Understanding, Preventing and Recovering from Negative Symptoms by John Watkins. Hill of Content Publishing, 1996.

Working with Voices by R Coleman and M Smith. Handsell Publishing, 1997
This is a workbook to help voice hearers manage their voices.

Human Voices: A Common Human Experience by John Watkins. Hill of Content Publishing, 1998

Delirium — F05

(Clinical term: Other mental disorders due to brain damage and dysfunction caused by physical disease Eu05)

Presenting complaints

- Families may request help because patient is suddenly more confused or becomes either much quieter or agitated and disturbed.
- Patients may appear uncooperative, fearful or tearful.
- Delirium occurs in many older patients hospitalized for physical conditions.

Diagnostic features

Acute onset, usually over hours or days, of:

- confusion (patient appears disoriented for time and place, may misidentify people and have a poor grasp of situations and surroundings)
- impairment of memory
- disturbance of conscious level with reduced ability to focus or shift attention and markedly diminished attention span.

May be accompanied by:

- agitation (hyperactive delirium) or, more commonly, apathy (hypoactive delirium)
- changes in mood, eg fearfulness, sadness
- perplexity and sometimes apathy
- illusions (misperceptions of normal stimuli)
- suspiciousness
- disturbed sleep (reversal of sleep pattern)
- disturbed thinking, often reflected in incoherent speech
- hallucinations (can occur in any sensory modality but visual hallucinations are most common)
- autonomic features (eg sweating, tachycardia, tachypnoea).

Symptoms often develop rapidly and may change from hour to hour. They are characteristically worse at night.

Delirium may occur in patients with previously normal mental function but is more common in those with previous degenerative brain disorder. Delirium may occur in patients with previously normal mental function or in those with dementia. People with chronic physical illnesses are also more vulnerable to delirium, and in these groups it might be precipitated by apparently innocuous things, including minor infections, changes to any drug treatment and changes in environment.

Differential diagnosis

'Acute psychotic disorders — F23' (if symptoms persist, delusions and disordered thinking predominate, and no physical cause is identified).

Delirium in the setting of dementia could be missed if the pre-existing dementia is not recognized. Some features of quiet delirium occur in acute dysphasias (stroke) and depression, and of hyperactive delirium in acute psychotic episodes (see below) or mania.

Essential information for family

- Strange behaviour or speech and sudden confusion can be symptoms of a medical illness, especially if the patient is elderly or has dementia.
- Seek help urgently if patient becomes confused.

General management and advice to family[64]

- Delirium is a medical emergency with appreciable mortality.
- Hospitalization might be required because of agitation or the physical illness that is causing delirum. Patients may need to be admitted to a medical ward in order to diagnose and treat the underlying disorder. In an emergency, where there is risk to life and safety, a medically ill patient may be taken to a general hospital for treatment under common law, without using the Mental Health Act. In such a case, a medical doctor may make this decision without involvement of a psychiatrist.
- Take measures to prevent the patient from harming themselves or others (eg remove unsafe objects, restrain if necessary).
- Supportive contact with familiar people can reduce confusion.
- Provide frequent reminders of time and place and minimize distracting stimuli to reduce confusion.
- Keep lighting levels bright to minimize visual illusions.
- Keep up fluid and food intake as much as possible.[65]
- Try and encourage mobility.[65]
- Try and encourage a restful sleep at night.

Medication[66]

- Avoid use of sedative or hypnotic medications (eg benzodiazepines) except for the treatment of alcohol or sedative withdrawal.
- Antipsychotic medication in low doses (*BNF* section 4.2.1) might sometimes be needed to control agitation, psychotic symptoms or aggression. Beware of drug side-effects (drugs with anticholinergic action and antiparkinsonian medication can exacerbate or cause delirium) and drug interactions.
- When drugs are required because of severe behavioural disturbance or risk to self and/or others, low-dose risperidone is the usual drug of first choice, except in alcohol or drug withdrawal states or in patients with liver disease in whom benzodiazepines are more appropriate. If oral medication is not possible, low-dose haloperidol might be helpful.
- If Lewy body dementia is suspected, benzodiazepines are preferred to antipsychotics, because the latter can be fatal (see **Dementia — F03**).[67]

Referral

Referral to secondary mental health services is rarely indicated. Referral to a physician is nearly always indicated if:

- the cause is unclear
- the cause is clear and treatable but carers are unable to support the patient or they are living alone
- drug or alcohol withdrawal or overdose or another underlying condition necessitating inpatient medical care is suspected.

Dementia — F03
(Clinical term: Dementia in Alzheimer's disease Eu00.)

Presenting complaints
- Patients may complain of forgetfulness, decline in mental functioning (eg getting muddled making phone calls, deciding which bus to catch, sorting out change at the checkout), difficulty finding words (especially names and nouns) or feeling depressed, but may be unaware of memory loss.
- Families may ask for help initially because of failing memory, disorientation, and change in personality or behaviour. In the later stages of the illness, they may seek help because of distressing or dangerous behaviour (eg aggression, wandering, incontinence or leaving the gas on unlit).
- Dementia may also be diagnosed during consultations for other problems, as relatives might confuse early dementia with natural ageing.
- Changes in behaviour and functioning (eg poor personal hygiene or social interaction) in an older patient should raise the possibility of a diagnosis of dementia.

Diagnostic features
- Decline in memory for recent events, thinking, judgement, orientation and language.
- Patients may have become apparently apathetic or disinterested, but might also appear alert and appropriate, despite deterioration in memory and other cognitive function.
- Decline in everyday function (eg dressing, washing and cooking).
- Changes in personality or emotional control — patients may become easily upset, tearful or irritable, as well as apathetic, and have persecutory delusions.
- Common with advancing age (5% over 65 years; 20% over 80 years); very rare in youth or middle age.

Dementia has a number of causes. The most common include Alzheimer's disease (60% of cases) characterized by a gradual progression; vascular dementia (20%) with a classically step-wise progression; and Lewy body dementia (15%) with fluctuating cognition, visual hallucinations and parkinsonism, but the clinical picture is often not clear cut.

Owing to the problems inherent in taking a history from people with dementia, it is very important that information about the level of current functioning and possible decline in functioning is obtained from an informant (eg spouse, child or other carer), together with the use of formal memory tests and assessment of activities of daily living.[1]

Tests of memory and thinking include the following:

- The ability to repeat the names of three common objects (eg apple, table, penny) immediately, and recall them after three minutes.
- The ability accurately to identify the day of the week, the month and the year.
- The ability to give their name and full, postal address.

A short screening test is set out in the resource section on the CD-ROM (R: 11–3).

Differential diagnosis
Examine and investigate for treatable causes of dementia. Common causes of cognitive worsening in the elderly are as follows:

- **'Delirium — F05'.** (Sudden increases in confusion, wandering attention or agitation will usually indicate a physical illness [eg acute infectious illness] or toxicity from medication.)

- 'Acute psychosis — F23'.
- 'Chronic (persistent) psychosis — F20#'.
- 'Depression — F32#'. (Depression may cause memory and concentration problems similar to those of dementia, especially in older patients, if low or sad mood is prominent, or if the impairment is patchy and has developed rapidly.)
- Common organic causes of impairment include metabolic and endocrine disorders, neoplasms, any drug treatments.

Helpful tests in distinguishing an organic cause include midstream urine sample (MSU), full blood count (FBC), vitamin B_{12}, folate, liver function tests (LFTs), thyroid function tests (TFTs), urea and electrolytes (U and E), Ca^{2+} and glucose.

Essential information for patient and family
- Dementia is frequent in old age but is not inevitable.
- Memory loss and confusion may cause behaviour problems, for example agitation, suspiciousness, emotional outbursts, apathy, disinhibition in aggression, inappropriate sexual behaviour, and an inability to take part in normal social interaction.
- Memory loss usually proceeds slowly, but the course and long-term prognosis vary with the disease causing dementia. Discuss diagnosis, likely progress and prognosis with the patient and family.
- Physical illness or other stress can increase confusion.
- The patient will have great difficulty in learning new information. Avoid placing patient in unfamiliar places or situations.
- Membership of a support group and information on dementia for the family can aid caring, although some carers might find this distressing in the short term.

Always give information about local services in addition to general advice about dementia.

General management and advice to patient and family[68]
- Regularly review the patient's ability to perform daily tasks safely, behavioural problems and general physical condition.
- If memory loss is mild, consider use of memory aids or reminders.
- Encourage the patient to make full use of remaining abilities.
- Encourage maintainance of the patient's physical health and fitness through good diet and exercise, plus swift treatment of intercurrent physical illness.
- Make sure the patient and family understand that the condition may impair the ability to drive. If the patient is incapable of understanding this advice, the GP should inform the DVLA immediately. In early dementia when sufficient skills are retained and progression is slow, a licence may be issued subject to annual review (car and motorbike drivers only).[3]
- Regularly assess risk (balancing safety and independence), especially at times of crisis. As appropriate, discuss arrangements for support in the home, community or day care programmes, or residential placement.
- Review how the carer is managing, especially if they live with the patient. Consider ways to reduce stress on those caring for the patient (eg self-help groups, home help, day care and respite care). Contact with other families caring for relatives with dementia may be helpful, although this can be distressing at first. An assessment of the patient's needs and those of the carer (under the Carer's Recognition and Services Act) can be requested from the local Social Services Department. Carers may need continuing support after the patient has entered residential care or has died.
- Discuss planning of legal and financial affairs with family members, including information on seeking 'power of attorney' and 'enduring power of attorney'. Attendance allowance and a discount on council tax bills can usually be claimed. An allowance (Invalid Carer's Allowance) can also be obtained by carers. An information sheet is available from the Alzheimer's Society (see below) and further information and help can be obtained through local Social Services.

- Non-pharmacological methods of dealing with difficult behaviour can be adopted. For example, carers may be able to deal with repetitive questioning if they are given the information that this is because of the dementia affecting the patient's memory.

Medication

- Antipsychotic medication in very low doses (*BNF* section 4.2.1) might sometimes be needed to manage some behavioural problems (eg aggression or restlessness). Behavioural problems change with the course of the dementia; therefore, withdraw medication every few months on a trial basis to see if it is still needed, and discontinue if it is not. Beware of drug side-effects (eg parkinsonian symptoms, anticholinergic effects) and drug interactions (avoid combining with tricyclic antidepressants, alcohol, anticonvulsants or L-dopa preparations.). Antipsychotics should be avoided in Lewy body dementia.[67]
- Avoid using sedative or hypnotic medications (eg benzodiazepines) if possible. If other treatments have failed and severe management problems remain, use very cautiously and for no more than two weeks; they may increase confusion.
- Aspirin in low doses can be prescribed in vascular dementia to attempt to slow deterioration.
- In Alzheimer's disease, consider referring to secondary care for assessment and initiation of anticholinesterase drugs, which may postpone the onset of more severe symptoms but do not affect the eventual outcome of the disease. NICE recommends that donepezil, rivastigmine and galantamine should be made available as part of the management of some people with mild-to-moderate Alzheimer's disease.[69] These drugs should be started by specialists and the patient assessed every six months by specialists or their GP following shared protocols.
- Memantine, which acts on the glutamate neuroreceptors, has been licensed in the UK for moderate to severe Alzheimer's disease, but the clinical evidence for its effectiveness is currently sparse.[70,71]

Referral

- Refer early to a specialist for assessment and possible treatment with anticholinesterase treatment in the case of early Alzheimer's.
- Consider referral to Social Services for practical help: needs assessment, formal care planning, home help, day care and help with placement and benefits.
- Refer to a physician if complex medical co-morbidity or sudden worsening of dementia.
- Refer to psychiatric services if there are intractable behavioural problems, unusually complex family relationships or if depressive or psychotic episode occurs.

Resources for patients and families

Alzheimer's Society 0845 300 0336 (helpline)
Email: helpline@alzheimers.org.uk; website: http://www.alzheimers.org.uk
Provides support to people with all forms of dementia — not just Alzheimer's — their family and friends, and supports research on education and training for primary care.

Age Concern http://www.ace.org.uk
England: 0800 009 966 (Information line 7am–7pm, seven days a week); Email: ace@ace.org.uk
Northern Ireland: 02890 245 729; Email: info@ageconcernni.org
Wales: 029 2037 1566; Email: enquiries@accymru.org.uk
Scotland: 0131 220 3345; Email: enquiries@acscot.org.uk
Provides information and advice relating to older people.

Help the Aged http://www.helptheaged.org.uk
England: 020 7278 1114; Email: info@helptheaged.org.uk
Wales: 02920 346 550; Email: infocymru@helptheaged.org.uk
Scotland: 0131 551 6331; Email: infoscot@helptheaged.org.uk
Northern Ireland: 02890 230 666; Email: infoni@helptheaged.org.uk
Provides advice and support to older people

Carers UK 0808 808 7777 (helpline 10am–12noon and 2–4pm, Monday–Friday)
Email: info@ukcarers.org.uk, website: http://www.carersonline.org.uk
Formerly the National Carers Association. Provides information and advice on all
aspects of care for both carers and professionals.

Counsel and Care 020 7485 1566 (10.30am–4pm, Monday–Friday)
Website: http://www.counselandcare.org.uk
Advice and information on home and residential care for older people.

Crossroads Association 0845 450 0350
Email: communications@crossroads.org.uk; website: http://www.crossroads.org.uk
Regional centres throughout the UK, providing practical support and help for
carers, including respite care, day centres, befriending and night care. There is also a
scheme for young carers.

Benefits Enquiry Line 0800 882 200
Advice and information for people with disabilities and their carers about benefits
and assistance with claim form completion.
Leaflets are available from the Royal College of Psychiatrists
(http://www.rcpsych.ac.uk):
*Memory and Dementia, Alzheimer's Disease and Dementia, Drug Treatment of
Alzheimer's.*
The Mental Health Foundation produces the information booklets *All About
Dementia* and *Because You Care* (which includes suggestions to carers about how to
deal with difficult behaviour in people with dementia). Publications, The Mental
Health Foundation, 7th Floor, 83 Victoria Street, London SW1H 0HW, UK. Tel: 020
7802 0304; website: http://www.mentalhealth.org.uk.

Alzheimer's at your Fingertips, 2nd edition, by Harry Cayton, Nori Graham and J
Warner. Class Publishing, 2002.
For patients and carers, this book answers commonly asked questions about all
types of dementia.

D

Depression — F32#
(Clinical term: Depressive episode Eu32)

Presenting complaints
The patient may present initially with one or more physical symptoms, such as pain or 'tiredness all the time'. Further enquiry may reveal low mood, loss of interest or irritability.

A wide range of presenting complaints may accompany or conceal depression. These include:

- anxiety or insomnia
- worries about social problems, eg financial or marital difficulties
- increased drug or alcohol use
- (in a new mother) constant worries about her baby or fear of harming the baby.

Diagnostic features
- Low or sad mood.
- Loss of interest or pleasure.

At least four of the following associated symptoms are present:
- disturbed sleep
- disturbed appetite
- guilt or low self-worth
- pessimism or hopelessness about the future
- fatigue or loss of energy
- agitation or slowing of movement or speech
- diurnal mood variation
- poor concentration
- suicidal thoughts or acts
- loss of self-confidence
- sexual dysfunction.

Symptoms of anxiety or nervousness and physical aches and pains are also frequently present.

Some groups are at higher risk, for example:

- those with adverse life events and social difficulties (eg the unemployed, single parents, the homeless, those living in care, those experiencing social isolation)
- those with a past history of depression and other psychiatric disorders
- those with chronic physical disorders
- women who have experienced recent childbirth (see **'Postnatal depression — F53'**).

It may be helpful to ask the following questions:

- During the past month, have you been bothered by little interest and pleasure in daily activities?
- During the past month, have you been bothered by feeling down, depressed and hopeless?

A negative answer to either of these questions makes depression unlikely.

Differential diagnosis and co-existing conditions
- **'Acute psychotic disorder — F23'** (if hallucinations [eg hearing voices] or delusions [eg strange or unusual beliefs] are present).
- **'Bipolar disorder — F31'** (if patient has a history of manic episodes [eg excitement, rapid speech and elevated mood]).

- 'Alcohol misuse — F10' or 'Drug use disorder — F11#' (if heavy alcohol or drug use is present).
- 'Chronic mixed anxiety and depression — F41.2'.
- 'Postnatal depression — F53'.
- 'Bereavement — Z63'.
- 'Adjustment disorder — F43.2'.
- 'Unexplained somatic complaints — F45'.
- 'Generalized anxiety — F41.1'.

Some medications might produce symptoms of depression (eg beta-blockers, other antihypertensives, H_2 blockers, oral contraceptives and corticosteroids).

Essential information for patient and family
- Depression is a common illness and effective treatments are available.
- Depression is not weakness or laziness.
- Depression can affect a person's ability to cope.
- Emotional and practical support from family and friends are very valuable.

Recommend information leaflets or audiotapes to reinforce the information (R: 6–1).

General management and advice to patient and family[72]
- Assess suicidal intent — see 'Self-harm'. The belief that enquiring about suicidal ideation may prompt some people to consider self-harm is not supported by research findings or clinical experience. Placed in the context of asking people about symptoms of depression, such questions feel less awkward for the interviewer; for example, 'It sounds as if you have been feeling very down recently; has there ever been a time when you have felt as though you couldn't be bothered carrying on?' 'Have you ever felt that life was not worth living/that you would be better off if you were dead?' 'Have you ever thought of harming yourself in any way?' Close supervision by family or friends or hospitalization may be needed.
- Consider high-risk groups, for example older people, men, those with physical illness, substance abuse, a family history of suicide and those who have previously demonstrated self-harm.
- Identify current life problems or social stresses, including precipitating factors. Focus on small, specific steps patients might take towards reducing or improving management of these problems. Avoid major decisions or life changes (R: 1–1).
- Plan short-term activities which give the patient enjoyment or build confidence. Exercise may be helpful.[73]
- If appropriate, advise reduction in caffeine intake[74] and drug and alcohol use.[75]
- Support the development of good sleep patterns and encourage a balanced diet.[76]
- Encourage patient to resist pessimism and self-criticism, not to act on pessimistic ideas (eg ending a marriage or leaving a job), and not to concentrate on negative or guilty thoughts.
- If physical symptoms are present, discuss the link between these and mood (see 'Unexplained somatic symptoms — F45').
- Involve the patient in discussing the advantages and disadvantages of available treatments. Inform them that medication usually works more quickly than psychotherapies.[77,78] Arrange another appointment to monitor progress one to two weeks later, whether or not on medication.
- After improvement, plan with the patient the action to be taken if signs of relapse occur.
- Patients might find it helpful to keep a mood diary, rating mood changes between 1 and 10 and noting down any external influencing factors. This can be practically useful in identifying patterns.

Medication[72]

Consider antidepressant drugs if sad mood or loss of interest are prominent for at least two weeks, preferably four weeks, and if four or more of the following symptoms are present (every day for most of the day), accompanied by significant impairment of functioning:

- fatigue or loss of energy
- disturbed sleep
- guilt or self-reproach
- poor concentration
- thoughts of death or suicide
- disturbed appetite
- agitation *or* slowing of movement and speech.

There is no evidence that people with recent onset of only few or very mild depressive symptoms respond to antidepressants.[79] There *is* evidence that persistent mild depression, lasting two years or more, responds to antidepressants.[55]

Consider delaying medication until the second or subsequent visit because there is a high rate of spontaneous recovery (see again within a week to reassess).

There is no evidence to suggest that any antidepressant is more effective than others;[77,80] however, their side-effect profiles differ, and therefore some drugs will be more acceptable to particular patients than others (*BNF* section 4.3).

Choice of medication:

- If the patient has responded well to a particular drug in the past, use that drug again.
- If the patient is older or physically ill, use medication with fewer anticholinergic and cardiovascular side-effects.
- If the patient is suicidal, avoid tricyclics and consider dispensing a few days' supply at a time.
- If the patient is anxious or unable to sleep, use a drug with more sedative effects, but warn of drowsiness and problems driving.
- If the patient is unwilling to give up alcohol, choose one of the SSRI antidepressants that do not interact with alcohol (eg fluoxetine, paroxetine and citalopram; *BNF* section 4.3.3).

Explain to the patient that:

- the medication must be taken every day (poor adherence is very common, particularly in pregnancy and breastfeeding)
- the drug is not addictive in that higher and higher doses are not required, but withdrawal symptoms may occur if drugs are stopped suddenly
- improvement in mood will start two to three weeks after starting the medication
- side-effects occur from the beginning but usually fade in seven to ten days with SSRIs; they may be more persistent with tricyclic antidepressants
- individuals vary in their reaction to different drugs, including absorption time, which will influence the appropriateness and timing of taking drugs with a sedative profile.

Stress that the patient should consult the doctor before stopping the medication. The drug should never be stopped abruptly (withdrawal symptoms may then occur). All antidepressants should be withdrawn slowly, preferably over four weeks in weekly decrements.

Continue full-dose antidepressant medication for at least four to six months after the condition improves to prevent relapse.[81,82] Review regularly — at least monthly — during this time to monitor response, side-effects and adherence. Consider, jointly with the patient, the need for futher continuation beyond four to six months. If the patient has had several episodes of major depression, consider carefully long-term, prophylactic treatment.[83] Obtain a second opinion at this point.

If sleep problems are very severe, consider a sedative antidepressant, for example a tricyclic.

If using tricyclic medication, build up over seven to ten days to the effective dose (eg dothiepin: start at 50–75 mg and build to 150 mg nocte; or imipramine: start at 25–50 mg each night and build to 100–150 mg).[84] It is reasonable to treat with doses of between 75 and 100 mg a day if the patient is responding.[85]

Withdraw antidepressant medication slowly, and monitor for withdrawal reactions and to ensure remission is stable. Gradual reduction of SSRIs can be achieved by using syrup in reducing doses or taking a tablet on alternate days.

Hypericum perforata (known as St John's Wort and available from health food stores) is efficacious for mild to moderate symptoms of depression, both acute and chronic, but not significant major depression.[86] GPs should enquire whether patient is taking St John's Wort because it is widely available and might interact with prescribed medication and diet (eg oral contraceptives, warfarin).[87–89] Over-the-counter formulations are very variable in dosage.

Referral

The following structured therapies, delivered by appropriately trained practitioners, are effective for some people with depression:[90]

- Cognitive behavioural therapy (CBT)
- Behaviour therapy
- Interpersonal therapy
- Structured problem-solving.

Patients with chronic, relapsing depression might benefit more from CBT or a combination of CBT and antidepressants than from medication alone.[91,92] Counselling might be helpful, especially in milder cases and if focused on specific psychosocial problems related to the depression (eg relationships, bereavement).[14] In the short term, it may have some advantages over normal GP care, and patients like it, but after 12 weeks there are no benefits.[14]

Referral to secondary mental health services is advised:

- as an emergency if there is a significant risk of suicide or danger to others, psychotic symptoms or severe agitation
- as a non-emergency, if significant depression persists despite treatment in primary care. (Antidepressant therapy has failed if the patient remains symptomatic after a full course of treatment at an adequate dosage. If there is no clear improvement after four weeks with the first drug, it should be changed to another class of drug.)

If drug or alcohol misuse is also a problem, see guidelines for these disorders.

Recommend voluntary/non-statutory services in all other cases where symptoms persist, where the patient has a poor or non-existent support network, or where social or relationship problems are contributing to the depression.[93]

Resources for patients and families

Resource leaflets: 1–1 *Problem-solving*, 6–1 *Depression and how to cope with it*, and 6–3 *Dealing with depressive thinking*

Depression Alliance http://www.depressionalliance.org
England: 020 8768 0123
Wales: 029 2069 2891 (10am–4pm, Monday–Friday)
Scotland: 0131 467 3050
Provides information and self-help groups.

Aware Defeat Depression Ltd 02871 260602
Email: info@aware-ni.org; website: http://www.aware-ni.org
Provides information leaflets, lectures and runs support groups for sufferers and relatives.

Samaritans 08457 909 090 (24-hour helpline)
Email: jo@samaritans.org; website: http://www.samaritans.org.uk
Offers confidential emotional support to any person who is despairing or suicidal.

Calm 0800 585858 (helpline 5pm–3am)
Helpline for young men who are depressed or suicidal.

SAD (Seasonal Affective Disorder) Association 01903 814 942
Website: http://www.sada.org.uk
Information about seasonal affective disorder (SAD). Offers advice and support to members.

UK Register of Counsellors 01788 568 739
Provides a list of BAC-accredited counsellors.
Leaflets are available from the Royal College of Psychiatrists
(http://www.rcpsych.ac.uk): Antidepressants, Depression
The Mental Health Foundation produces the information booklet *All About Depression*. Publications, The Mental Health Foundation, 7th Floor, 83 Victoria Street, London SW1H 0HW, UK. Tel: 020 7802 0304; website:
http://www.mentalhealth.org.uk.

Overcoming Depression by Paul Gilbert. Constable & Robinson, 2000
Self-help book.

Overcoming Depression by Chris Williams. Arnold Publishing, 2001
Self-help book (also available as a CD-ROM; see below).

Mind over Mood by Dennis Greenberger and Christine Padesky. New York, Guilford Press, 1995
Self-help manual designed to be used as an adjunct to therapy (a clinician's guide is also available).

The Feeling Good Handbook by David D Burns. Avon Books, 1989
A self-help manual.

Depression — the Way Out of your Prison, 2nd edn by Dorothy Rowe. London: Routledge, 1996
An explanatory book.

Coping with Depression. Talking Life, 1A Grosvenor Rd, Hoylake, Wirral CH47 3BS, UK. Tel: 0151 632 0662; website: http://www.talkinglife.co.uk.
Tape programme, produced with The Royal College of Psychiatrists' Defeat Depression initiative, describes strategies for coping with all types of depression using cognitive techniques.

Overcoming Depression. University of Leeds Media Innovations Ltd., 3 Gemini Business Park, Sheepscar Way, Leeds LS7 3JB, UK. Tel: 0113 262 1600; website: http://www.calipso.co.uk.
A CD-ROM self-help package.

Beating the Blues. Ultrasis UK Ltd, 4th Floor, 13/17 Long Lane, London EC1A 9PN, UK. Tel: 020 7600 6777; website: http://www.ultrasis.com.
Interactive multi-media programme designed for use in primary care setting, with practitioner assessment and progress review each week.

Dissociative (conversion) disorder — F44

[Clinical term: Dissociative (conversion) disorders Eu44]

D

Presenting complaints

Patients exhibit unusual or dramatic physical symptoms, such as seizures, amnesia, trance, loss of sensation, visual disturbances, paralysis, aphonia, identity confusion and 'possession' states. There is no evidence that the patient is intentionally producing the symptom.

Diagnostic features

Physical symptoms that are unusual in presentation and not consistent with known disease.

Onset is often sudden and related to psychological stress or difficult personal circumstances.

In acute cases, symptoms may:

- be dramatic and unusual
- change from time to time
- be related to attention from others.

In more chronic cases, patients might appear inappropriately calm in view of the seriousness of the complaint.

Differential diagnosis

Carefully consider physical conditions that might cause symptoms. A full history and physical (including neurological) examination are essential. Early symptoms of neurological disorders (eg multiple sclerosis) may resemble conversion symptoms.

- If other unexplained physical symptoms are present, see **'Unexplained somatic complaints — F45'**.
- **'Depression — F32#'** (atypical depression may present in this way).

Essential information for patient and family

- Physical or neurological symptoms often have no clear physical cause. Symptoms can be brought about by stress.
- Symptoms usually resolve rapidly (from hours to a few weeks), leaving no permanent damage.

General management and advice to patient and family

- Encourage the patient to acknowledge recent stresses or difficulties (although it is not necessary for the patient to link the stresses to current symptoms).
- Advise the patient to take a brief rest and relief from stress, then return to usual activities.
- Give positive reinforcement for improvement. Try not to reinforce symptoms. Encourage problem-solving for current stresses and difficulties.
- Advise against prolonged rest or withdrawal from activities.
- Discuss plan with patient's family (but care is required because in some instances family problems may have precipitated the episode).

Medication

Avoid anxiolytics or sedatives.

In more chronic cases with depressive symptoms, antidepressant medication may be helpful.

D

Referral

See general referral criteria.

Non-urgent referral to secondary mental health services is advised if confident of the diagnosis:

- if symptoms persist
- if symptoms are recurrent or severe
- if the patient is prepared to discuss a psychological contribution to symptoms.

If unsure of the diagnosis, consider referral to a physician before referral to secondary mental health services.

Resources for patients and families

BACP (British Association for Counselling and Psychotherapy) 0870 443 5252
Website: http://www.counselling.co.uk.
Provides advice on sources of individual counselling and family therapy in the UK.

Domestic violence or partner abuse

Patients may be fearful and reluctant to disclose domestic violence and abuse. Professionals should be particularly sensitive and empathetic in their approach.

Presenting complaints
The patient may present with:

- physical injuries: bruising, cuts, burns, broken bones
- increased rate or severity of injuries, especially located on the abdomen, during pregnancy
- physical complaints: headaches, chronic pain, pelvic inflammatory disease, pelvic pain, sexual dysfunction
- psychiatric symptoms: depression, anxiety, suicidality, Post-traumatic stress disorder, alcohol or drug abuse
- comments about relationship problems or jealousy by the partner
- complaints of being hit or harmed by the partner
- fearfulness
- a partner who insists on being present at appointments; a partner who intimidates or controls the patient.

Diagnostic pointers
- Dysjunction between physical signs and reported mechanism and history of injury should increase the index of suspicion.
- Physical, sexual or emotional abuse perpetrated by a spouse or partner. Both men and women can be victims, but female victims of male partners experience more severe injury and greater depression. (Partner abuse also occurs in gay and lesbian relationships.)
- Behavioural changes such as hypervigilance, submissive behaviour in the presence of the abuser, partner speaks or responds on behalf of patient.

Co-existing conditions
- Domestic violence is associated with high rates of mental health problems, which also need to be assessed and treated:
  — 'Self-harm' and 'Depression — F32#' are among the most common mental health sequelae of partner abuse.[94] Living with violence can exacerbate a predisposition to depression, but a woman's first exposure to abuse can also cause subsequent depression. Depression may improve as time passes after abuse.
  — Battered women are nearly four times more likely to suffer from 'Post-traumatic stress disorder — F43.1', directly related to the experience of partner violence.
  — 'Alcohol misuse — F10' and 'Drug use disorders — F11#' occur in higher rates in abused women, with evidence that it may be a consequence and not just an association with partner violence.
  — Higher levels of 'Generalized anxiety — F41.1' and 'Phobic disorders — F40' occur, as well as worse long-term physical health.
- Children witnessing domestic violence might present with symptoms related to this experience. For example, young children might experience tummy aches, difficulty in sleeping, regression tantrums, and enuresis; boys might present with aggression, disobedience, truancy or substance misuse, girls with withdrawal from others, anxiety and depression, low self-esteem, vague physical symptoms. Girls are also more likely to develop eating disorders or deliberate self-harm tendencies. Schooling might be affected and children can exhibit symptoms of Post-traumatic stress disorder (nightmares, flash backs, easily startled).

- Children living in the home are also at higher risk of being assaulted or abused by the perpetrator. See **'Child abuse and neglect'**.

Essential information for patient and family

Domestic violence is a universal problem: one in four British women and one in seven men are physically assaulted by a partner in their lives.[95] Rates are higher if forms of emotional abuse are included.

- The effects of domestic violence go beyond physical injury.
- The risk of attack is increased for women when they try to leave. The woman should have safety awareness and be encouraged to seek appropriate support (see Resources below).
- Children who witness or experience domestic violence are also directly affected and are at risk.

General management and advice to patient

- **Assess immediate risk.** Ask if patient feels she or her children might be in danger when she returns home today. Detailed risk assessment questions are probably not appropriate within primary-care consultations. However, encourage the woman to protect herself and her children. Reassure her that seeking help does *not* mean that her children will be taken in to care. Encourage her to talk to the children about how they feel.
- Abused women report that they feel they can confide in their GP, yet often feel ashamed to disclose their situation. Most women experiencing partner abuse are not recognized within primary care.[96] Although there is debate about routine screening,[97] having a low threshold for asking direct questions about domestic violence is necessary to identify cases.
- The higher prevalence of current or past abuse in women with mental health problems is a compelling reason for asking about abuse routinely in such cases.
- In the absence of visible injury, the practitioner can lead up to explicit enquiry about abuse with a statement like, 'Because conflict or violence is so common in the lives of women, we have begun to ask routinely about abuse in relationships'. If the presenting complaint is anxiety or depression, exploration of stressors should include enquiry about partner abuse. The following questions (HARK — humiliation, afraid, rape, kick) can be used to ask about past abuse:
  - **Humiliation:** Within the past year, have you been humiliated or emotionally abused in other ways by your partner, ex-partner or anyone close to you?
  - **Afraid:** Within the past year, have you been afraid of your partner, ex-partner or anyone close to you?
  - **Rape:** Within the past year, have you been raped or forced to have any kind of sexual activity by your partner, ex-partner or anyone close to you?
  - **Kick:** Within the past year, have you been kicked, hit, slapped or otherwise physically hurt by your partner, ex-partner or anyone close to you?
  If the answer to any of these question is 'yes', with the woman's permission summarize information in the medical record, including a description of the abuse and any related symptoms. A more detailed record can be made at a subsequent consultation.
- **Documentation**: Good records might prove invaluable in future legal proceedings, as well as in alerting other colleagues with whom the woman might consult.
- **Confidentiality** is crucial; accidental access to the record by the partner can place the woman at greater risk — information should *not* be entered into hand-held records (eg antenatal or child health records), and care should be taken in entering an identifiable term on a computer summary that might be visible to the partner if he attends a consultation.
- After disclosure, or in the absence of disclosure if the practitioner still suspects abuse, give a contact number for local agencies that provide advocacy (see Resources

below). Evaluations of advocacy projects in the UK are positive and, generally, abused women find referral to advocacy acceptable.[98]

- Cognitive behaviour therapy interventions are effective in improving the mental health of abused women.[99]

Referral

After disclosure of a history of partner abuse by a patient and contact with an advocacy agency, further follow-up for mental health sequelae by the primary care clinician is recommended. This might result in referral to a therapist.

Resources for patients and families

Contact the Police Domestic Violence Officer to discuss safety and options.

Women's Aid Federation
National Domestic Violence helpline (24-hour)
England: 08457 023 468
Wales: 029 2039 0874
Northern Ireland: 01232 249 041/358
Scotland: 0131 221 0401
Website: http://www.womensaid.org.uk
Support, advice, information and referrals for women experiencing domestic violence.

Zero Tolerance 0800 028 3398 (helpline)
Website: http://www.domesticviolenceprevention.com
Support, advice and information for women experiencing domestic violence.

Rape Crisis Federation 020 7837 1600 (24-hour helpline)
Website: http://www.rapecrisis.co.uk

Victim Support 0845 3030 900 (Support line 9am–9pm, Monday–Friday; 9am–7pm, Saturday/Sunday; 9am–5pm, bank holidays; see telephone directory for local branch)
Provides emotional support and practical information for anyone who has suffered the effects of crime, regardless of whether the crime has been reported.

Refuge 0870 599 5443 (24-hour national crisis line)
Offers support, information and referrals. It runs its own refuges in London and the South East.

Kiran — Asian Women's Aid 020 8558 1986; Email: kiranawa@talk21.com
Advice, support and refuge for Asian women, and women from other cultures (eg Turkey, Iran, Morocco and Malaysia, etc.)

Everyman Project 020 7737 6747
Counselling, support and advice to men who are violent or concerned about their violence, and anyone affected by that violence.

Relate 01788 573 241/456 1310
Website: http://www.relate.org.uk
Counselling for adults with relationship difficulties, whether married or not.

Parentline 01702 559 900 (helpline)
Offers help and advice to parents on bringing up children and teenagers.

The Suzy Lamplugh Trust Website: http://www.suzylamplugh.org.uk
Works to minimize the damage caused to individuals and to society by aggression in all its forms.

For legal advice (eg child custody, restraining injunctions):
The National Council for Civil Liberties 020 7378 8659 (advice line)
Citizens' Advice Bureau (see telephone directory for local branch)
Rights of Women 020 7251 6575
Leaflets are available from the Royal College of Psychiatrists
(http://www.rcpsych.ac.uk): Fact sheet 18, for parents and teachers. Domestic violence — its effects on children.

Drug use disorders — F10–19

(F10 alcohol, F11 opioids, F12 cannabinoids, F13 sedatives or hypnotics, F14 cocaine, F15 other stimulants including coffee, F16 hallucinogens, F17 tobacco, F18 volatile solvents, F19 multiple drug use and use of other psychotic substances)
(Clinical term: Mental and behavioural disorders due to use of opioids — Eu11)

Presenting complaints

- Patients may have depressed mood, nervousness or insomnia.
- Patients might present with a direct request for help to withdraw from or to stabilize their drug use.
- Patients might present in a state of intoxication or withdrawal, or with physical complications of their drug use (eg abscesses or thromboses).
- Patients may present with social or legal consequences of their drug use (eg debt or prosecution).
- Occasionally, covert drug use may manifest itself as bizarre, unexplained behaviour.

Signs of drug withdrawal include the following:

- Opioids: nausea, sweating, restlessness, goose bumps, diarrhoea (cold turkey), hallucinations.
- Sedatives: anxiety, tremors, insomnia, hallucinations (rare).
- Stimulants (cocaine, crack, amphetamine, ecstasy): depression, moodiness, irritability.

The family may request help before the patient (eg because the patient is irritable at home or missing work).

Whatever their motivation for seeking help, the aim of treatment is to assist the patient to remain healthy until, if motivated to do so and with appropriate help and support, they can achieve a drug-free life.

Diagnostic features

- Drug use has caused physical harm (eg injuries while intoxicated), psychological harm (eg symptoms of mental disorder due to drug use), or has led to harmful social consequences (eg loss of job, severe family problems, criminality).
- Habitual and/or harmful or chaotic drug use.
- Difficulty controlling drug use.
- Strong desire to use drugs.
- Tolerance (can use large amounts of drugs without appearing intoxicated).
- Withdrawal (eg anxiety, tremors or other withdrawal symptoms after stopping use).

Diagnosis is aided by the following:

- History: including reason for presentation, past and current (ie in the past four weeks) drug use, routes of use, past medical and psychiatric history, social (and especially child care) responsibilities, forensic history and past contact with treatment services. Poly-drug use/misuse/abuse is common and current and previous history should be elicited.
- Examination: motivation, physical (needle tracks or complications, eg thrombosis or viral illness), mental state.
- Investigations (haemoglobin, liver function tests [LFTs] including gamma-glutamyl transferase [GGT], urine drug screen, Hepatitis B and C]).

Differential diagnosis and co-existing conditions

- 'Alcohol misuse — F10' often co-exists. Poly-drug use is very common.

- Symptoms of anxiety or depression may also occur with heavy drug use. If these continue after a period of abstinence (eg about two to three weeks), see **'Depression — F32#'**, **'Generalized anxiety — F41.1'** and **'Phobic disorders — F40'**.
- **'Psychotic disorders — F23, F20#'**.
- Acute organic syndromes.
- Presentation of other psychiatric disorders should trigger inquiry about alcohol and drug misuse history.

Essential information for patient and family

- Drug misuse can be a chronic behavioural disorder. Controlling or stopping use often requires several attempts. Relapse is common.
- Abstinence should be seen as the long-term goal. Harm reduction (especially reducing intravenous drug use) might be a more realistic goal in the short to medium term.
- Stopping or reducing drug use can result in psychological, social and physical benefits.
- Using some drugs during pregnancy risks harming the baby.[100]
- For intravenous drug-users, there is a risk of contracting and/or transmitting HIV infection, hepatitis or other infections carried by body fluids. Discuss appropriate precautions (eg use condoms and do not share needles, syringes, spoons, water or any other injecting equipment).

General management and advice to patient and family

Advice should be given according to the patient's motivation and willingness to change.[101] For many patients with chronic, relapsing opioid dependence, the treatment of choice is maintenance on long-acting opioids.[102]

In assessing patients with alcohol or other type of addictive behaviour, the framework of cycles of change can be helpful in assessing the patient's readiness for change. A patient may be:

- pre-contemplative, ie not considering any change
- contemplative, ie considering change or prepared to change behaviour, or
- in an action phase where they are actually in the process of change.

Of course, because of the relapsing nature of these disorders, patients may shift from an action phase back to a pre-contemplative phase and then move through the phases of change. Assessment can be a prompt for some to move into a contemplative or action phase.

For all patients:

- Discuss costs and benefits of drug use from the patient's perspective.
- Feedback information about health risks, including the results of investigations.
- Emphasize personal responsibility for change.
- Give clear advice to change.
- Assess and manage physical health problems (eg anaemia, chest problems) and nutritional deficiencies.
- Consider options for problem-solving, or targeted counselling, to deal with life problems related to drug use.
- Goal setting needs to be negotiated and matched to individual needs and assessment, as well as overall pattern of drinking and dependence.

For patients not willing to stop or change drug use now:

- Do not reject or blame.
- Advise on harm-reduction strategies (eg if the patient is injecting, advise on needle exchange, not injecting alone, not mixing alcohol, benzodiazepines and opiates) (R: 7–1).

- Clearly point out medical, psychological and social problems caused by drugs.
- Make a future appointment to re-assess health (eg well-woman checks, immunization) and discuss drug use.

If reducing drug use is a reasonable goal (or if a patient is unwilling to quit):

- Negotiate a clear goal for decreased use and regularly review progress.
- Discuss strategies to avoid or cope with high-risk situations (eg social situations, stressful events).
- Introduce self-monitoring procedures (eg diary of drug use) (R: 7–2) and safer drug-use behaviours (eg time restrictions, slowing down rate of use).
- It is useful to set agreed rights and responsibilities for both patient and healthcare team. This may include a contract, which you both sign, clearly setting out your and the patient's responsibilities and the consequences of non-adherence.
- Consider options for referral to appropriate statutory or voluntary services for increased support, eg counselling and/or rehabilitation.

If maintenance on substitute drugs is considered a reasonable goal (or if a patient is unwilling to quit):

- Negotiate a clear goal for less harmful behaviour. Help the patient develop a hierarchy of aims (eg reducing injecting behaviour, stopping illicit use and maintenance on prescribed, substitute drugs).
- Discuss strategies to avoid or cope with high-risk situations (eg social situations or stressful events).
- Consider withdrawal symptoms and how to avoid or reduce them. Provide information on the recognition and management of methadone toxicity.
- Consider options for referral to appropriate statutory or voluntary (including NAO) services for increased support, eg counselling and/or rehabilitation.

For patients willing to stop now:

- Set a definite day to quit.
- Consider withdrawal symptoms and how to manage them.
- Emphasize importance of planning ahead to cope with difficulties (see below). If patient is unclear what their coping strategies are, consider deferring 'quit date' and work on coping strategies.
- Discuss strategies to avoid or cope with high-risk situations (eg social situations or stressful events).
- Make specific plans to avoid drug use (eg how to respond to friends who still use drugs).
- Identify family or friends who will support stopping drug use.
- Consider options for referral to appropriate statutory or voluntary (including NAO) services for increased support, eg counselling or rehabilitation or both.

For patients who do not succeed or who relapse:

- Identify and give credit for any success.
- Discuss situations which led to relapse.
- Return to earlier steps.

Self-help organizations are often helpful (see below).

Medication

To withdraw a patient from benzodiazepines, convert to a long-acting drug such as diazepam and reduce gradually (eg by 2 mg a fortnight) over a period of two to six months (*BNF* section 4.1). Benzodiazepine prescribing should be undertaken with caution, and long-term prescribing is now rarely initiated.[103,104]

Withdrawal from stimulants or cocaine is distressing and may require medical supervision under a shared-care scheme.

Both long-term maintenance of a patient on substitute opiates (eg methadone) and withdrawal from opiates should be done as part of a shared-care scheme.[105] A multidisciplinary approach is essential and should include drug counselling/therapy[106] and possible future rehabilitation needs.[107] The doctor signing the prescription is solely responsible for prescribing; this cannot be delegated. Doctors prescribing methadone should be familiar with the Department of Health's document entitled *Drug Misuse and Dependence: Guidelines on Clinical Management*.[108]

- Careful assessment, including urine or saliva analysis and, where possible, dose assessment is essential before prescribing any substitute medication, including methadone. Dosages will depend on the results of this assessment.
- For long-term maintenance or stabilization prior to gradual withdrawal, the dose should be titrated up to that needed both to block withdrawal symptoms and block craving for opiates.[109]
- For gradual withdrawal, after a period of stabilization, the drug can be slowly tapered (eg by 5 mg each fortnight).
- Daily dispensing (using blue FP 10 prescription forms) and, where available, supervised ingestion are recommended, especially in the first three months of treatment. Record exact details of the prescription, frequency and chemist in case the patient presents to a colleague.
- In the UK, Methadone Mixture BNF at 1 mg/ml is the most often-used substitute medication for opioid addiction[110] (*BNF* section 4.10). Newer drugs have become available (eg buprenorphine[111]) and can be considered as alternatives to methadone.
- Withdrawal from opiates for patients whose drug use is already well controlled can be managed with lofexidine[112,113] (*BNF* section 4.10).
- Wherever possible, treatment should be undertaken in the context of shared care.

Referral

Help with life problems, employment and social relationships is an important component of treatment.[114]

Shared care between all agencies (non-statutory agencies, NHS mental health and drug misuse services) and professionals involved is essential. Clarity on who is responsible for prescribing and for the physical care of the patient is crucial.

Resources for patients and families

Resource leaflets: 7–1 *Harm minimization advice* and 7–2 *Drug use diary*

Narcotics Anonymous UK 020 7730 0009
Email: helpline@ukna.org; website: http://www.ukna.org
A network of recovering addicts supporting each other to live without drugs.

CITA (Council for Involuntary Tranquilliser Addiction) 0151 949 0102 (helpline 10.00am–1.00pm, Monday–Friday; emergency weekend number available)
Offers advice on withdrawing from tranquillisers and help with anxiety and depression.

ADFAM National 020 7928 8900 (helpline 10am–5pm, Monday, Wednesday–Friday; 10am–6.45pm, Tuesday)
Website: http://www.adfam.org.uk
Confidential support and information for families and friends of drug users.

National Drugs Helpline/Talk to Frank 0800 776 600 (24-hour)
Website: http://www.talktofrank.com
Provides free, confidential advice, including information on local services.

Release 020 7603 8654 (24-hour helpline), 020 7729 9904 (advice line, 10 am–6 pm), 0808 8000 800 (Drugs in School helpline, 10 am–6 pm)

Email:info@release.org.uk; website: http://www.release.org.uk.
Advice, support and information to drug users and their friends and families on all aspects of drug use and drug-related legal problems.

National Institute on Drug Abuse (NIDA) Website: http://www.nida.nih.gov
A useful American site with lots of information and leaflets to download.

Families Anonymous 020 7498 4680 (1pm–5pm, Monday–Friday)
Email: office@famanon.org.uk, website: http://www.famanon.org.uk
Runs self-help groups in the UK for families and friends of those with a drug problem.

Leaflets are available from the Royal College of Psychiatrists
(http://www.rcpsych.ac.uk): *Alcohol and Other Drug Misuse*, *Drug and Alcohol Misuse*

Coping with Tranquilliser Addiction, produced in association with CITA. Talking Life, 1A Grosvenor Rd, Hoylake, Wirral CH47 3BS, UK. Tel 0151 632 0662; website: http://www.talkinglife.co.uk.
Self-help cassette.

Eating disorders — F50
(Clinical term: Eating disorders Eu50)

Presenting complaints

The family may ask for help because of the patient's loss of weight, refusal to eat, vomiting or amenorrhoea. Earlier stages may include levels of dietary restriction that cause alarm within the family.

The patient may engage in extreme dietary restriction, binge eating, and various forms of extreme weight-control behaviour, such as self-induced vomiting, driven exercising or laxative misuse. Both anorexia nervosa and bulimia nervosa may present as physical disorders:

- Non-specific symptoms: abdominal pain, bloating, constipation, cold intolerance, light-headedness, hair, nail or skin changes.
- Food allergy/intolerance and chronic fatigue syndromes sometimes precede the development of an eating disorder and may cause diagnostic confusion.
- Amenorrhoea, fertility problems, gastrointestinal and oropharyngeal problems.
- Low mood, anxiety/irritability.

Although the range of physical presenting complaints is large, in practice the most important task for the practitioner in primary care is to be alert to the possibility of an eating disorder and to enquire further in a sensitive manner.

Diagnostic features

Common features are:

- unreasonable fear of being fat or gaining weight
- self-evaluation almost exclusively based on shape and weight
- extensive efforts to control/reduce weight (eg strict dieting, vomiting, use of purgatives, excessive exercise)
- denial that weight or eating habits are a problem (anorexia nervosa)
- obsessional symptoms
- relationship difficulties
- increasing withdrawal
- school and work problems.

Patients with **anorexia nervosa** typically show:

- severe dietary restriction despite very low weight (body mass index $<17.5 \text{ kg/m}^2$)
- morbid fear of fatness
- distorted body image (ie an unreasonable belief that one is overweight)
- amenorrhoea
- a proportion of patients binge and purge.

Patients with **bulimia nervosa** typically show:

- binge-eating (ie discrete episodes of uncontrolled overeating)
- purging (attempts to eliminate food by self-induced vomiting or via diuretic or laxative use)
- strict dieting and other compensatory measures such as excessive exercise
- self-evaluation based on shape and weight.

A patient may show both anorexic and bulimic patterns at different times. In addition, full criteria for anorexia or bulimia nervosa are not fulfilled by 30–50% of patients with clinically significant eating disorders (these patients are said to have atypical eating disorders or eating disorders not otherwise specified [EDNOS]).

Differential diagnosis and co-existing conditions

- Physical illness (eg malabsorption syndrome, chronic inflammatory intestinal diseases, tumours, tuberculosis, vasculitis and diabetes mellitus) may cause weight loss or vomiting, although it is not self-induced.
- There may be co-existing problems, such as **'Depression —F32#'**, **Generalized anxiety — F41.1'**, **'Obsessive-compulsive disorder — F42'**, **'Drug use disorders — F11#'** or **'Self-harm'**.

The differential diagnosis of weight loss is large, but when an appropriate history is taken with corroboration, it is unusual for diagnostic difficulty to occur. It is important not to delay diagnosis by over-investigation and referral, which may render the doctor complicit with the anorexic denial of the patient.

Medical consequences of severe weight loss include impaired attention and concentration, impaired visuo-spatial abilities and poor memory, hypotension, bradycardia, ECG alterations, arrhythmias, mitral valve prolapse, bone marrow suppression, osteoporosis, low glucose, amenorrhoea, muscle weakness, impaired gastric emptying, constipation.

Medical complications of purging include dental problems, salivary-gland swelling, upper and lower gastrointestinal bleeding, dehydration and electrolyte imbalance, cardiac arrhythmias and epileptic seizures.

Essential information for patient and family

- Purging and severe starvation may cause serious physical harm. Anorexia nervosa can be life-threatening.
- Purging and severe dieting are ineffective ways of achieving lasting weight-control.
- Information leaflets, self-help books and self-help organizations such as the Eating Disorders Association may be helpful in explaining the diagnosis and available treatment options, providing information about what practical steps the person can take to overcome their difficulties and putting patients and their families in touch with other patients.

General management and advice to patient and family[115,116]

The GP can undertake straightforward steps to treat eating disorders with the help of the practice counsellor, practice nurse and/or a dietician, although most cases will be referred on for specialist treatment.

It is important to support the family and to engage them constructively in management.

In anorexia nervosa:

- It is helpful to see the patient without, as well as with, the family.
- Expect denial and ambivalence. Elicit the patient's concerns about the negative effects of the eating problem on aspects of their life. Ask the patient about the benefits that their eating has for them (eg the feeling of being in control, feeling safe, being able to get care and attention from family). Do not try to force the patient to change if he/she is not ready.
- Educate the patient about food and weight.
- Weigh the patient regularly and chart his/her weight. Set manageable goals in agreement with the patient (eg aim for a 0.5 kg weight increase per week [this requires a calorie intake of about 2500 kilocalories per day]). A supportive family member may be able to help the patient achieve this. Consultation with a dietician may be helpful to establish normal calorie and nutrient intake and regular patterns of eating. If after four to eight weeks this approach is not succeeding, refer the patient to a specialist.
- A return to normal eating habits may be a distant goal.
- Encourage the family to be patient and consistent.

In bulimia nervosa:

- Use a collaborative approach.
- Ask the patient to obtain one of the readily available cognitive behavioural self-help books (see below).[117] These provide reliable sources of information and specific guidance for overcoming the eating disorder. Encourage the patient to follow the advice contained in the book and see them at one- to two-week intervals to oversee their use of the book. If after eight weeks this approach is not succeeding, refer the patient to a specialist.
- Discuss the patient's biased beliefs about weight, shape and eating (eg carbohydrates are fattening) and encourage review of rigid views about body image (eg patients believe no one will like them unless they are very thin). Do not simply state that the patient's view is wrong.

Medication[115,116]

- In bulimia nervosa, antidepressants (eg fluoxetine at 60 mg mane) are effective in reducing binging and vomiting in a proportion of cases;[118] however, compliance with medication may be poor, and long-term benefit uncertain (*BNF* section 4.3). Any beneficial effects will be evident within two to four weeks. If after eight weeks this approach is not succeeding, refer the patient to a specialist.
- No pharmacological treatment for anorexia nervosa has been established to date.[119] Psychiatric conditions (eg depression) might co-occur and may respond to pharmacological treatment, although effectiveness may be reduced while at low weight.
- Order blood tests for urea and electrolytes with patients who are vomiting frequently or regularly misusing laxatives.

Referral

Refer to secondary mental health services for non-urgent assessment if there is a lack of progress in primary care (see above), despite the measures described. If available, consider family therapy for anorexic patients (under 18 years),[120] individual psychotherapy for anorexic patients over 18,[121] and cognitive behavioural therapy[122] for those with bulimia nervosa.

Consider non-statutory/voluntary services/self-help organizations, such as the Eating Disorders Association.

Refer for urgent assessment (if possible, to secondary mental health services with expertise in eating disorders) if physically unwell.[123]

Resources for patients and families

Eating Disorders Association (EDA) 01603 621 414 (helpline: 9am–6.30pm)
Email: info@edauk.com; website: http://www.edauk.com.
Self-help support groups for sufferers, their relatives and friends. It assists in putting people in touch with sources of help in their own area.

Centre for Eating Disorders (Scotland) 0131 668 3051 (helpline)
Psychotherapy for individuals, self-help manuals and information packs.

Anorexia Bulimia Careline (Northern Ireland) 02890 614 440 (helpline)
Leaflets are available from the Royal College of Psychiatrists (http://www.rcpsych.ac.uk): Anorexia and Bulimia, Changing Minds: Anorexia and Bulimia, and Worries about Weight.

Bulimia nervosa and binge eating disorders:
Bulimia Nervosa — A Cognitive Therapy Programme for Clients by Myra Cooper *et al.* Jessica Kingsley, 2000.
Self-help manual.

Bulimia and Binge Eating by P Cooper. Constable & Robinson, London, 1995.
Self-help manual.

Overcoming Binge Eating by Christopher Fairburn. New York: Guilford Press, 1995.
Self-help manual.

Overcoming Bulimia. University of Leeds Media Innovations Ltd, 3 Gemini Business
Park, Sheepscar Way, Leeds LS7 3JB. Tel: 0113 262 1600; website
http://www.calipso.co.uk.
A CD-ROM self-help package.
The Mental Health Foundation produces the information booklet *All About Bulimia
Nervosa.* Publications, The Mental Health Foundation, 7th Floor, 83 Victoria Street,
London SW1H 0HW. Tel: 020 7802 0304; website: http://www.mentalhealth.org.uk.

Anorexia nervosa:
Overcoming Anorexia Nervosa. A Self-Help Guide Using Cognitive Behavioural Techniques
by Christopher Freeman. London: Constable & Robinson, 2002.
Self-help manual.

Getting Better Bit(e) by Bit(e) by Ulrike Schmidt and Janet Treasure. Psychology Press,
1997.
Self-help manual.

Anorexia Nervosa — The Wish to Change, 2nd edition, by AH Crisp *et al*. Psychology
Press, 1996.
Self-help manual.

Overcoming Anorexia. University of Leeds Media Innovations Ltd, 3 Gemini Business
Park, Sheepscar Way, Leeds LS7 3JB. Tel: 0113 262 1600; website:
http://www.calipso.co.uk.
A CD-ROM self-help package. Available early 2004.

Anorexia Nervosa: A Survival Guide for Families, Friends and Sufferers by Janet Treasure.
Psychology Press, 1997.
The Mental Health Foundation produces the information booklet *All About Anorexia
Nervosa.* Publications, The Mental Health Foundation, 7th Floor, 83 Victoria Street,
London SW1H 0HW. Tel: 020 7802 0304; website: http://www.mentalhealth.org.uk.

Epilepsy — G40.9
(Clinical term: Epilepsy F25)

Presenting complaints
- Usual presentation is sudden collapse associated with loss of consciousness and a convulsion.
- A range of phenomena may also be epileptic in origin, although frequently are not recognized as such by patients: repetitive psychological sensations (such as déjà vu), motor phenomena, brief loss of consciousness and sudden muscle jerks.

Diagnostic features
Epilepsy is the tendency to have repeated seizures that originate in the brain.

The lack of a comprehensive diagnostic test, and the similarity of presentation of many other conditions, can lead to diagnostic inaccuracies.[124] Diagnosis should be established by a physician/paediatrician with training and expertise in epilepsy.

Epilepsy is primarily diagnosed on the basis of an accurate description of the seizure. As the patient is frequently unconscious, a witness history is absolutely essential.

- Partial (focal) seizures:
  — simple partial: no loss of consciousness
  — complex partial: commonly impaired consciousness, 'dazed' with automatisms such as lick-smacking or fumbling with fingers
  — simple or complex partial evolving to secondarily generalized — as above but progresses to generalized convulsive seizure.
- Generalized seizures:
  — absence: brief loss of consciousness.
  — myoclonic: brief sudden jerking of limbs, often in the morning
  — clonic: rhythmic jerking
  — tonic: stiffness of body
  — tonic–clonic: classical stiffening then jerking of body and fall to ground, often with incontinence and tongue biting; so-called 'grand mal'.

Epilepsy may affect any patient group throughout the lifespan. High-risk groups include those with an intellectual disability, traumatic brain injury and cerebrovascular disease.

Differential diagnosis
Thirty to forty percent of epilepsy has a recognizable cause. For example, intrauterine and perinatal factors; infections leading to brain damage; tumours, primarily intracerebral or metastases from extracerebral sites; injury to the brain or surgical intervention; degenerative brain disease; metabolic disorders including liver/kidney diseases; hypoglycaemia; drugs and alcohol in both intoxication and withdrawal states; prescribed medication, including psychotropic medication reducing threshold of seizures.

Epileptic seizures need to be distinguished from other causes of impairment of consciousness or episodic neuropsychiatric dysfunction:

- Certain physical conditions (eg syncope, transient ischaemic attacks [TIAs], migraine, acute confusional states).
- Certain psychiatric illnesses, for example acute episodes of anxiety symptoms, particularly autonomic symptoms, somatoform disorders including conversion and dissociative disorders, psychotic illnesses including schizophrenia-like psychotic symptoms, organic confusional states.

The seizure type, epilepsy syndrome and aetiology should be determined because correct classification has important implications for treatment and prognosis. Further investigations (EEG/CT-MRI, as appropriate) should be done in the evaluation of a suspected epileptic seizure (defined on basis of a careful history) to aid diagnosis, classification and prognosis.

Essential information for patient and family

- Epilepsy is a common condition; 0.5–1.0% of the population in the UK has epilepsy.
- Epileptic seizures are usually self-remitting and brief.
- Rarely, status epilepticus develops, ie ongoing seizures one after another or an unusually prolonged seizure of four to five minutes or longer. Status can be a potentially dangerous situation and an ambulance should be called to seek professional treatment. Injectable medication by the paramedics might be required, or the patient may be taken to hospital for further treatment.
- At the time of the seizure, ensure that the patient does not come to any harm because of the manifestations of loss of consciousness, eg injury caused by a fall.
- Most patients achieve seizure freedom.
- A three- to five-year seizure-free period with anticonvulsant medication is considered to be a good result. Consideration can be given to reduction/withdrawal of anticonvulsant medication if this is achieved, particularly where side-effects have been an ongoing issue.
- Continued seizures place individuals at some risk — eg bathing, driving — which need careful explanation.
- Psychiatric symptoms can occur secondary to epilepsy and during or between seizures: neurotic, psychotic or cognitive symptoms. Complex partial seizures are particularly relevant in this case.
- A long history of seizures and prolonged use of anticonvulsants can sometimes both individually or together lead to cognitive impairment.
- Women with epilepsy need careful pre-conceptual counselling.[125]

General management and advice to patient and family[126]

- Because 30–40% of epilepsy has a recognizable cause, a new case needs to be investigated to find the cause. This is more likely to be relevant for adult-onset epilepsy.
- During a seizure, the best intervention from the family is to ensure that the patient is protected from injury during the period of impaired consciousness. The patient should be placed on a comfortable surface in the coma position and any hard objects removed from the vicinity.
- Recording frequency and types of seizures in a diary is very helpful for determining treatment.
- Psychosocial aspects of treatment include clear and supportive education to patient and family. Essential limitation of activities that may increase risk of injury to the patient must be advised appropriately (eg driving, swimming, use of stairs or crossing streets with traffic).
- Engagement with support groups might be useful for both patient and family.
- You should enquire about the contraceptive method used by women of childbearing age and on carbamazepine, phenytoin, topiramate or phenobarbitone, and pre-conceptual counselling and advice on childbearing given.
- The DVLA must be notified in all cases. Licences for motor vehicles can be restored after one year seizure-free or after three years if the seizures are uniquely nocturnal; for LGV/PCV drivers, licences can be restored after 10 years if the patient has been seizure-free and has not taken antiepileptic drugs for that time.[3]

Medication[126,127]

- Antiepileptics are the mainstay of treatment. Seizure type affects the choice of treatment. The antiepileptic drug should be gradually increased to a maximum tolerable dose, if necessary, to control of seizures completely (*BNF* section 4.8).

- The decision to start antiepileptic treatment should be made by a doctor skilled in the management of epilepsy, along with the patient.
- To ensure compliance with medication, it is important to educate the patient about possible precipitants of seizures (eg missing doses, alcohol, photosensitivity, sleep deprivation and even emotional states).
- Good compliance ensures earlier control of seizures and thus reduced doses of medication, risk of side-effects and any long-term effects on cognitive functioning. It also lessens the damaging effects of prolonged seizures on confidence and psychosocial skills.

The following clinical scenarios are faced in the management of epilepsy.

- *Single seizure.* A single seizure is predictive of further seizures in the individual (in 30–40% of cases).[128] Risk of recurrence is higher in those with a congenital neurological deficit or EEG abnormalities. In general, management is an individual decision, and the wishes and circumstances of the patient must be taken into consideration.
- *Subsequent seizures.* An attempt should be made to control seizures with monotherapy. Treatment choice is influenced by seizure type and gender. Patient concerns over side-effects are of major importance and decisions should be based on the fully informed choice of patients and their families.
  — Seizure type: for patients with partial epilepsy, carbamazepine (starting dose 200 mg, maintenance 400–1600 mg), lamotrigine (starting dose 25 mg, maintenance 100–400 mg) and valproate (starting dose 200–500 mg, maintenance 500–3000 mg) are the treatments of choice (*BNF* section 4.8).[129] For patients with generalized epilepsy (or where classification is not possible), valproate and lamotrigine are preferred.
  — Gender: women of childbearing age who have epilepsy face very specific risks from epilepsy treatments, for example interference with contraceptive treatment and teratogenic effects of anticonvulsants.
- *First drug failure.* Patients who fail with their first anticonvulsant, owing either to poor seizure control or intolerable side-effects, should be switched to an alternative monotherapy.
- *Monotherapy failure.* If monotherapy is not completely successful, try combinations with second-line drugs. Drug interactions are complex and mainly relate to liver enzyme effects. Serum level monitoring becomes relevant when it is proving difficult to balance therapeutic benefit with side-effects and in renal/hepatic disease and pregnancy. Again, treatment choice is influenced by gender and seizure type:
  — partial: gabapentin, levetiracetam, tiagabine and topiramate
  — generalized: topiramate and possibly levetiracetam. Ethosuxamide can be used in patients with absence epilepsy.
- *Refractory epilepsy.* Patients with drug-resistant epilepsy should have:
  — reassessment of diagnosis
  — reassessment of drug therapy
  — assessment of compliance
  — assessment of precipitants
  — assessment of suitability for epilepsy surgery.
- *Antiepileptic drug withdrawal*:
  — Three to five years of complete control is generally considered sufficient to justify reductions or trial of cessation of medication.[130]
  — Risk of re-occurrence of seizures has to be balanced against the hazards of continuing medication, including effect on psychosocial aspects of a patient's life.

Referral

Referral to neurology or other epilepsy services (including those for people with intellectual disability) is essential for:

- a new diagnosis
- initiation of treatment
- pre-conceptual counselling
- refractory epilepsy assessment
- withdrawal of antiepileptic drugs
- epilepsy surgery.

Some psychiatric services have specialist neuropsychiatry/epilepsy clinics, with specialist nurses for counselling. Psychotherapeutic services especially geared for epilepsy are not yet widely established.

Referral to Social Services can be considered for specific benefits relating to a patient's disability.

Resources for patients and families

Epilepsy Action 0808 800 5050 (helpline 9am–4.30pm, Monday–Thursday; 9am–4pm, Friday)
Email: helpline@epilepsy.org.uk; website: http://www.epilepsy.org.uk.
Epilepsy Action is the working name for the British Epilepsy Association.

National Society for Epilepsy 01494 601 400 (helpline 10am–4pm, Monday–Friday)
Website: http://www.epilepsynse.org.uk.

Epilepsy Youth in Europe (EYiE)
Website: http://www.eyie.org.
Provides an opportunity for young people to discuss epilepsy and its effect on their lives.

Epilepsy Bereaved 01235 777 2852.
Email: http://dspace.dial.pipex.com/epilepsybereaved/eb/ebhome.htm.

Generalized anxiety — F41.1
(Clinical term: Generalized anxiety disorder Eu41.1)

Presenting complaints
Tension-related symptoms, eg headache, pounding heart, insomnia, complaint of 'stress'. Enquiry reveals prominent anxiety.

Diagnostic features
Multiple, persistent and uncued anxiety or tension including:

- autonomic arousal (eg dizziness, sweating, fast or pounding heart, dry mouth, stomach pains)
- mental tension (eg undue worry, feeling tense or nervous, poor concentration, sense of foreboding)
- physical tension (eg restlessness, headaches, tremors, cannot relax, chest pain or constriction).

Symptoms may last for months and recur regularly, and are often worsened by stressful events in those prone to worry.

Co-existing disorders
If the disorders listed below are the most prominent feature (see appropriate guidelines), treat accordingly:

- 'Depression — F32#'
- 'Panic disorder — F41.0'
- 'Phobic disorders — F40'
- 'Post-traumatic stress disorder — F43.1'
- 'Alcohol misuse — F10' or 'Drug use disorders — F11'.

Certain physical conditions (eg thyrotoxicosis), medications (eg methylxanthines, beta-agonists) or street drugs (stimulants) may cause anxiety symptoms.

Essential information for patient and family
- Anxiety has both physical and mental effects.
- The ability to reduce anxiety can be learned.[131]

General management and advice to patient and family[132]
- Explain the link between the physical and psychological symptoms of anxiety.
- Encourage use of relaxation methods daily to reduce anxiety (R: 1–2).
- Cut down caffeine consumption (coffee, tea, stimulant drinks).
- Avoid using alcohol, tobacco and street drugs to cope with anxiety.
- Tell about practice or non-statutory resources for problem-solving, relaxation and yoga.
- Regular physical exercise is often helpful.
- Use self-help publications to develop psychosocial strategies to cope with anxiety (see below).
- Encourage engagement in activities that are pleasurable or have previously reduced anxiety.
- Encourage simple cognitive strategies:
  — identify undue worries (eg when daughter is five minutes late from school, mother worries that she may have had an accident)
  — discuss ways to question these undue worries when they occur (eg when the mother starts to worry about daughter, she could tell herself, 'I'm starting to be caught up in worry again. She's only a few minutes late and should be home

soon. I won't call her school to check unless she's an hour late'. Explore alternative explanations (R: 4–2).

- Structured problem-solving methods can ease current life problems that contribute to anxiety:[133] (R: 1–1)
  - identify triggers of undue worry (eg a woman presents with worry, tension, nausea and insomnia, which began after her son was diagnosed with asthma and worsens when he has asthmatic episodes). Ask the patient to:
    - list every solution they can think of (eg meet the nurse to learn about asthma management, read leaflets about it, discuss concerns with other parents of asthmatic children, write down a management plan for son's asthma episodes)
    - list the pros and cons of each possible solution (try this between appointments)
  - help the patient to choose their preferred approach (not necessarily the first that comes to mind)
  - help the patient to work out the steps necessary to achieve the plan
  - set a date to review the plan. Work out and encourage what is working.

Medication[132]

The longer-term outcome seems better after psychosocial treatment than with drug treatment. Medication is a secondary treatment in managing generalized anxiety.[131,134] It may be used if significant anxiety persists despite the measures described above.

- Anti-anxiety medication[135] (*BNF* section 4.1.2): avoid short-acting benzodiazepines; they should not be used *for less than two weeks.*
- Antidepressant drugs (*BNF* section 4.3), for example tricyclics or SSRIs, may help, especially if depression is present.[136] Discontinuation should be gradual over a month.

Beta-blockers may reduce physical symptoms such as tremor in particular settings.[137]

Liaison and referral

See general referral criteria.

Liaison or non-urgent referral to secondary mental health services is advised if anxiety is sufficiently severe or enduring to interfere with social or work functioning.

Consider cognitive/behavioural therapy or anxiety management.[135] Self-care classes and 'assisted bibliotherapy' can also be effective in primary care for milder anxiety.[138,139]

Resources for patients and families

Resource leaflets: 1–1 *Problem-solving*, 1–2 *Learning to relax*, 4–1 *Anxiety and how to reduce it* and 4–2 *Dealing with anxious thoughts*

No Panic 01952 590 545 (helpline 10 am–10 pm); 0808 808 0545 (gives numbers of volunteers for the day)
Website: http://www.no-panic.co.uk.
Helpline, information booklets, local self-help groups (including telephone recovery groups) for people with anxiety, phobias obsessions, panic.

Triumph Over Phobia (TOP) UK 01225 330 353
Email: triumphoverphobia@compuserve.com; website:
http://www.triumphoverphobia.com.
Structured self-help groups for sufferers from phobias or obsessive-compulsive disorder. It produces self-help materials.

Stresswatch Scotland 01563 528 910 (helpline 10am–1pm, Monday–Friday, excluding Wed)

Advice, information, materials on panic, anxiety, stress phobias.

The Mental Health Foundation produces the information booklet *All About Anxiety*. Publications, The Mental Health Foundation, 7ᵗʰ Floor, 83 Victoria Street, London SW1H 0HW. Tel: 020 7802 0304. website: http://www.mentalhealth.org.uk.

Mind Publications produces the booklet *How To Cope With Panic Attacks*. MIND, Granta House, 15–19 Broadway, London E15 4BQ, Tel: 020 8519 2122, and The Mental Health Foundation, 7th Floor, 83 Victoria Street, London SW1 0HW. Tel: 020 7802 0300.

Living with Fear, 2nd edition, by Isaac M Marks. McGraw Hill, 2001. Tel: 01628 252 700; Email: orders@mcgraw-hill.co.uk.
Self-help manual.

Overcoming Anxiety: a Self-Help Guide Using CBT by Helen Kinnerly. Constable and Robinson, 1997.
Self-help manual.

Learn to Relax by Mike George. Duncan Baird, 1998.
Relaxation exercises (also available as a cassette).

Coping with Anxiety. Talking Life, 1A Grosvenor Rd, Hoylake, Wirral CH47 3BS. Tel: 0151 632 0662; website: www.http://www.talkinglife.co.uk.
A cassette package describing three strategies for relieving anxiety.

Overcoming Anxiety. University of Leeds Media Innovations Ltd, 3 Gemini Business Park, Sheepscar Way, Leeds LS7 3JB. Tel: 0113 262 1600; website: http://www.calipso.co.uk.
A CD-ROM self-help package.

Fear Fighter http://www.fearfighter.com
Self-help guidance plus option of live helpline advice if you get stuck.
Yoga and meditation classes, as part of adult education programmes, are provided at most Colleges of Further Education.

Headache — R51

(Migraine G43.9, Tension headache G44.2, Cluster headache G44.0)
(Clinical term: Headache R040)

Presenting complaints

Most people have occasional headache and regard it as normal. Headache becomes a problem at some time in the lives of about 40% of people in the UK. The patient with headache presents with bothersome recurrent or unremitting headache, which may be associated with other symptoms.

Such headaches:

- are debilitating and disabling
- impair quality of life
- engender fears of serious pathology.

The headache disorders encountered in general practice are:

- *Migraine*, affecting 12–15% of the UK population, in more women than men (ratio of 3:1).[140]
- *Tension-type headache*, which affects >80% of people from time to time[141] but recurs frequently in a small minority. In 2–3% of adults it is chronic,[142] occurring on most days each week.
- *Cluster headache*, an intense and frequently recurring but short-lasting headache affecting 1 in 1000 men and 1 in 6000 women.
- *Medication-overuse headache*, a chronic daily headache occurring in up to 3% of adults, affecting 5 women to each man, and some children. This is a secondary headache, but it occurs only as a complication of a pre-existing primary headache disorder (usually migraine).
- A large number of other *secondary headaches*, some serious but which overall account for <1% of presenting patients.

Diagnostic features

There are no diagnostic tests for any of the primary headache disorders. The history is all-important. Once serious causes have been ruled out, a headache diary kept over a few weeks can clarify the pattern of headaches and medication usage.

Questions to ask in the history[143]

- How many different headache types does the patient experience?
  A separate history is needed for each.
- Time questions
  — Why consulting now?
  — How recent in onset?
  — How frequent and what temporal pattern (episodic or daily and/or unremitting)?
  — How long lasting?
- Character questions
  — Intensity of pain?
  — Nature and quality of pain?
  — Site and spread of pain?
  — Associated symptoms?
- Cause questions
  — Predisposing and/or trigger factors?
  — Aggravating and/or relieving factors?
  — Family history of similar headache?

- Response questions
  - What does the patient do during the headache?
  - How much is activity (function) limited or prevented?
  - What medication has been and is used and in what manner?
- State of health between attacks
  - Completely well, or residual or persisting symptoms?
  - Concerns, anxieties, fears about recurrent attacks, and/or their cause?

Migraine
Adults with migraine typically describe:

- recurrent episodic moderate or severe headaches
- often unilateral and/or pulsating
- lasting from four hours to three days
- gastrointestinal symptoms (anorexia, nausea and sometimes vomiting)
- limited functional activity and preference of dark and quiet
- freedom from symptoms between attacks.

In children:

- attacks may be shorter-lasting
- headache is more commonly bilateral
- gastrointestinal disturbance is more prominent.

Migraine with aura affects one-third of migraine patients and accounts for 10% of attacks overall. It is characterized by aura preceding the headache, consisting of reversible neurological symptoms lasting 10–60 minutes. During the aura patients experience:

- hemianopic visual disturbances, or a spreading scintillating scotoma (patients may draw a jagged crescent if asked)
- and/or unilateral paraesthesiae of hand, arm and/or face
- and/or (rarely) dysphasia.

Typical aura may occur without headache especially in middle-aged men. Rare families carry the dominant gene(s) of *familial hemiplegic migraine* in which aura includes motor weakness.

Tension-type headache (TTH)
There are two subtypes.

- Episodic tension-type headache: occurs in attack-like episodes lasting hours up to a few days and with variable frequency; can be unilateral but is more often generalized; is typically described as pressure or tightness, like a vice or tight band around the head, and commonly spreading in to or arising from the neck; lacks the associated symptom complex of migraine.
- Chronic tension-type headache: occurs by definition on >15 days a month; may be daily and unremitting.

Cluster headache (CH)
Cluster headache mostly affects smokers but can also occur in children. More men are affected than women. It manifests as strictly unilateral, excruciating pain around the eye, typically once or more daily (commonly at night) for 30–60 minutes. There are highly characteristic associated autonomic features:

- the eye is red and waters
- the nose runs or is blocked on the same side
- ptosis may occur.

Cluster headache causes marked agitation — the patient, unable to stay in bed, paces the room and may even go outdoors.

This highly recognizable condition also has in two subtypes.

- Episodic cluster headache: occurs in bouts (clusters), typically of 6–12 weeks' duration, once every year or two years.
- Chronic cluster headache: is less common; has no remissions between clusters; patients may develop a continuous milder background headache and also may develop from and/or revert to episodic CH.

Medication-overuse headache (MOH)

Chronic overuse of medication taken for headache can cause daily headache.[144] All acute headache medications are implicated.[145] MOH does not develop when analgesics are regularly taken for another indication. Frequency of intake is important: use of simple analgesics on ≥ 15 days a month, or opioids, ergotamine or triptans on ≥ 10 days a month, carries a clear risk.[146]

Medication overuse headache:

- occurs daily or near-daily
- is present, and often at its worst, on awakening in the morning
- is oppressive
- increases after physical exertion
- is *confirmed* only when symptoms improve within two months of withdrawing the overused medication.

Physical examination of headache patients

All these headaches are diagnosed solely on history, with diagnostic signs present in CH patients if they are seen during attacks.

Physical examination reassures often worried patients and so has therapeutic value. It can exclude (or may confirm) secondary headache when the history is suggestive. Examination *must* include the optic fundi, *should* include blood pressure measurement, and *may* include the head and neck — muscle tenderness, stiffness, limitation in range of movement and crepitation are common and do not necessarily indicate headache causation.

Investigation of headache patients

Investigations, including neuroimaging, are indicated *only* when history or examination suggest headache may be secondary to some other condition.

Differential diagnosis

- Each of the primary headaches is in the differential diagnosis of each of the others.
- Transient ischaemic attack is in the differential diagnosis of typical migraine aura without headache, especially as it most often occurs in middle-aged men.
- Otherwise, the differential diagnosis includes a small number of serious secondary headaches:[143]
  — intracranial tumours
  — meningitis
  — subarachnoid haemorrhage
  — temporal arteritis
  — primary angle-closure glaucoma
  — idiopathic intracranial hypertension
  — carbon monoxide poisoning.

New or recently changed headache calls for careful assessment.

Essential information for patient and family

Many headache disorders, but especially migraine, impact on a range of people other than the patient,[147] including the family.[148] Recurrent disabling headaches often lead to lifestyle compromises in response to attacks or in a bid to avoid them. Episodic headache can thus have continuous impact.

The mechanisms of many headaches are not well understood. Although patients want to know the cause of their headache, or identify triggers to avoid and thus be cured, this are rarely possible.

Optimal management requires an individualized approach and almost always the use of drugs. Treatment needs may change over time.

Advice and support for patient and family

Many people with recurrent headache, and their families, wrongly fear underlying disease. *Reassurance* is important in migraine, and should never be omitted. Episodic TTH is self-limiting and rarely raises anxieties about its causation or prognosis. Provided that patients are not at risk of escalating medication consumption, little more need be done. *Explanation* that the 'treatment' of headache is the cause of it is vital to the successful management of MOH.

Underlying contributory factors

TTH may be stress-related or associated with functional or structural cervical or cranial musculoskeletal abnormality. These aetiological factors are not mutually exclusive and, quite often, neither is in evidence.

Most CH sufferers are, or have been, smokers — many of them heavy smokers. Advice to stop smoking is invariably good advice. However, the effect of stopping on the future course of CH has not been well studied.

Predisposing and trigger factors

These are generally more important in migraine than in other headache disorders.

Predisposing factors are not always avoidable but may be treatable. They include:

- stress
- depression/anxiety
- menstruation
- menopause
- head or neck trauma.

Trigger factors are important in some patients.[143] Diaries may be useful in detecting them, but triggers appear to be cumulative, jointly contributing to a 'threshold' above which attacks are initiated. Triggers are not always avoidable. Recognized triggers include:

- Stress, anxiety and emotion. Stress may induce other triggers such as missed meals and poor sleep. Bright lights, loud noise and strenuous unaccustomed exercise (all perhaps stress-inducing) are triggers in some people.
- Relaxation after stress, especially at weekends or on holiday.
- Other change in habit, eg missing meals, missing sleep, lying in late, long distance travel. The cause of the change (stress, relaxation) may be the true trigger.
- Dietary sensitivities (usually to certain alcoholic drinks, mature cheeses, citrus fruits) affect, at most, 20% of migraine sufferers. The foods may not always trigger an attack but tip the balance when a person is vulnerable. Dietary triggers, if real, are usefully avoided. Excluded foods should be reintroduced if there is no significant improvement. Alcohol, even in small quantities, potently triggers cluster headache during cluster bouts.
- Hormonal changes commonly influence migraine without aura,[149] with many women more susceptible during menstruation. Nonetheless, menstrual migraine (occurring regularly on day 1 of menstruation ± 2 days and at no other time) is uncommon.[150]

Hormonal contraception, pregnancy and HRT

Headache is often a side-effect of combined oral contraceptives (COCs) and many women report onset of migraine after starting them. Others report improvement of pre-existing migraine. The following advice may be given:[143]

- Both migraine and the ethinyloestradiol component of COCs are independent risk factors for stroke in young women. COCs should be avoided in:[151, 152]
  — migraine with aura
  — migraine without aura in the presence of additional risk factors for stroke
  — migraine treated with ergots (but not triptans).
- Progestogen-only contraception is acceptable with any subtype of migraine.
- Most women who suffer from migraine find they improve during pregnancy.
- Hormone replacement therapy (HRT) is not contraindicated: the menopause commonly exacerbates migraine and symptoms can be relieved with HRT (best provided by percutaneous or transdermal delivery systems used continuously).

Non-drug treatments and self-help

Improving physical fitness may reduce susceptibility to migraine and TTH. Physical therapy (massage, mobilization, manipulation and correction of posture) may be helpful where a specific indication exists (eg neck dysfunction). A therapist with specific training is more likely to achieve good results than a generalist. Psychological therapies (relaxation therapy, stress reduction and coping strategies) are first-line treatments where a specific indication exists (eg anxiety, stress). Biofeedback techniques have some support from clinical trials. Patients with chronic TTH may benefit from cognitive therapies. Transcutaneous electrical nerve stimulation (TENS) may help in chronic TTH when other options fail.

Many patients enquire about any or all of the following:

- *Acupuncture*: of uncertain value generally, but some people appear to benefit. It may be worth a try in frequent episodic or chronic TTH when other treatment options fail.
- *Dental treatment* including splints and bite-raising appliances to correct malocclusion: of unproven value in migraine but occasional patients claim benefit.
- *Hypnotherapy*: of unproven value.
- *Herbals*: not recommended. Feverfew preparations are highly variable in content; their toxicity is not well understood. Feverfew *is unsuitable for children*.
- *Homoeopathy*: of no value generally. Its basis calls for expert prescribing; there is no case for over-the-counter sales of homoeopathic remedies.
- *Reflexology*: has no scientific basis.
- *Devices*: many are on the market, some costly and promoted with unsupportable claims of efficacy. 'Testimonials' can be attributed to placebo effect and should be disregarded.

Medication

Drug treatment is in accordance to the diagnosis (hence the diagnosis must be right). Acute and/or preventive medication may be appropriate.[143]

Migraine

Acute intervention

Drug treatment should be selected for each patient according to his or her need and response to it. Since little basis other than trial and error exists for achieving this, patients should climb a treatment ladder (stepped management). This is a reliable strategy for achieving correctly individualized care:

- Step one:
  — simple oral analgesia (aspirin 900 mg [adults only], paracetamol 1000 mg, ibuprofen 400–600 mg) in soluble or mouth-dispersible formulations taken early in the attack
  — plus, if necessary, metoclopramide 10 mg or domperidone 20 mg as antiemetics and to promote gastric emptying.
- Step two:
  — parenteral administration to bypass the stomach

— diclofenac suppositories 100 mg for pain plus domperidone suppositories 30 mg (if needed) for nausea/vomiting.
- Step three:
  — triptans should be offered, unless contraindicated, to all patients failing steps one and two
  — available triptans differ somewhat,[153] but there are unpredictable individual variations in response to them — patients should try several, and choose the most effective
  — triptans are associated with return of symptoms within 48 hours (relapse) in up to 40% of patients who initially had responded to treatment

Triptans include:

- *Sumatriptan* tablets (50 mg and 100 mg), nasal spray (10 mg [licensed for adolescents] and 20 mg) or self-administered subcutaneous injection (6 mg). The last is appropriate when a rapid response is important above all, or if vomiting precludes oral therapy.
- *Zolmitriptan* tablets (2.5 mg), mouth-dispersible tablets (2.5 mg) (two of either may be taken if needed) or nasal spray (5 mg). The last may be useful despite vomiting since absorption is through the nasal mucosa.
- *Rizatriptan* tablets (5 mg [to be used when propranolol is being taken] and 10 mg) or mouth-dispersible wafers (10 mg).
- *Naratriptan* tablets (2.5 mg). It has slower onset of effect but may be appropriate when other triptans cause undue side-effects.
- *Almotriptan* tablets (12.5 mg).
- *Eletriptan* tablets (20 mg and 40 mg: 2 x 40 mg may be taken if needed). Unlike other triptans, eletriptan exhibits a clear dose–response relationship for efficacy, in the range 20–80mg.
- *Frovatriptan* tablets (2.5 mg).

Contraindications: there are specific precautions attached to some triptans. As a class, triptans should be avoided in:

- uncontrolled hypertension
- coronary heart disease, cerebrovascular disease and peripheral vascular disease
- presence of risk factors for coronary or cerebrovascular disease.

Treatment of relapse: a second dose of a triptan is usually effective for relapse. The second dose may lead to further relapse — in some people, repeated dosing gives rise to repeated relapse.[145] Diclofenac may be an effective alternative or ergotamine tartrate, with prolonged duration of action, may be useful but it should not be used within 12 hours of any triptan.

Prophylaxis

Prophylactic therapy is added when the best acute therapy gives inadequate symptom control. The judge of this is usually the patient. In children, an index is frequency of absence from school.

Over-frequent use of acute therapy is also a criterion for prophylaxis, but prophylactic drugs are inappropriate and will be ineffective for medication overuse headache.

Poor compliance is a major factor impairing efficacy of migraine prophylactics. Once-daily dosing is preferable. Otherwise, there are no sound criteria for choice of prophylactic drug except those of comorbidity and contraindications. The dose of each drug should, usually, start low in the suggested range and be increased in the absence of troublesome side-effects.

- *Beta-adrenergic blockers* without partial agonism:[154] atenolol 25–100 mg bd, propranolol LA 80 mg od–160 mg bd. Avoid in asthma, heart failure, peripheral vascular disease and depression. Propranolol has the best evidence of safety during pregnancy and lactation.[155]

- *Sodium valproate* 0.6–2.5 g daily.[156] Avoid during pregnancy and when pregnancy may occur, and use with care in children.
- *Pizotifen* 1.5 mg at bedtime. Avoid when weight gain is undesirable.
- *Amitriptyline* 10–150 mg at bedtime (or 2–4 hours before). Use when migraine coexists with TTH, depression or sleep disturbance. It may be used concomitantly with a beta-blocker. Explain the choice of this drug to patients who do not consider themselves depressed or they may reject it.
- *Methysergide* 1–2 mg tds (hospital use only). This is held in reserve because of its association with retroperitoneal fibrosis but seems not to have this side-effect in courses of less than six months.
- *In children*: beta-blockers or pizotifen (available as an elixir) may be tried. Some paediatricians use sodium valproate or amitriptyline. Dosage is adjusted according to age.

Duration of use of prophylaxis: prophylaxis is required for periods of exacerbation. If effective it should be continued for 4–6 months, then withdrawn (abruptly or tapered) to establish continued need. Prophylactic drugs that are apparently not effective should not be discontinued too soon as patients be labelled as non-responders prematurely; 3–4 weeks may be the minimum treatment time.

If prophylaxis fails, review the diagnosis, compliance and concordance. It is also important to review other medication, especially for overuse. If prophylaxis still fails to have measurable benefit, discontinue it.

Tension-type headache
Drug therapy has limited scope but is effective in some patients:

- symptomatic treatment with over-the-counter analgesics is appropriate for episodic TTH occurring on less than two days per week: use aspirin 600–900 mg,[157] ibuprofen 400 mg or paracetamol 1000 mg
- codeine and dihydrocodeine should be avoided
- as the frequency of headaches increases, so does the risk of medication overuse
- these treatments are inappropriate in chronic TTH, but a three-week course of naproxen 250–500 mg bd may interrupt frequently recurring or unremitting headaches
- amitriptyline is otherwise the prophylactic treatment of choice for frequent episodic or chronic TTH; intolerance is reduced by starting at 10 mg at night and incrementing by 10–25 mg each 1–2 weeks, usually into the range 50–150 mg at night
- sodium valproate 0.6–2.5 g daily is an alternative; avoid during pregnancy and use with care in children.

Duration of use of prophylaxis — withdrawal may be attempted after improvement has been maintained for 4–6 months.

If prophylaxis fails — failure may be due to subtherapeutic dosage or insufficient duration of treatment. Review compliance and concordance: patients who are not informed that they are receiving medication often used as an anti-depressant, and told why, may default when they find out. Review other medication, especially for overuse. When prophylaxis still fails to have measurable benefit, discontinue it.

Cluster headache
The objective in both episodic and chronic CH, not always achievable, is total attack suppression. In most cases, preventive drugs are the mainstay of treatment.
Acute therapies:

- *sumatriptan* 6 mg subcutaneously is the only proven highly-effective acute treatment
- *oxygen* 100% at 7 l/min (requires a special mask and regulator) helps some people
- analgesics have no place in treating CH.

Prophylaxis

Prophylaxis of episodic CH should begin early after the start of a new cluster bout. The following are used by specialists. Failure of one drug does not predict failure of others. Combinations may be tried,[158] but the potential for toxicity is obviously high:

- *verapamil* 240–960 mg/day[159]
- *prednisolone* 60–80 mg/day for 2–4 days, discontinued by dose reduction over 2–3 weeks
- *lithium carbonate* 600–1600 mg/day
- *ergotamine* 2–4 mg/day per rectum, usually omitted every seventh day
- *methysergide* 1–2 mg tds

Duration of use of prophylaxis: apart from prednisolone, treatment should be discontinued two weeks after full remission.

Medication-overuse headache

Prevention is ideal, with education the key factor. Once MOH has developed, early intervention is important since the long-term prognosis depends on the duration of medication overuse.[160]

- Treatment is withdrawal of the suspected medication(s).
- Although this will lead initially to worsening headache, with forewarning and explanation it is probably most successfully done abruptly.[161]
- Within 2–3 weeks, usually, the headache shows signs of improvement. Patients should be reviewed at this time to ensure withdrawal has been achieved.
- Improvement may be slow but continues for weeks and then months.
- 50–75% of patients revert to their original headache type, which may be migraine (usually) or TTH. This headache should be reviewed after 2–3 months and managed appropriately.
- Most patients require extended support. The relapse rate is around 40% within five years.

Referral

Most primary headaches, and MOH, are best managed in primary care. The following are reasons for specialist referral:

- diagnostic uncertainty after due enquiry
- suspicion of secondary headache, especially those listed above as serious; referral may need to be immediate
- cases where serious pathology is in the differential diagnosis:
  — migraine aura without headache, especially in older men
  — migraine aura including motor weakness
  — newly occurring 'thunderclap' headache
  — headache associated with unexplained physical (especially neurological) signs
- persistent management failure
- cluster headache is usually best managed by specialists
- the presence of risk factors for coronary heart disease occasionally warrants referral to a cardiologist prior to use of triptans
- comorbid disorders requiring specialist management.

Resources for patient and family

Migraine Action Association 01536 461333 (9am–5pm Monday–Friday)
Website: http://www.migraine.org.uk
A membership organization for people affected by migraine, producing a quarterly newsletter and other information leaflets. It runs a telephone help-line. It has local branches, some of which meet regularly.

Migraine Trust 020 7436 1336
Website: http://www.migrainetrust.org
An organization supporting scientific research and also providing information for headache sufferers in the form of a newsletter, booklets and factsheets. It gives financial support to a number of specialist headache clinics.

Organisation for the Understanding of Cluster Headaches (OUCH) 0161 272 1702
Website: http://www.clusterheadaches.org.uk
A membership organization specifically for those affected by CH. It provides information, holds an annual conference and supports patient-involvement in research. OUCH also offers high-flow oxygen regulators on loan, which otherwise must be purchased at high cost.

World Headache Alliance
Website: http://www.w-h-a.org
A world umbrella organization, registered as a charity in the UK, of which all the above are members. It supports its member organizations in 26 countries. The website carries information for those affected by headache and links to many other helpful sites.

Motor neurone disease — G12.2
(Clinical term: Motor neurone disease F152)

Presenting complaints

Motor neurone disease (MND) is the third most common neurodegenerative disease of adult onset. It tends to occur in middle aged or older people, with an average age of onset of 55 years. It is more common in men, with a male:female ratio of 1.6:1.

- MND tends to be focal in onset, affecting a particular group of muscles, eg one hand, one leg or the bulbar muscles at first, with gradual progression of the neuromuscular problems.
- With an upper-limb presentation, early symptoms include weakness or loss of dexterity of one hand. The patient may have noticed muscle wasting, commonly affecting the intrinsic hand muscles, and muscle twitching or fasciculation.
- Presenting symptoms in the lower limbs include unilateral foot drop, a sensation of heaviness affecting one or both legs, or a tendency to trip. Difficulty in running, excessive fatigue when walking, or difficulty in climbing the stairs are also common early symptoms.
- Bulbar onset disease occurs in approximately 20% of cases and this presentation is common in elderly women. The first symptom is usually slurring of speech caused by impairment of tongue movement. This problem is often initially misdiagnosed as a 'slight stroke', but a careful history will reveal that the problem has been of gradual onset and is progressive. Dysphagia usually develops after the onset of dysarthria.
- Common general symptoms at the time of presentation include fatigue and weight loss.
- Occasionally patients will present with symptoms resulting from weakness of respiratory muscles including dyspnoea on exertion or on lying flat. Sleep-related symptoms may also occur as a result of neuromuscular respiratory compromise, including apnoeic spells, frequent arousals, unrefreshing sleep, early morning headaches, daytime sleepiness and anorexia.
- Clinical examination will often reveal the presence of lower motor neurone (muscle weakness, wasting and fasciculation) signs and upper motor neurone (increased tone, brisk reflexes, extensor plantar responses) signs, which may initially be confined to one limb or segmental region. Pain, sensory abnormalities and sphincter dysfunction are usually absent.
- Patients will most commonly have features of both upper and lower motor neurone damage at the time of presentation, ie the amyotrophic lateral sclerosis (ALS) variant of MND. Sometimes patients present with problems confined to the bulbar musculature (progressive bulbar palsy variant); to lower motor neurones within the spinal cord (progressive muscular atrophy variant) or to upper motor neurones (primary lateral sclerosis variant). Later in the disease most patients will have features of ALS.

Diagnostic features

- As yet, no disease-specific test for MND exists and the diagnosis is based on the clinical findings supported by neurological investigations.
- The 'El Escorial' criteria, agreed in 1994, stratify patients into categories of diagnostic certainty, ie definite, probable, possible and suspected MND.[162] Essentially the diagnosis can be made if evidence of mixed upper and lower motor neurone damage in the absence of sensory abnormalities is shown on clinical examination. These signs must show progressive spread within a region or to other regions of the body over a period of time, and electrophysiological or neuroimaging abnormalities that might otherwise explain the clinical picture must be absent.

- In approximately 5–10% of cases it may not be possible to be confident about the diagnosis until several months have elapsed.
- The most important investigation to confirm the diagnosis of MND is neurophysiological assessment with electromyography (EMG) and nerve conduction studies. Imaging of the brain and spinal cord may be necessary to exclude other diagnoses. Most haematological and biochemical investigations are normal, although the serum creatine kinase level may be modestly elevated.

Differential diagnosis

It is important to exclude other conditions that may mimic the early stages of MND. These include:

- degenerative or compressive disease of the spine with radiculomyelopathy
- multifocal cerebrovascular disease
- myasthenia gravis (particularly bulbar presentation)
- other motor neuropathies, especially multifocal motor neuropathy with conduction block
- muscle disease, eg polymyositis, inclusion body myositis
- syringomyelia, syringobulbia
- metabolic disorders, eg hyperthyroidism, hypercalcaemia
- other motor neurone disorders, eg Kennedy's disease or spinal muscular atrophy
- post-poliomyelitis syndrome
- benign cramp fasciculation syndrome.

Useful investigations to exclude other disorders which may mimic MND include brain and/or spinal MRI scan; electromyography and nerve conduction studies; tensilon test and acetylcholine receptor antibody titres; and blood tests including thyroid function, serum calcium and creatine kinase. Muscle biopsy may be required in occasional patients.

Essential information for patients and family members

- Motor neurone disease is one of the three commonest adult-onset neurodegenerative disorders. These three are a group of conditions caused by damage and cell death of particular groups of cells in the nervous system.
- Motor neurones are a group of large cells in the brain and spine, which form a connection between the brain and the muscles, allowing voluntary movement to occur. In MND muscle weakness, stiffness and wasting occur because damage to motor neurones means that the muscles are no longer properly connected to the nervous system.
- In the majority of people who develop MND, other non-motor functions of the nervous system, including intellect, memory, vision, sensation, control of bladder and bowel function, are not significantly affected.
- The symptoms resulting from MND do tend to progress over time, but it is important to be aware that the speed of this progression varies between different individuals. In some people the symptoms change only very gradually over a period of years.
- Curative treatment is not available for MND at the present time. However, much can be done to alleviate the symptoms which may arise during the course of the condition. In addition, one treatment, riluzole, has a modest effect in slowing the progression of the disease. Several other potential disease-modifying therapies are currently being tested in experimental clinical trials.
- Further information and advice about MND is available through the Motor Neurone Disease Association (MNDA), and they will also be able to advise you of the nearest specialist MND care Centre.

Advice and support for patients and family members

- Patients and families may receive advice and support from the Motor Neurone Disease Association and its network of regional care advisors.
- Clinical care and support of patients and families is now usually delivered through multidisciplinary teams which link hospital-based and community care. These teams may include the following professionals: neurologist, general practitioner, specialist nurse, district nurse, physiotherapist, occupational therapist, speech therapist, dietician and social worker.
- Many hospital-based neurological centres now have specialist clinics for patients with neuromuscular disorders including MND. A network of specialist clinics has been established with support from the MNDA. In the UK at present MND clinics are established in Belfast; Birmingham, Cardiff, Liverpool, London, Manchester, Newcastle, Oxford, Preston and Sheffield. Some of these clinics offer a helpline service. Contact details can be obtained via the MNDA.

Medication and other therapies

There are two aims in the treatment of MND. The first is the alleviation of symptoms to maintain the highest quality of life for as long as possible. The second is to slow the progression of motor neurone degeneration and protect motor neurones from further injury.[163]

Symptomatic therapy[164]

Listed below are common symptoms, which may develop during the course of MND, and symptomatic therapies that may be helpful.

- Muscle weakness:
  — physiotherapy to prevent muscle contractures and joint stiffness
  — devices to maintain mobility and independence, eg walking aids, ankle foot orthoses, wheelchairs, supporting collars, mobile arm supports.
- Muscle cramps:
  — quinine sulphate.
- Muscle fasciculations:
  — low-dose diazepam, baclofen or phenytoin.
- Spasticity:
  — anti-spasticity agents, eg baclofen or tizanidine, with careful titration of the dose as loss of tone can sometimes worsen mobility.
- Dysphagia:
  — advice on food consistency and swallowing technique
  — nutritional supplements
  — consider percutaneous endoscopic gastrostomy (PEG) tube insertion.[165]
- Drooling of saliva:
  — anticholinergic agents, eg hyoscine transdermal patches, amitriptyline or atropine
  — portable suction device
  — consider low-dose parotid irradiation if drug treatments fail.
- Difficulty coughing up secretions:
  — carbocisteine as a mucolytic agent.
- Emotional lability:[166]
  — amitriptyline or selective serotonin reuptake inhibitor (SSRI).
- Dysarthria:
  — advice from a speech therapist
  — communication aids, eg light-writer.
- Depression and anxiety:
  — tricyclic anti-dperessants or SSRI's
  — benzodiazepine.

- Sleep disturbance:
  — common causes in MND include respiratory insufficiency, anxiety, depression, muscle cramps and immobility. Treatment should be directed at the underlying cause.
- Constipation:
  — review medication and ensure adequate fluid intake
  — bulk-forming or osmotic laxatives, glycerol suppositories.
- Musculoskeletal pain:
  — analgesia, non steroidal anti-inflammatory agent, physiotherapy
  — consider steroid injection for painful frozen shoulder.
- Breathlessness:
  — early recognition and treatment of aspiration pneumonia
  — upright sleeping position
  — consider nocturnal non-invasive ventilation (NIV).[167]
- Terminal care:
  — involvement of palliative care team
  — opiate and anxiolytic therapy as required to ensure comfort and alleviation of distress.

Neuroprotective therapy
- Scientific insights into the mechanisms of motor neurone degeneration have led to the development of a number of compounds that protect motor neurones in experimental models of MND.
- Over 50 potential neuroprotective agents have been tested in clinical trials in MND. One of these, riluzole, has been shown to slow disease progression significantly and is currently the only drug licensed as a neuroprotective agent in MND. It is a sodium-channel blocker whose primary action is thought to reduce the toxic effects that result from excessive activation of glutamate receptors in the nervous system.
- Two double-blind placebo-controlled trials of riluzole have been undertaken, which included more than 1000 patients. A Cochrane review of riluzole therapy in MND concluded that there was a significant, although modest, effect in prolonging survival.[168] In the UK, prescribing of riluzole is undertaken under guidelines issued by the National Institute for Clinical Excellence.[169]
- Multiple other potential neuroprotective agents are currently under investigation in clinical trials.

Referral
- Patients with suspected motor neurone disease should be referred urgently to a neurologist for assessment and further investigation.
- Delays may occur in establishing the diagnosis where the initial referral is made to a non-neurological clinic; however, local clinic waiting times may influence the referral decision. Patients with dysarthria should ideally be referred to a neurologist rather than an ENT surgeon and patients with painless foot drop or wasting and weakness of the hand should be referred to a neurologist rather than an orthopaedic surgeon.
- Consider referral to social services for practical help, needs assessment, formal care planning, home help and help with application for benefits once the patient has developed significant neuromuscular disability.
- Referral for other specialist help, eg to a gastroenterologist for PEG tube insertion, to a respiratory physician for consideration of non-invasive respiratory support or to the local hospice/palliative care services in the later stages of the disease, may be appropriate for some patients.

Resources for patients and families

Motor Neurone Disease Association 01604 250505, Helpline 08457 626262
Email: helpline@mndassociation.org
PO Box 246, Northampton NN1 2PR
Access via the MND Association to:

- the national network of Care and Research centres
- a variety of publications, booklets, information sheets
- regional care advisors
- regional MNDA branches
- equipment

Scottish Motor Neurone Disease Association 0141 945 1077
Email: info@scotmnd.sol.co.uk
76 Firhill Road, Glasgow G20 7BA
The ALS Association (USA) +1 800-7824747
Website: http://www.alsa.org/als/
The ALS Association National Office, 27001 Agoura Road, Suite 150, Calabasas
Hills, CA 91301-5104, USA

Multiple Sclerosis — G35

(Clinical term: Multiple Sclerosis F20)

M

Presenting complaints

Patients present with either sub-acute, episodic neurological symptoms (85%), termed relapsing remitting Multiple Sclerosis (MS); or a minority present with steadily progressive neurological symptoms from onset (15%), termed primary progressive MS. Over time most patients with relapsing remitting MS acquire residual disability from relapses and enter a later 'secondary' progressive phase of the disease.[170]

In relapsing remitting MS symptoms tend to evolve over days to weeks and resolve over weeks to months. Common presenting symptoms include:

- unilateral visual loss or blurring with prominent loss of colour vision and pain on eye movement (optic neuritis)
- sensory loss, parasthaesia or weakness in one or more limbs (partial transverse myelitis)
- double vision (brain-stem syndromes).

Primary progressive MS generally presents with progressive gait disturbance, with a progressive spastic paraparesis being by far the most common finding. In occasional patients ataxia, sphincter or cognitive symptoms may be more prominent.

Diagnostic features

Relapsing remitting MS:

- more common in caucasian populations, peak onset between age 20–40 years, with a female predominance
- episodic neurological symptoms disseminated both in time and within the central nervous system
- spontaneous early remissions, sometimes of many years
- symptoms are often associated with prominent physical fatigue.

Primary progressive MS:

- becomes more common in older patients (mean age of onset of 40, can present up to age 60 or very occasionally older), with no sex predominance
- typically progressive gait disturbance. Patients will generally complain of fatigable lower limb weakness, stiffness or 'heaviness', often associated with early bladder symptoms of urgency or frequency, and/or erectile dysfunction in men.

MS remains a clinical diagnosis, there is no 'gold standard' investigation although magnetic resonance imaging (MRI) scans will reveal typical white matter or spinal changes in the vast majority of patients (>95%). Nevertheless a number of other conditions can mimic MS both clinically and radiologically and the diagnosis is one of exclusion, assuming that no better explanation can be found for the patient's symptoms and neurological signs.[171]

Differential diagnosis

Most structural conditions, such as cervical myelopathy or syringomyelia, which at one time formed a major part of the differential diagnosis, will be identified by MRI. Although brain scanning will generally reveal the periventricular and sub-cortical changes associated with MS, imaging of the spinal cord is essential in those patients presenting with primarily spinal symptomatology, particularly in late-onset progressive disease where the differential is wide.

Other systemic inflammatory conditions, such as the connective tissue disorders and sarcoid, need to be considered and a careful history to include both previous minor neurological symptoms (which have often been forgotten or overlooked) and systemic features (rash, joint disease, etc) is required.

Where clinical or imaging findings are atypical or equivocal further investigations, such as lumbar puncture for oligoclonal bands in the spinal fluid and visual evoked potentials, are often undertaken to substantiate or exclude the diagnosis. Blood tests, eg inflammatory markers, immunology and B12 and folate, will generally be performed as part of the process of exclusion of other causes of CNS disease.

Essential information for the patient and their family
- MS has a very variable clinical course; at 15 years from onset most patients remain independently mobile, and for up to 20% of patients the disease has a benign course over 20 years or more.
- Life expectancy is not substantially affected for most patients.
- Although there is a degree of genetic susceptibility to the disease it is not strongly hereditary and the risk to other close relatives is of the order of 2–4%.

Contact details for the local MS specialist nurse service should be given to all patients and their families.

General management advice to the patient and family
- Patients should be encouraged to maintain their general health and routine activities. Regular exercise, a healthy diet (emphasizing polyunsaturated rather than saturated fats) and prompt treatment of other illness are appropriate.
- Although fatigue is a very common feature (>80% patients), this tends to be improved by regular physical activity and its impact can be limited by pacing of day-to-day activities and maintenance of a good sleep pattern
- Although relapses are often unpredictable, they are more common in the weeks following infection and possibly at times of emotional stress.
- For many patients MS symptoms are temporarily exacerbated by heat (Uhtoff's phenomenon).
- Pregnancy does not adversely affect the natural history of MS. Relapses tend to be less frequent in the later stages of pregnancy, with a rise in disease activity in the six months post-partum. Epidurals, anaesthesia, operative delivery and breast feeding do not influence the risk of relapse. The major issue to consider in relation to pregnancy is the inevitable uncertainty about long-term physical disability.
- Patients should be told to notify the DVLA and their insurers about their diagnosis — in general this will not result in any restriction to their driving licence unless there are specific physical disabilities (eg visual field loss, poor acuity, severe tremor). If there are concerns about driving ability a formal driving assessment at a recognized centre should be suggested.
- Regular medical review of symptoms and their treatment should be encouraged for most patients, ideally by a member of a multidisciplinary team familiar with the disease and current management strategies.
- The impact of the disease on other family members, particularly children, should be acknowledged and support offered where appropriate.
- For patients with moderate or severe disability timely access to appropriate community therapy and social services should be facilitated.

Medication
Relapse

- Short course of corticosteroids (Methylprednisolone 500 mg–1g, IV or oral for 3–5 days) accelerate recovery from relapse and should be considered for any attacks resulting in significant disability. Steroids do not appear to influence long-term outcome from relapse and there is no role for long-term oral steroids.

Disease management

- In ambulant patients with active relapsing remitting MS (two significant relapses in the last two years) referral to secondary or tertiary care should be discussed for consideration of disease-modifying agents.[172] Interferon beta-1a/b and glatiramer acetate are licensed for the treatment of relapsing remitting MS. In most patients treatment will reduce relapse rate and may delay development of fixed disability. All treatments are given by injection, varying from weekly I/M to daily s/c dependent upon particular product. Initiation of treatment will normally be supervised by MS nurse specialists. Good patient ducation on the role and likely side-effects of treatment and good patient support in the early stages are imperative to ensure compliance.
- In secondary progressive MS there is much more limited evidence for a role of disease-modifying agents. Current guidelines (www.theabn.org) suggest that treatment should be considered in ambulant secondary progressive patients with frequent disabling relapses, although such patients are rare as relapses tend to be less frequent in more advanced disease. Again, assessment by local neurology services is appropriate.
- No treatment has been found to date to alter the natural history of primary progressive MS.
- In very active MS there may be a role for more potent immunosuppressive treatment under the guidance of specialist neurology services.

Symptom management

- Careful consideration should be given to the use of symptomatic treatments, particularly in patients on multiple drug treatments. Both drug interactions and impact on other symptoms need to be considered (eg worsening of fatigue or impaired balance with carbamazepine given for neuropathic pain).[173]
- Symptomatic treatment should be regularly reviewed in the light of fluctuations or progression of disease, occasional careful withdrawal of individual drugs may be appropriate to confirm the continued need for treatment
- Symptomatic spasticity (painful spasms, disturbed sleep by spasm) should be treated with anti-spasmodics (baclofen, tizanidine). Side-effects can include exacerbation of weakness or impairment of function by alleviation of 'useful' spasticity (eg in the patient who uses the lower limb spasticity to allow them to briefly stand and transfer).
- Neurogenic bladder symptoms of detrusor instability (usually urgency or frequency) can be suppressed with anticholinergics. A significant post-micturition residual (usually >100 mls), suggesting detrusor/sphincter dysnergia, should be excluded as this will tend to be worsened by treatment. Incomplete bladder emptying is best managed by clean intermittent self-catheterization by patients or carers, usually once or twice daily.
- Mood disturbance, particularly depression, is common (up to 50% of patients experience it at some point in their illness) and both are under-recognized and under-treated. Standard treatment with a tricyclic (which may also improve neurogenic bladder instability) or SSRI should be considered.
- Persistent pain occurs in around 30% of patients and may be neuropathic or musculoskeletal, secondary to abnormal gait or limited mobility. Neuropathic pain (generally described with terms such as burning, sharp, stabbing) can be treated with low-dose amitryptiline or anticonvulsants.
- Erectile dysfunction occurs in up to 50% of male patients and should be actively identified. It is particularly likely to occur in conjunction with other symptoms of spinal disease (lower limb weakness and spasticity, bladder dysfunction). Treatment with sildenafil (Viagra) or tadalafil is generally effective; if not, consideration should be given to referral to secondary care for assessment.

Referral

- Patients with active relapsing remitting MS should be referred to a neurologist with an interest in MS for consideration of disease-modifying therapy.
- Consider referral to community occupational therapy or social services for those patients with impaired mobility or more significant disability.
- Review the need for additional therapy or specialist referral at the time of acute relapse.
- In patients with complex disability consider involvement of local neuro-rehabilitation services.

Resources for patients and families

The Multiple Sclerosis Society 0800 800 8000 (national helpline)
Website: http://www.mssociety.org.uk
E-mail: info@mssociety.org.uk
Provides information, support and extensive literature to patients and their families through a national centre and local branch structure. The society supports development of MS nurse posts through the MS Nurse fund and is the largest funding body for MS research in the UK

Multiple Sclerosis Trust 01462 476700
Spirella Building, Bridge Road, Letchworth Garden City, Hertfordshire, SG6 4ET
Website: http://www.mstrust.org.uk
E-mail: info@mstrust.org.uk
Carers UK 0808 808 7777 (helpline 10am–12pm, 2–4pm Monday–Friday)
Website: http://www.carersonline.org.uk
E-mail: info@ukcarers.org.uk

Obsessive-compulsive disorder (OCD) — F42

(Clinical term: Obsessive compulsive disorder Eu42)

Presenting complaints
- Commonly concern avoidance and thoughts of 'contamination' by objects or situations, and repetitive cleaning and washing rituals to dispel the contamination.
- Also common are intrusive thoughts of doubt and repetitive checking to prevent harm to self or others, or urges to obtain order or precision or follow a strictly personal routine.

Patients often conceal their symptoms (because of their perceived silly or shameful nature) for fear of ridicule or other unpleasant consequences and so seek help only many years after their problem began.

Diagnostic features
- Obsessions: recurrent intrusive, unwanted, nonsensical thoughts, images or impulses that the patient knows are 'silly' but cannot banish. The obsessions relate to the presenting complaint and usually cause anxiety or other discomfort.
- Compulsions: repetitive rituals performed to reduce anxiety from obsessions by warding off the imagined dreaded consequences. Common rituals are repetitive checking, washing or cleaning, or repetitive rearranging and ordering of objects. Other compulsive behaviours include hoarding of objects and extreme slowness in carrying out every day activities.
- Most patients have both obsessive thoughts and compulsive rituals.
- Most patients have or have had insight into their obsessions and compulsions (although this can depend on when you ask them and how anxious they are) and regard them as 'silly' and resist them.

Symptoms should last for at least two weeks and the patient should have insight into at least one of the symptoms (ie obsessions or compulsions) as being excessive or unreasonable.

Differential diagnosis and co-existing conditions
- 'Phobias — F40' — phobics fear phobic objects more directly than the imagined consequences characteristically seen in OCD.
- Hypochondriasis — the fear is of an illness rather than contamination *per se*.
- 'Depression — F32#' — common co-existent condition.
- 'Generalized anxiety — F41.1' — worries are less stereotyped than in obsessions.
- Other conditions in which stereotyped repetitive behaviour may be seen are:
  - 'Eating disorders — F50'
  - 'Autism spectrum disorders — F84'
  - Tourettes syndrome
  - 'Psychosis — F23, F20#'.

Essential information for patient and family
- Patients and their relatives need to understand (as the symptoms can be bizarre and nonsensical) that OCD is well known and can be overcome by systematic self-help involving exposure and ritual prevention.
- Patients often pressure their families to participate in their rituals (eg cleaning, checking, etc.) and to give reassurance about their doubts.
- Such demands can be very frequent and insistent and can become a source of conflict and stress within the family.

General management and advice to patient and family[174]

- Patients and their relatives can understand the problem better and how to help it by reading and implementing a self-help manual (see below).
- The doctor should explain to them together that giving reassurance or help with rituals may transiently relieve the patient's anxiety but worsens their problems.
- The doctor can help the patient and family start treatment by agreeing that if the patient seeks reassurance or help with rituals, the family will reply, 'The doctor says no answer'.
- Exposure to stimuli triggering obsessional thoughts and response prevention (ie prevention of performance of rituals) is effective[175–177] and the improvement lasts longer than that observed with drug treatment.[178,179]
- Cognitive therapy involves correcting faulty interpretations and beliefs about thoughts and their consequences[175–177,180] and is as effective as behaviour therapy.[181]

Medication[174]

- Drug treatment might be indicated where patients are unwilling to engage in behaviour or cognitive therapy, or where expertise to deliver such therapies is not available.
- Clomipramine and SSRIs (eg fluoxetine, fluvoxamine, sertraline and citalopram) are effective in the treatment of OCD. An adequate trial of treatment usually requires moderate to maximum *BNF* dose and a duration of about 12 weeks[179] (*BNF* 4.3.1 and 4.3.3).
- Discontinuation of drug after improvement often results in relapse within weeks so long-term maintenance treatment with medication may be required.[179]

Referral

See general referral criteria. These particularly apply where there are co-existing disorders.

Special considerations for children and adolescents

- In children, care needs to be taken to distinguish between normal rituals, which are common up to the age of about 10 years, and OCD.
- Parents are often involved in maintaining the rituals by providing reassurance.
- Children and adolescents may not recognize the excessive or unreasonable nature of their thoughts and rituals and may not wish to engage in therapy.
- Very few drug treatments are licensed for children in the UK.
- In children cognitive behaviour therapy has been shown to be as effective as clomipramine.[182]

Resources for patients and families
OCD Action 020 7226 4000 (9.30am–5pm, Tuesday, Wednesday, 11am–5pm, Thursday)
Email: info@ocdaction.org.uk; website: http://www.ocdaction.org.uk
Provides information, advice and support for people with obsessive compulsive disorder and related disorders such as body dysmorphic disorder and trichotillomania

Triumph over Phobia 01225 330 353
Email: triumphoverphobia@compuserve.com; website:
http://www.triumphoverphobia.com
Structured self-help groups for sufferers from phobias or obsessive-compulsive disorder. Produces self-help materials.

Living with Fear, 2nd edition, by Isaac M Marks. McGraw-Hill, 2001. Tel 01628 252700; Email: orders@mcgraw-hill.co.uk
Self-help manual.

Getting Control: Overcoming Your Obsessions and Compulsions by Lee Baer. Brown & Co, 1991.
Self-help manual.

The Imp of the Mind: Exploring the Silent Epidemic of Obsessive Bad Thoughts by Lee Baer. Penguin & Dutton Books, 2001.
Self-help manual.

Obsessive-Compulsive Disorder — the Facts, 2nd edition, by Padmal de Silva and Stanley Rachman. Oxford University Press, 1998.

Understanding Obsessions and Compulsions. A Self-Help Manual by F Tallis. Sheldon Press, 1992.

Obsessive Compulsive Disorder by Stuart Montgomery and Joseph Zohar. Martin Dunitz, 1999.

Panic disorder — F41.0

(Clinical term: Panic disorder [episodic paroxysmal anxiety] Eu41.0)

Presenting complaints

One or more unexplained sudden physical symptoms (eg chest pain, dizziness, shortness of breath) or intense fear of impending collapse, heart attack or stroke.

Diagnostic features

Spontaneous episodes of severe anxiety that start suddenly, rise rapidly, and last from a few minutes to an hour. Such panic 'attacks' occur with physical sensations such as palpitations, chest pain, sense of choking, churning stomach, dizziness, feelings of unreality, or impending disaster (losing control, going mad, sudden death, heart attack). The patient fears further panics and avoids places where they have occurred.

Differential diagnosis and co-existing conditions

Many medical conditions can cause panic-like symptoms (eg arrhythmia, cerebral ischaemia, coronary disease, asthma, thyrotoxicosis) and can also co-exist with panic. History and physical examination should exclude many of these. Investigate any physical symptoms until confident there is no physical cause. Repeating investigations can increase anxiety and should be avoided.

- Drugs may induce panic, as may withdrawal from drugs such as benzodiazepines.
- 'Phobic disorders — F40' (when panics occur in particular situations).
- 'Depression — F32#' (if low or sad mood is present). Depression may co-exist with panic.

Essential information for patient and family

- Panics are common and can be treated.
- Anxiety often causes frightening physical symptoms (eg chest pain, dizziness, shortness of breath) which do not indicate physical illness and will pass when anxiety subsides. Explain how the body's arousal causes these symptoms and how anxiety about them can create a vicious cycle.
- Panic causes frightening thoughts (eg fear of dying, that one is going mad or will lose control) and *vice versa*. These pass when anxiety subsides.
- Mental and physical anxiety reinforce each other.
- Withdrawing from or avoiding situations where panics occur may give immediate relief ('a quick fix') but worsen the problem in the long run.

General management and advice to patient and family[129]

- Advise the patient to learn to spot early warning signs of impending panic and do the following at their start:
  - If it is practical to do so, stay where you are until the panic passes, which may take up to an hour (eg if you're in a car on a busy road, pull over and park where it is safe to do so; if panic starts on a train platform as your train comes in, get onto the train and complete your journey). Do not rush to a place of 'safety'.
  - Tell yourself that the frightening thoughts and sensations are a sign of panic and will eventually pass. Note the time passing on your watch. It may feel like an eternity but it will usually only last a few minutes. Focus thinking on something visible and non-threatening (eg if in a supermarket, look at booklets there).
  - Breathing too rapidly (hyperventilation) can worsen panic. Start slow deep breathing, counting slowly 'one-two-three' on each breath in and on each breath out.

- Notice what you fear during a panic (eg that you're having a heart attack) and challenge it (eg remind yourself, 'This is not a heart attack; it is a panic that will pass in a few minutes').
- Alternatively, some patients improve by thinking the very worst and trying hard to faint on the spot, which they won't be able to do (paradoxical intention).
- Cut down caffeine intake (coffee, tea, street drugs).
- Avoid using alcohol or cigarettes to cope with anxiety.
- Self-help groups, books, tapes or leaflets may help people manage panic and overcome fears[183] (R: 4–1, 4–2).
- A few minutes of cognitive behavioural therapy advice improves panic patients enduringly.[183]

Medication[184]

Most patients benefit from the measures described above and need no medication, unless their mood is very low.

- If there is marked depression, tricyclics or SSRIs may help after some weeks[185] (*BNF* section 4.3).
- It is best to face fears without medication or alcohol or street drugs. If the feared situation is rare (eg flying for someone who flies rarely), occasional short-term beta-blockers might help.
- Relapse is higher after discontinuation of an antidepressant or SSRI[186,187] or a benzodiazepine[188] than after discontinuation of pill placebo or of cognitive behaviour therapy.

Referral

See general referral criteria.

Avoid unnecessary medical referral and investigations for physical symptoms if the diagnosis is clear.

Consider self-help/voluntary/non-statutory services.

Resources for patients and families

Resource leaflets: 4-1 *Anxiety and how to reduce it*, 4-2 *Dealing with anxious thoughts*, 1-1 *Problem-solving* and 1-2 *Learning to relax*

Triumph Over Phobia (TOP) UK 01225 330 353
Email: triumphoverphobia@compuserve.com; website: http://www.triumphoverphobia.com.
Structured self-help groups for sufferers from phobias or obsessive-compulsive disorder. It produces self-help materials.

No Panic 01952 590 545 (helpline 10am–10pm), 0808 808 0545 (gives numbers of volunteers for the day)
Website: http://www.no-panic.co.uk
Helpline, information booklets, local self-help groups (including telephone recovery groups) for people with anxiety, phobias obsessions and panic.

Social Anxiety UK
Website: http://www.social-anxiety.org.uk.
Information and support for sufferers of social anxiety and related problems. The site has a chat room and details of local meetings across the UK.

First Steps to Freedom 01926 851 608 (24-hour helpline)
Email: info@firststeps.demon.co.uk; website: http://www.first-steps.org
Runs self-help groups.

Stresswatch Scotland 01563 528 910 (helpline 10am–1pm, Monday–Friday, excluding Wednesday)
Advice, information, materials on panic, anxiety, stress and phobias.

Living with Fear, 2nd edition, by Isaac Marks. McGraw-Hill, 2001. Tel: 01628 252 700; Email: orders@mcgraw-hill.co.uk.
Self-help manual.

Overcoming Panic — A Self-Help Guide Using CBT by Derrick Silove and Vijaya Manicavasagar. Constable & Robinson, 1997.
Self-help manual.

Who's Afraid...? Coping With Fear, Anxiety and Panic Attacks by Alice Neville. Arrow Books, 1991.
Mind Publications produces the booklet *How To Cope With Panic Attacks*. MIND, Granta House, 15–19 Broadway, London E15 4BQ, tel: 020 8519 2122, and The Mental Health Foundation, 83 Victoria Street, London SW1H 0HW. Tel: 020 7802 0300.

Parkinson's disease — G20

(Secondary Parkinsonism — G21.9, Secondary Parkinsonism due to drugs — G21.1, Essential tremor — G25.0, DSM — IV 294.1 Dementia due to Parkinson's disease)

Parkinson's disease (PD) is the second most common neurodegenerative disease after Alzheimer's disease. The prevalence rate in the UK for PD is approximately 100–200 per 100 000 of the population. The prevalence increases above the age of 50 years to 500/100,000 (one in 200), giving estimates of around 100 000 patients with PD in the UK.

Diagnostic features

The clinical diagnosis of Parkinson's disease is based entirely on clinical history and examination. Although the majority of cases are correctly diagnosed, there are inconsistencies between the clinical diagnosis and the neuropathological diagnosis in 20–25% of patients.

The diagnosis requires a combination of:

- bradykinesia – poverty of movement
- tremor – typically at rest affecting the upper limbs and 'pill-rolling'
- rigidity – increase in tone (either lead pipe or cogwheel due to superimposed tremor)
- postural instability – usually a feature of the illness after several years.

Symptoms usually begin unilaterally in PD, although asymmetric onset is neither sensitive nor specific as a marker for PD.

Nonmotor clinical features develop in PD. These features are common and include:

- Dementia – cognitive deficits occur later in the disease course in 30–40% of patients; typically seen in older rather than younger patients.
- Autonomic disturbances – PD patients may demonstrate gastrointestinal or urinary dysfunction (often constipation and urgency with urge incontinence respectively), orthostatic hypotension and sexual dysfunction. Prominent autonomic symptoms suggest that the diagnosis may be an atypical parkinsonism, such as multiple system atrophy (MSA).
- Depression – may occur in 40% of patients.
- Pain and sensory symptoms – occur in up to 50% of patients and are often related to the degree of motor impairment.

Differential diagnosis

The presence of atypical clinical features suggests other neurodegenerative disorders, often termed Atypical Parkinsonism. Errors in the diagnosis of PD are more likely in the early stages of the illness when atypical features may not have yet developed. Therefore it is prudent to review the diagnosis should this occur.

- Essential tremor (ET): the tremor is usually upper limb, symmetrical and worse with posture and action as compared to at rest in PD. It may also involve the head and voice. ET is dominantly inherited and may respond to beta-blockade or primidone, but patients *should not* be given levodopa.
- Drug–induced parkinsonism: neuroleptic medication used for psychiatric illness, such as chlorpromazine, haloperidol and other major tranquillizers, can cause a parkinsonism that may be difficult to distinguish from PD. Conventional anti-emetics (prochlorperazine, metoclopramide) and drugs that deplete dopamine (such as tetrabenazine) may result in a similar parkinsonian syndrome.
- Parkinsonism 'plus': the term is used when the clinical state has additional features to the parkinsonism. The most commonly recognized are multiple system atrophy (MSA) and progressive supranuclear palsy (PSP) (also known as

Steele–Richardson–Olszweski disease). In these conditions there is additional pathology in multiple regions other than the substantia nigra. Both conditions respond relatively poorly to conventional therapy used in PD and shorten life expectancy. In MSA there can be severe autonomic disturbances, while PSP commonly presents with early postural instability, speech and swallowing difficulties, and dementia of variable severity.

Essential information for patients and family.

The clinical management of PD is dependent on three main principles:

i) accurate diagnosis of the parkinsonian state
ii) symptomatic therapy when needed to reduce functional disability and handicap in the community
iii) planning of treatment for each individual over the long term.

Parkinson's disease is more common in the elderly but can affect younger people too. The progression of the disease is variable — there is as yet no proven therapy that significantly delays disease progression. Although life expectancy is shortened by the illness, most patients can live a good quality life with modern therapy. The principle of management is not just pharmacological. Remaining physically active with advice from a physiotherapist, occupational therapist and speech therapist when needed can help to maintain independence.

Advice and support for patient and family

The majority of patients with Parkinson's disease do not have a family history of the illness. However, in those with a family history of PD there is an increased risk of PD occurring in other family members.

Although PD usually presents with a disorder of movement, non-motor symptoms may occur particularly as the disease progresses. These include neurobehavioural problems, such as depression, personality change, sleep disorders (eg vivid dreams) and psychosis. It can be difficult to separate the effects of medication from that of the disease with, for example, neuropsychiatric effects. Such symptoms should be reported and discussed with the physician.

The management of PD involves a dialogue between patient and family and the doctor (with nurse practitioner) in order to establish individual needs. The pharmacological management can be complicated using several different agents in order to achieve control of symptoms throughout the day with the minimum of side-effects.

Medication

The vast majority of patients with PD respond to levodopa-based therapy. The foundation of treatment for patients with disabling motor symptoms is dopaminergic in the early stages of the disease. An inability to tolerate the drugs or lack of a significant relief of symptoms in response to levodopa-based therapy should lead to the diagnosis being reassessed.

There are many different drugs available to treat symptoms of PD. Traditional drugs such as anticholinergics have little place in modern therapy due to potential side-effects. Fluctuations in the motor response can occur in up to 50% of patients after 5 years of the illness — sparing the total daily dosage of levodopa therapy with the use of long-acting dopamine agonists can reduce the frequency and duration of the fluctuations and associated dyskinesia (involuntary movements). Taking medication at regular intervals throughout the day can help to reduce the incidence of fluctuations.

Early recognition and effective treatment of non-motor symptoms, such as depression, can relieve distress to the patient and their family/carer. Sleep disorders are very common in PD. Nocturnal akinesia and rigidity may respond to a long-acting levodopa therapy. Sleep attacks with sudden drowsiness may be related to the use of dopaminergic therapy. Patients should be told of the risk of such attacks. Should they occur, adjustment of medication can be tried. The patient with sleep attacks should avoid situations of risk, eg stopping driving.

Parkinsonian psychosis can be very disabling and distressing. Management includes review of medication, looking for secondary causes of confusion such as infection, and if necessary the use of atypical neuroleptic medication (such as quetiapine). There is an increased risk of dementia in PD particularly, in the elderly. This may necessitate alteration to drug therapy (which could then have a detrimental effect on the motor state) in order to reduce confusion, hallucinations and nightmares. It is important to recognize the effects of the disease, in particular dementia, on the health and welfare of other family members and carers.

Referral

Referral to a Neurologist, or health care of the elderly physician with an interest in movement disorders is essential for:

- correct diagnosis
- discussion of the disease and prognosis
- initiation of appropriate medication to meet the needs of the patient
- referral to therapists and social services if needed to maintain independence
- an understanding of the range of presentations as the disease progresses and intervention when necessary
- becoming a point of contact for support, education and advice.

Operative treatment

Deep brain stimulation has become a therapeutic alternative in some patients, especially those with fluctuating symptoms who do not respond well to levodopa.

References

References 189–194 (see pages 268–269) are articles that give an overview of the evidence base for this subject.

Resources for patients and families

Parkinson's disease at your fingertips. 2nd Edition. Oxtoby M, Williams A. London: Class Publishing, 1999.
Understanding Parkinson's disease. Pearce JMS. A Family Doctor Publication in association with the BMA, July 2000.

Parkinson's Disease Society 020 7931 8080, Fax: 020 7233 9908
Website: http://www.parkinsons.org.uk
215 Vauxhall Bridge Road, London SW1V 1EJ.

Personality (behavioural) disorders — F60

(Clinical term: Disorders of adult personality and behaviour Eu60)

Some people find the term 'Personality disorder' inflammatory, and it is therefore perhaps preferable to talk to the patient about their 'personality difficulties'.

Presenting complaints

Patients may present in a variety of ways:

- Constantly worrying or displaying excessive dependence on the primary care team
- Repeated consultations, including for unexplained physical symptoms
- Threatening self-harm or aggressive behaviour
- Intense and superficial relationships
- With complaints of another mental disorder: depression, anxiety, eating disorders and addictions are all more prevalent
- Impulsive or threatening behaviours, eg repeated self-harm.

These patients are usually difficult, with multiple social problems; and they may have a previous history of problematic dealings with the health service. They are more likely to attend in a crisis but may then fail to re-attend for follow-up appointments.

Alternatively, the patient may come to the attention of the primary care team because of the impact their behaviour is having on others:

— Family and carers may express concern about the patient's behaviour (eg threatening behaviour, self-harm).

— Through their antisocial behaviour, in which case they may be referred by the Criminal Justice System.

Diagnostic features

- Maladaptive patterns of behaviour, thinking and control of emotions.
- Disturbance is enduring and not limited to episodes of mental illness.
- Disorder leads to considerable personal distress and/or significant problems in occupational and social functioning.
- Early manifestations (eg conduct disorder) may appear in childhood, but Personality disorder should not be diagnosed in someone under the age of 18.

ICD-10 recognizes nine subcategories of Personality disorder, each with its own set of diagnostic criteria. They fall into three groups:

- Group A: Paranoid and schizoid; characterized by oddness, difficulty mixing with others and paranoid thinking.
- Group B: Dissocial, emotionally unstable (impulsive type and borderline type) and histrionic; characterized by problems with impulse control, affect regulation and relationship instability.
- Group C: Anankastic, anxious and dependent; characterized by anxiety, excessive dependency on others and obsessional behaviour.

Differential diagnosis

Although other mental disorders can occur in the context of a personality disorder, a primary diagnosis of personality disorder should only be made in the absence of mental illness. If possible, obtain an informant's account of the patient's personality.

Consider the following, particularly when behaviour is 'out of character':

- 'Depression — F32#'
- 'Acute to chronic (persistent) psychotic disorder — F23, F20#'
- Anxiety disorders

- **'Drug use disorders — F10–19'**; these commonly occur in people with dissocial and emotionally unstable personality disorders
- A medical condition causing personality change (eg head injury, acute confusional state, **'Dementia — F03'**).

Essential information for patient and family
- Mental illness and addictions occurring in people with personality disorders are treatable.
- Modification of problematic behaviour is possible, but the patient must be motivated to change his/her behaviour.
- Specialist treatment consists of a combination of psychological treatments (including group and individual psychotherapies) reinforced by drug therapy at critical times.
- Treatment of any sort (including for associated conditions) requires the patient's active involvement. The relationship with the professional concerned is crucial.

General management and advice to patient and family[195]
- Consistency and continuity in approach, basic problem-solving techniques, and assistance in containing psychological stress form the foundation for the clinical approach to these patients.
- Difficulties with others can be minimized, if the person is taught to avoid situations that lead them into conflict with others (eg avoiding group living if mixing with others makes them anxious).
- Ensure that both the patient and others involved in their care understand the treatment plan and aims.
- The practitioner needs to be very clear about his/her role and its boundaries.
- The practitioner needs to communicate effectively with others in their team. If several health professionals are involved in the patient's care, ensure that a consistent approach is adopted.
- Professional disputes about patient care (which commonly occur with this patient group) can be minimized by holding regular meetings with those involved with the patient.
- Establish a clear protocol for how all members of the team will respond to the patient during a crisis. Crisis contacts should be brief, focused and goal-oriented. If possible, give the patient some responsibility for resolving the crisis.
- Treat co-morbid conditions.
- Focus on immediate, everyday problems. The aim is not to cure the personality disorder but to help the patient deal with everyday life. Behavioural disturbances associated with Personality disorder tend to improve with advancing age.
- Specialist treatment of personality disorders consists of a combination of psychological treatments reinforced by drug therapy.
- Personality-disordered patients can be supported by a primary care team in conjunction with input from specialist psychiatric services where appropriate. The support generally needs to be long-term and the style of consultation needs to be adapted to the type of personality disorder that the patient has.

Medication[195]
- Medication, while of some benefit, is not the mainstay of treatment.
  - Antidepressant medication: SSRIs have a growing evidence base in the management of impulsive behaviour.[1]
  - Low-dose atypical antipsychotic medication: may help to reduce paranoid ideation and the level of arousal experienced by some personality-disordered patients. However, the long-term effectiveness is not yet established.
  - Mood stabilizers: may help to ease the affective instability experienced by those with an emotionally unstable personality disorder.
- Be mindful of the possibility of overdose in this group of patients.

Referral

Referral to a community mental health team for an assessment can be helpful under the following circumstances:

- For diagnostic clarification
- If there is a risk of harm to self or others
- For treatment of co-morbid mental illness
- For specialist treatment of the underlying personality disorder.

The referral might, however, be unsuccessful, either because the patient does not want to be referred, does not attend for assessment or fails to co-operate with the treatment offered. Increasingly, it is the case that community mental health teams (whose main remit is to deal with severe mental illness) do not have the resources or expertise to manage personality-disordered patients. The need for specialist psychiatric services for this group of patients has recently been acknowledged by the Department of Health.[195]

Resources for patients and families

Borderline http://www.BPDcentral.com
This site is mainly for families of people with Borderline personality disorder.

Borderline UK http://www.borderlineuk.co.uk
A national user-led network of people within the UK who have been diagnosed with Borderline personality disorder. The site provides detailed information on Borderline personality disorder.

Borderline Personality Disorder Research Foundation
http://www.borderlineresearch.org
Provides details of research and other information

Understanding Personality Disorders. Available from MIND Publications, 15–19 Broadway, London E15 4BQ, tel: 020 8519 2122.
Leaflet with straightforward explanations. Useful for family members, staff and others.

Phobic disorders — F40

Includes agoraphobia, social phobia, and specific phobia
(Clinical code: Phobic anxiety disorders Eu40)

Presenting complaints
Patients may fear and/or avoid activities such as going outside their home, shopping, visiting friends, or other situations that trigger panic.

While in or thinking about the feared situation, patients may complain of palpitations, dizziness, inability to breathe properly, or other physical symptoms of anxiety.

Ask 'Is there anything you tend to avoid or fear more than most people do?'

Diagnostic features
Unreasonably strong fear and/or avoidance of people, places, or events.
Commonly feared/avoided situations include:

- leaving home, or being alone at home
- crowds or public places
- travelling by bus, train, plane or car
- open spaces
- performing in public
- social events
- other, such as animals, darkness, heights, blood, etc.

Differential diagnosis
- **'Panic disorder — F41.0'** (if panics are prominent and not brought on by anything in particular).
- **'Depression — F32#'** (if low or sad mood is prominent).

Essential information for patient and family
- Patients can treat their phobia successfully.
- Avoiding feared situations feeds the fear.
- By facing the fear systematically, one overcomes it.

General management and advice to patient and family[129] (R: 4–1, 4–2, 4–3, 4–4)
- Does the patient understand the problem and want to deal with it?
- Encourage the patient and his/her relatives to read and follow self-exposure instructions from an appropriate manual or website.
- Suggest that the patient list all situations that he/she fears and avoids although other people do not.
- Help the patient to plan progressively more challenging exposure steps so he/she can gradually get used to each feared situation in turn (R: 4–3):
  — Find a first small step towards whatever frightens him/her (eg if afraid of leaving home, take a short walk away from home with a relative).
  — Practise this small step of facing a feared situation for an hour each day until it becomes boring rather than frightening.
  — Say that success involves learning to experience and stay with panic. While performing the step say to yourself 'If I face my panic (in whatever place frightens me) by remaining there rather than running away, and practise slow, deep breathing, the fear will start to die down within 30–60 minutes'. See advice on **'Panic disorders — F41.0'**.
  — The patient should not leave the feared situation until the fear starts to subside.

121

- Once doing that step feels fairly comfortable, go on to a slightly more difficult step and repeat the procedure (eg spend a longer time away from home; then do this alone).
- If exposure to real feared situation(s) is hard to arrange, the patient should instead write and read, or tape record and listen to, long scenarios of exposure to that situation(s).
- The patient should take no alcohol, anti-anxiety medication or street drugs for at least four hours before practising these steps.
• The patient should ask a friend or relative to help plan his/her exercises to face and overcome the fear (R: 4–4). Self-help groups can assist in this.
• The patient should keep a diary of the 'face-the-fear' exercises described above, to fine-tune step-by-step management.

Medication

By facing their fear systematically, many patients will need no medication.[129]

• Where patients only meet their real phobic situation rarely (eg flying or speaking in public), occasional short-term anti-anxiety or beta-blocker drugs can help.[137,196] Regular use is undesirable and fear is likely to return when the drug is stopped.
• If exposure is refused or fails after a daily hourly trial for four weeks, or depression is also present, tricyclic or SSRI medication may be indicated.

Referral

See general referral criteria.

Resources for patients and families
Resource leaflets: 4–1 *Anxiety and how to reduce it*, 4–2 *Dealing with anxious thoughts*, 4–3 *How to overcome a phobia* and 4–4 *Helping someone else to overcome a phobia*

Triumph Over Phobia (TOP UK) 01225 330 353
Email: triumphoverphobia@compuserve.com.
Structured self-help groups for sufferers from phobias or Obsessive-compulsive disorder. It produces self-help materials.

Stresswatch Scotland 01563 528 910 (helpline 10am–1pm, Monday–Friday, excluding Wednesday)
Advice, information, materials on panic, anxiety, stress and phobias.

Fear Fighter http://www.fearfighter.com.
Self-help guidance plus option of live helpline advice if you get stuck.
Leaflets are available from the Royal College of Psychiatrists
(http://www.rcpsych.ac.uk): Anxiety and Phobias, and Social Phobias.

Living With Fear, 2nd edition, by Isaac Marks. McGraw Hill, 2001, tel: 01628 252700,
Email: orders@mcgraw-hill.co.uk.
Self-help manual.

Painfully Shy: How to Overcome Social Anxiety by B Markway. Griffin, 2001
Triumph Over Shyness: Conquering Shyness & Social Anxiety by M Stein. McGraw–Hill, 2003
Available as an *e* book, which can be downloaded from Amazon.

Post-traumatic stress disorder (PTSD) — F43.1
(Clinical code: Post-traumatic stress disorder Eu43.1)

Presenting complaints
Physical symptoms (eg various pains, poor sleep or fatigue) and various anxiety and depressive symptoms linked to a particular trauma, of more than a month's duration.

Diagnostic features
- History of an exceptionally traumatic event (brief, prolonged or repeated) that would probably distress almost anyone.
- Intrusive memories, flashbacks and nightmares.
- The patient avoids thoughts, activities and situations reminding him/her of the trauma; sense of 'numbness'; emotional blunting and detachment from other people; unresponsive to surroundings; no longer enjoys anything (anhedonia).
- Autonomic arousal, hypervigilance, increased startle, insomnia, irritability, excessive anger, impaired concentration and/or memory.

Differential diagnoses and co-existing conditions
- 'Depression — F32#' (if showing preoccupation with and rumination about a past traumatic event that emerged during a depressive episode).
- 'Phobic disorders — F40' (if patient avoids particular objects, situations or activities after a traumatic event, but has no non-phobic distress).
- 'Adjustment disorder — F43.2' (if the patient only partly fulfils criteria or the problem followed an event that was not especially traumatic).
- 'Generalized anxiety — F41.1' (if there are no intrusions and/or avoidance). ˙

Essential information for patient and family
- Traumatic events often have psychological effects. For the majority, symptoms subside with no intervention. (R: 2)
- Once symptoms have continued for over a month, treatment can be effective.
- The patient needs support and understanding, not to be told to 'snap out of it'.

General management and advice to patient and family[197]
- Educate the patient and family about PTSD to help them understand the patient's altered attitude and behaviour.
- Most people find it helpful to discuss the event unhurriedly with sympathetic friends and family. Explain that avoidance of cues associated with the trauma strengthens and maintains fears and distress. Encourage the patient to face avoided activities and situations gradually (see 'Phobic disorders — F40').
- Ask about suicide risk (see Self-harm).
- Avoid using alcohol, tobacco or street drugs to cope with anxiety.
- Single session intervention is not needed for everyone after a trauma.[198]
- Provide a few sessions of cognitive behaviour therapy from about a month after the trauma benefit patients.[199–201]
- The evidence for a benefit from eye movement desensitization and reprocessing remains controversial.[202]
- Other psychological therapies, including group and psychodynamic therapies, are of unknown effectiveness.[200]

Medication
The long-term outcome appears better after psychosocial approaches than after drug treatment.

Antidepressants might help, especially if depression is prominent.[203] Drugs for PTSD are generally needed in higher doses and for longer than when used for depression. Improvement may take up to eight weeks to manifest.

Referral

See general referral criteria.
If available, consider behaviour therapy (exposure) or cognitive techniques.[199–201]

Resources for patients and families

Medical Foundation for the Care of Victims of Torture
Website: http://www.torturecare.org.uk
Provides survivors of torture with medical treatment, social assistance and psychotherapeutic support.

CombatStress 01372 841 600
Email: contactus@combatstress.org.uk; website: http://www.combatstress.com.
Supports men and women discharged from the armed services and merchant navy who suffer from mental health problems, including post-traumatic stress disorder. Has a regional network of welfare officers who visit people at home or in hospital.

Refugee Support Centre 020 7820 3606
Counsels refugees, asylum seekers. Gives training and information to health and social care professionals on psychosocial needs of refugees.

Victim Support 0845 3030 900 (support line 9 am–9pm, Monday–Friday; 9am–7pm, Saturday and Sunday; 9am–5pm, bank holidays)
Email: contact@victimsupport.org.uk; website: http://www.victimsupport.org.uk
Provides emotional support and practical information for anyone who has suffered the effects of crime, regardless of whether the crime has been reported.

Rape Crisis Federation 0115 900 3560 (9am–5pm, Monday–Friday)
Email: info@rapecrisis.co.uk; website: http://www.rapecrisis.co.uk

Women against Rape 020 7482 2496
Email: war@womenagainstrape.net; website: http://www.womenagainstrape.net

Fear Fighter http://www.fearfighter.com
Self-help guidance plus the option of live helpline advice, if you get stuck.

Living With Fear by Isaac Marks, 2nd edition. McGraw Hill, 2001, tel: 01628 252 700; Email: orders@mcgraw-hill.co.uk.
Self-help manual. Includes help with fear and avoidance symptoms of PTSD.

Overcoming Traumatic Stress by Claudia Herbert and Ann Wetmore. London: Robinson Publishing, 1999.

Postnatal depression — F53
(Closest equivalent clinical term: Neurotic depression of reactive type Eu204)

Presenting complaints
Women may present with one of three distinct syndromes — in descending order of severity:

- Baby blues — normally occurs in the week after birth, and tends to be mild. Women with baby blues do not usually present, because the condition is short-lived, but it can develop into postnatal depression. A new mother presenting with depression should never be dismissed as having 'just the baby blues'.
- Postnatal depression — presents with mild/moderate to severe depression, usually 4–12 weeks after birth but may be up to six months after the birth.
- Puerperal psychosis — pronounced disturbance of mood, presenting in the first few weeks after birth.

Diagnostic features
Baby blues:

- emotional lability, crying, irritability, tiredness and feelings of inadequacy.

Postnatal depression:

- tearfulness, which may be worse at particular times of the day
- irritability, agitation, poor concentration
- anxiety (the mother might be afraid to be alone with the baby)
- sleep difficulties (even if baby is sleeping)
- appetite disturbance
- guilt
- ambivalence about the baby
- low self-esteem, indecisiveness
- exhaustion and general inability to cope
- thoughts of self-harm and suicide
- vague physical symptoms.

Risk factors include a previous history of depression or postnatal depression, poor relationship with partner, adverse social circumstances, an unplanned pregnancy and perinatal death.

Puerperal psychosis:

- pronounced disturbance of mood — either consistently low or high, or fluctuating unpredictably between the two, and sometimes interspersed with periods of normal mental state
- extreme irritability
- delusions (often taking the form of irrational preoccupations concerning the baby) and hallucinations
- onset within the first few weeks after birth.

Risk factors include a previous or family history of psychosis, and young age.
    In different cultures, pregnancy and childbirth are associated with widely differing traditions and rituals, as well as differences in the concept of depression.

Differential diagnosis and co-existing conditions
- 'Panic disorder — F41.0'.
- 'Generalized anxiety — F41.1'.

Depression following childbirth is essentially the same condition as depression at any other time. There is a risk that normal physical or emotional changes following childbirth may be mistaken for depression or alternatively may mask depressive symptoms.

Essential information for patient and family

- Baby blues affects up to 50% of new mothers and is usually self-limiting.
- Postnatal depression is common, affecting 10–15% of new mothers; puerperal psychosis is a much rarer condition (0.5–1.0% of all births).
- It can be very difficult for new mothers to admit that they are not coping or feeling depressed at a time they perceive should be happy.
- Mothers may be concerned that if they are honest about their feelings their baby will be taken into care.
- Mothers with postnatal depression do not usually harm their babies; babies may be at risk from mothers suffering from puerperal psychosis.
- Emotional *and* practical support from family and friends is very valuable.[204]
- The outcome for most mothers with postnatal depression is very good, provided they receive appropriate care.
- If untreated, postnatal depression can be prolonged and can have an effect on mother–baby attachment and in turn on the child's educational, emotional and behavioural experiences.

General management and advice to patient and family

Postnatal depression:

- The Edinburgh Postnatal Depression Scale (EPDS) is an effective tool for screening and monitoring progress;[205] it is not a diagnostic tool.
- If available, non-directive counselling, interpersonal psychotherapy and cognitive behavioural therapy are effective.[206–208]
- Postnatal groups run by health visitors and mental health nurses are effective.
- Provision of social support, for example a home help or child care, may be helpful.

Puerperal psychosis:

- Very close monitoring of mother and baby is essential, which usually requires admission, preferably to a specialist unit.
- Medication is always required.
- Psychological therapies are likely to be helpful after the acute phase.
- Electroconvulsive therapy may occasionally be necessary.

Medication

- Antidepressants: the response in mothers suffering postnatal depression is usually good.[209] Antidepressants should continue to be taken for up to six months after recovery.
- SSRIs are the treatment of choice. Fluoxetine is contraindicated in breastfeeding mothers (*BNF* 4.3.3).
- Antipsychotic medication and mood stabilizers might be needed for puerperal psychosis.

Referral

- Preconceptual referral is recommended for women:
  — with a history of bipolar disorder or other psychosis, including a previous puerperal episode, who have a high risk of puerperal psychosis
  — taking any mood stabilizers or long-term antipsychotics.[210]
- Refractory cases of depression should be referred to the community mental health team.
- In severe cases, referral to inpatient services might be necessary, ideally to a specialist mother and baby unit (babies should not be admitted to general psychiatric wards).

Resources for patients and families

The Association for Post Natal Illness (APNI) 020 7386 0868
Email: info@apni.org; website: http://www.apni.org
Provides information on postnatal depression. APNI will put affected mothers in touch with others who have had similar experiences.

National Childbirth Trust (NCT) 0870 444 8707
Website: http://www.nctpregnancyandbabycare.com
Provides information and support on all aspects of pregnancy and childbirth, with local groups around the country.

Meet-a-Mum Association (MAMA) 01525 217 064
Email: meet-a-mum.assoc@blueyonder.co.uk; website: http://www.MAMA.org.uk
Local self-help groups for pregnant women and those with young children.

Fathers Direct http://www.fathersdirect.com

The Samaritans 08457 909090 (helpline: 24-hour, everyday)
Email: jo@samaritans.org; website: http://www.samaritans.org.uk
Offer confidential emotional support to any person who is despairing or suicidal.

Depression Alliance http://www.depressionalliance.org
England: 020 8768 0123
Wales: 029 2069 2891 (10am–4pm, Monday–Friday)
Scotland: 0131 467 3050
Provides information and self-help groups.

Aware Defeat Depression Ltd 02871 260 602
Email: info@aware-ni.org; website: http://www.aware-ni.org
Provides information leaflets, lectures and runs support groups for sufferers of depression and their relatives.
Leaflets are available from the Royal College of Psychiatrists
(http://www.rcpsych.ac.uk): Postnatal Depression — Help is at Hand, Mental Illness after Childbirth.

Postnatal Depression: Facing the Paradox of Loss, Happiness and Motherhood by Paula Nicholson. Wiley, 2001

Maternal Distress and Postnatal Depression: The Myth of Madonna by J Littlewood and N McHugh. Macmillan, 1997

Coping with Postnatal Depression by Fiona Marshall. Sheldon Press, SPCK Mail Order, 36 Steep Hill, Lincoln LN2 1LU, UK.

Self-harm — X60–X84
(Clinical term: Self-harm U2...)

Presenting complaints
The majority of people who present either to Accident and Emergency or to primary care following non-fatal self-harm do so after:

- an overdose
- an episode of self-cutting
- other more violent forms of deliberate self-harm, such as asphyxiation or self-poisoning using car exhaust fumes (these suggest a high degree of suicidal intent).

Best practice suggests that GPs should try to contact and assess their patients when notified that they have self-harmed, although current evidence does not yet show that this significantly reduces repetition rates.

Assessment
There are three assessment tasks:

- To assess and manage the current episode
- To identify and manage any associated conditions
- To prevent repetition of the self-harm.

Assessing and managing the current episode
- Pay prompt attention to any medical sequelae, including long-term physical damage (eg liver damage from overdose).
- Identify relevant/ongoing trigger(s) (note that precipitating events that surround episodes of self-harm are poor predictors of suicide risk, making the notion of a 'suicidal gesture' following interpersonal crisis difficult to sustain).
- Assess suicidal intent, including:
  — deliberate isolation at time of self-harm
  — precautions made against discovery
  — 'final acts' in anticipation of death, for example giving possessions away, making a will
  — communication of intent before the attempt and self-report of motivation for self-harm (to solve a problem or escape a situation)
  — patient's perceptions of barriers/incentives, for example, 'I could never actually kill myself because of the children' (generic, therefore safer) or 'I'll kill myself if she doesn't come back by next Monday' (specific, therefore riskier).
- Assess background history, including past and current contact with mental health services, social problems and substance misuse problems.
- Note that socio-demographic groups at increased risk include men, those aged 15–25 or over 55, those who are widowed, separated or divorced, those who are socially isolated, unemployed, those with a family history of suicide and a previous history of self-harm.
- Note that rates of suicide are particularly high in the period following discharge from psychiatric hospital, release from prison, and in the months following an episode of non-fatal self-harm. (The suicide rate increases 100-fold in the year following an episode of self-harm.) Patients who regularly present with self-harm have an even higher rate of eventual suicide.
- Note that the most important risk factor for suicide is the presence of depression, drug/alcohol abuse, or other mental health problems (see below).
- Identify current life problems, social stresses and precipitating factors. Episodes often occur in the context of multiple social difficulties and interpersonal problems. It

is therefore important to assess the nature and extent of unresolved problems and how the patient would cope with future crises (see below). Focus on small, specific steps the patient might take towards reducing or improving management of these problems. Avoid major decisions or life changes.
- Support the family. It is likely to be very distressing to discover that a family member is self-harming.

Identification and management of any associated conditions
- Mental disorders, most commonly '**Depression — F32#**', '**Alcohol misuse — F10**' or '**Drug use disorders — F11#**', but also psychoses.
- '**Bereavement and loss — Z63**'.
- Painful, disabling or life-threatening physical illnesses.
- Being the victim or perpetrator of violence (see '**Domestic violence or partner abuse**').

Prevention of repeated self-harm
This requires a thorough assessment of suicidal intent:

- Does the patient think that life is not worth living?
- Does the patient have a sense of hopelessness?
- Does the patient have a suicide plan and the (immediate) means to carry it out?
- Is the patient likely to act on the plan?

The belief that enquiring about suicidal ideation might prompt some people to consider self-harm is not supported by research findings or clinical experience. Placed in the context of asking people about symptoms of depression, such questions feel less awkward for the interviewer; for example, 'It sounds as if you have been feeling very down recently; has there ever been a time when you have felt as though you couldn't be bothered carrying on?' 'Have you ever felt that life was not worth living/that you would be better off if you were dead?' 'Have you ever thought of harming yourself in any way?'

Some people self-harm by repeatedly cutting or — more rarely — burning themselves.

- Cutting usually occurs when the person is experiencing strong feelings, such as tension or frustration. Patients often report that cutting provides temporary relief from distress.
- Patients usually deny having thoughts of suicide.
- Some patients lead ordinary lives and they feel their experience of self-cutting is not a major problem; for others it is part of a wider problem that includes long-standing feelings of low self-esteem and deep-rooted sadness, and is associated with other forms of self-harm, such as alcohol abuse or drug problems.

Essential information for patient and family
- Patient confidentiality may be particularly sensitive when patients present with self-harm. It might be necessary (and appropriate) to override patient confidentiality when that patient's life is at risk.
- It can come as a great shock to family members that a relative is experiencing thoughts of self-harm.
- Feelings of self-harm are common among people who experience mental distress and only a small proportion of people with suicidal thoughts actually act on them.
- The family should take any possible specific steps to reduce the opportunity for further self-harm — for example, by removing weapons, drugs, etc.
- Patients and family members may be reassured by knowing about help lines and local services that are available 24 hours a day, for example the Samaritans.

General management and advice to patient and family[211]

- Assessment of suicidal ideation is an important part of the mental-state examination of anyone who presents with a mental health problem.
- Any underlying mental disorder needs to be treated.
- Patients who, as a result of assessment, are considered at risk of further self-harm should be reviewed regularly by the GP.
- Psychological treatments may help the person make sense of their difficulties without feeling the need to self-harm.[212] The approach that therapists usually use involves paying attention to how a person is feeling rather than concentrating directly on whether or not they are harming themselves.
- Clinicians managing complex or protracted cases of self-harm should consider seeking peer support or supervision.

Medication

Medication needs to be given as required for any underlying psychiatric disorder.

Use of antidepressants such as SSRIs, selective noradrenalin reuptake inhibitors (SNRIs) and lofepramine is recommended for all those who have depressive symptoms and are felt to be at risk of suicide, because they are relatively safe in overdose.

Referral

- Those with active suicidal intent or continuing suicidal ideation might need to be referred to specialist medical services.
- Where a mental disorder has been diagnosed, refer to the relevant guidelines for that disorder.
- Consider referral for psychological therapies, as appropriate.
- It has been argued that because of the rates of underlying mental disorder and greater risk of subsequent suicide in the elderly, all elderly people who present to primary care services following deliberate self-harm should be referred to secondary care services.

Resources for patients and families

Self Harm Alliance Helpline 01242 578820 (6pm–7pm, Tuesday, Sunday; 11am–1pm, Thursday)
Email: selfharmalliance@aol.com; website: http://www.selfharmalliance.org
Helpline, produces monthly newsletters, provides postal and email support, and offers an advocacy service.

Self Injury and Related Issues (SIARI)
Email: jan@siari.uk; website: http://www.siari.co.uk
Forum for self-harmers.

The Samaritans 08457 909 090 (24-hour helpline, everyday)
Email: jo@samaritans.org; website: http://www.samaritans.org.uk
Offers confidential emotional support to any person who is despairing or suicidal.

Cruse Bereavement Care 020 8940 4818 (for details of local services)
Helpline: 0870 167 1677 (9.30am–5.00pm, Monday–Friday)
Email: info@crusebereavementcare.org.uk; website:
http://www.crusebereavementcare.org.uk
Offers support, information, training and direct telephone help to anyone who has been affected by a death.

Bereavement Information Pack for those affected by a suicide. A copy of the booklet can be purchased from the Royal College of Psychiatrist, Book Sales, 17 Belgrave Square, London SW1X 8PG.

Sexual disorders (female) — F52
(Clinical term: Sexual dysfunction, not caused by organic disorder or disease Eu52)

Clinical judgements about sexual dysfunction should take into account the individual's ethnic, cultural, religious and social background, which may influence sexual desire, expectations and attitudes about performance.

Presenting complaints
- Patients may be reluctant to discuss sexual matters. They may instead complain of physical symptoms, depressed mood or relationship problems. It is important to be aware that patients with sexual problems may have a history of sexual abuse/assault (in childhood or later).
- Patients may present sexual problems during a routine cervical-smear test, well-woman clinic or when discussing contraception.

Diagnostic features
Sexual dysfunction can cause marked distress and interpersonal difficulty. Common sexual disorders presenting in women are:

- lack or loss of sexual desire, sexual aversion
- sexual arousal disorder (inability to attain/maintain an adequate physiological response to sexual excitement)
- sexual pain disorders:
  — vaginismus (involuntary spasm of vaginal muscles on attempted penetration accompanied by a fear or phobia — the phobia can rarely occur without the spasm)
  — dyspareunia (recurrent genital pain associated with sexual intercourse — superficial vulval, vaginal or deep pelvic)
- orgasmic disorder (delay in, or absence of, orgasm or climax).
  — Distinguish between lifelong versus acquired, generalized versus situational, and psychological versus combined factors.

Differential diagnosis and co-existing conditions
When the sexual dysfunction can be better accounted for by another axis 1 disorder, or is due to the direct physiological effects of a substance/medication, or a general medical condition; that is:

- If low or sad mood is prominent, see **'Depression — F32#'.** Depression may cause low desire, or may result from sexual and relationship problems.
- Relationship problems. If persistent discord in the relationship is the primary problem, relationship counselling should precede specific psychosexual treatment of the sexual dysfunction.
- Gynaecological disorders (vulval pain disorders [eg vulval vestibulitis], vaginal infections, pelvic infections [salpingitis] and other pelvic lesions [eg tumours or cysts]), although vaginismus rarely has a physical cause.
- Side-effects of medication, alcohol or drugs (eg SSRI antidepressants, oral contraceptives and beta-blockers).
- Physical illnesses that affect the sexual physiology — vascular, neurological or endocrine systems — might contribute (eg atherosclerosis, multiple sclerosis, diabetes).
- Note that more than one sexual dysfunction can co-exist.

131

Lack or loss of sexual desire

Essential information for patient and partner

Sexual desire varies at differing times in an individual's life and varies widely between individuals. Research shows that at any one time 30–40% of women will claim low sexual desire. Loss of or low sexual desire has many causes, including relationship problems, earlier traumas (eg sexual abuse/assault), fear of pregnancy, postnatal problems, loss and bereavement, physical and psychiatric illnesses, stress (including long working hours) and many more. Women with low/no libido do not usually initiate sexual activity or may only engage in it reluctantly when it is initiated by a partner.

General management and advice to patient and partner

Discuss patient's beliefs about sexual relations. Check whether the patient and/or the partner have unreasonable expectations. Ask the patient about traumatic sexual and relationship experiences and negative attitudes to sex. Accept that this may take more than one appointment.

If possible, see partners together as well as individually. Try to find out if this is a problem for the woman or the relationship. If the latter, consider a difference in sexual need rather than dysfunction. Suggest development of an understanding and acceptance of what each partner wants during intimacy and help them to communicate these wants. Suggest introducing this communication into intimacy in a planned way (ie 'I would like this…').

Over several weeks, encourage patient and partner to practise pleasurable physical contact without intercourse, commencing with non-genital touching and moving through mutual genital stimulation to a gradual return to full intercourse. Partners must take it in turns to be active and passive in terms of touching and to initiate/go second ('sensate focus' therapy).

Consider ways of building self-esteem (eg exercise, education) and advise time and space to herself.

Sexual arousal disorder

Essential information for patient and partner

The essential feature is an inability to achieve or maintain an adequate lubrication–swelling response of sexual excitement. It is often accompanied by sexual desire disorder and orgasmic disorder. Women may have little or no subjective sense of sexual arousal. Resulting problems include painful intercourse, sexual avoidance and relationship discord.

General management and advice to patient and partner

Advise similar strategies as in management of low sexual desire ('sensate focus' therapy) and anorgasmia, including self-pleasuring manually/with a vibrator and the use of sexual fantasy.

Vaginismus

Essential information for patient and partner

Vaginismus is an involuntary spasm of the pubococcygeal muscles, accompanied by intense fear of penetration and anticipation of pain. Sexual responses (eg desire, pleasure) may not be impaired unless penetration is attempted or anticipated. It is found more often in younger women than older ones, in women with negative attitudes to sex, and those with a history of previous sexual abuse/assault. Once vaginismus is established, it is usually chronic but it can be overcome with specific psychosexual therapy.

General management and advice to patient and partner

The patient needs to gain confidence and control over vaginal muscle spasm. Exercises (systematic desensitization) involving vaginal muscle relaxation (reverse Kegels) and the systematic introduction of graded trainers (fingers, tampons or vaginal dilators) are successful if coupled with addressing the fear or phobia. Control can then be shared with a partner. Treatment often requires long-term therapy but has a promising outcome. Avoidance of practice and low motivation are common problems.

Dyspareunia

Essential information for patient and partner

There are many physical causes, both of deep and superficial dyspareunia. Women typically seek treatment in general medical settings. Genital abnormalities are rarely found on examination. Exclude treatable causes. Pain can occur before, during and after intercourse. In some cases, however, anticipation, poor lubrication and muscle tension are significant factors. Even where there has been a physical cause and it has resolved, anticipation of pain may frequently maintain the dyspareunia. The use and understanding of pain cycles is very helpful and often the secret to success.

General management and advice to patient and partner

Treat any physical cause. Check if patient experiences desire/arousal/lubrication. Relaxation, good arousal, prolonged foreplay and careful penetration may overcome psychogenic problems. Referral to a gynaecologist or genito-urinary medicine (GUM) clinic or psychosexual service is advisable if simple measures are unsuccessful.

Anorgasmia

Essential information for patient and partner

Previous trauma, restrictive upbringing and negative attitudes to sex may have led to an inhibition of the normal sexual response. Many women are unable to experience orgasm during intercourse but can often achieve it by clitoral stimulation. Women may achieve sexual satisfaction without an orgasm.

General management and advice to patient and partner

Discuss the couple's beliefs and attitudes. Encourage self-pleasuring, manually or using a vibrator, and the use of sexual fantasy. The couple should be helped to communicate openly and to reduce any unrealistic expectations. Self-help books, leaflets or educational videos may be useful (see 'Resources' below).

Referral

Patients can refer themselves to:

- Relate
- BASRT (British Association for Sexual and Relationship Therapy)-registered psychosexual therapists
- Brook Advisory Centres
- Family planning clinics
- Genito-urinary medicine (GUM) clinics.

Consider referral to a psychosexual specialist if patient and doctor are unable to enter into a programme of treatment or if primary care treatment has failed.

Resources for patients and partners

Relate 0845 1304 010/4561 310 (helpline)
Website: http://www.relate.org.uk
Counselling for adults with relationship difficulties, whether married or not.

BASRT (British Association for Sexual and Relationship Therapy) 020 8543 2707
Email: info@basrt.org.uk; website: http://www.basrt.org.uk
Registered therapists are multidisciplinary, and work in the NHS as well as
privately.

Brook Advisory Centres 020 7617 8000 (24-hour helpline)
Email: admin@brookcentres.org.uk; website: http://www.brook.org.uk
Free counselling and confidential advice on contraception and sexual matters,
especially for young people (under 25).

AVERT http://www.avert.org.uk
Includes useful lesbian and young people's sections, which give basic information
on homosexuality and sexual health.

Lovelife http://www.lovelife.uk.com
Designed for 16–24-year-olds, includes a list of GUM and family planning clinics
around the country.

Dr Miriam Stoppard's Everywoman's Life Guide by Miriam Stoppard. Profile Pursuit
Ltd, 2002

Embarrassing Problems: Straight-Talking Good Advice by M Stern. Health Press, 1995

Painful Sex: A Guide to Causes, Treatment and Prevention by M Goldsmith. Thorsons,
1995

Becoming Orgasmic: A Sexual Growth Program for Women by JR Heiman and J
LoPiccolo, Prentice-Hall, 1988
Self-help exercises for anorgasmia.

A Woman's Guide to Overcoming Sexual Fear and Pain by Goodwin and Aurelie Jones,
New Harbinger Publications, 1997

Sexual disorders (male) — F52
(Clinical term: Sexual dysfunction, not caused by organic disorder or disease Eu52)

Clinical judgements about sexual dysfunction should take into account the individual's ethnic, cultural, religious, and social background, which may influence sexual desire, expectations, and attitudes about performance. Sexual problems in non-Western patients are often somatized; expectations may be unrealistic and psychological explanations and therapies may not be readily accepted.

Presenting complaints
Patients may be reluctant to discuss sexual matters. They may instead complain of physical symptoms, depressed mood or relationship problems.

Diagnostic features
Sexual dysfunction may cause marked distress and interpersonal difficulty. Common sexual disorders in men are as follows:

- erectile dysfunction or impotence
- premature ejaculation
- retarded ejaculation or orgasmic dysfunction (intravaginal ejaculation is greatly delayed or absent but can often occur normally during masturbation)
- lack or loss of sexual desire.

Distinguish between lifelong versus acquired, generalized versus situational, and sexual dysfunction caused by psychological versus combined factors.

Differential diagnosis and co-existing conditions
When the sexual dysfunction can be better accounted for by another axis 1 disorder, or is caused by the direct psychological effects of a substance/medication, or a general medical condition; that is:

- 'Depression — F32#'.
- Problems in relationships with partners frequently co-exist and may contribute to sexual disorder, especially those of desire. Where there is persistent discord in the relationship, relationship counselling should precede specific treatment of the sexual dysfunction.
- Specific organic pathology is a rare cause of orgasmic dysfunction or premature ejaculation.
- Physical factors frequently contribute to erectile dysfunction, including diabetes, hypertension, alcohol abuse, smoking, medication (eg antidepressants, antipsychotics, diuretics and beta-blockers), multiple sclerosis and spinal injury. (Important clue: inability to achieve erection at *any* time — nocturnal, morning, masturbation, etc.)
- Patients may have unreasonable expectations of their own performance.
- Note that more than one sexual dysfunction can co-exist.

Erectile dysfunction (failure of genital response; impotence)

Essential information for patient and partner
Erectile dysfunction is the persistent or recurrent inability to attain or maintain an adequate erection. It is often a temporary response to stress or loss of confidence and responds to psychosexual treatment, especially if morning erections occur. It is frequently associated with sexual anxiety, fear of failure, concerns about sexual

135

performance, and a decreased subjective sense of sexual excitement and pleasure. It may also be caused by physical factors (problems with the blood vessels or nerves) or by medication.

General management and advice to patient and partner[213]
Advise patient and partner to refrain from attempting intercourse for several weeks. Encourage them to practise pleasurable physical contact without intercourse during that time, commencing with non-genital touching and moving through mutual genital stimulation to a gradual return to full intercourse at the end of that period. Partners must take it in turns to be active and passive in terms of touching, and to initiate/go second ('sensate focus' therapy).

Progression along this continuum should be guided by the return of consistent, reliable erections. A book containing self-help exercises (see 'Resources' below) might be helpful. Inform patient and partner of the possibilities of physical treatment by penile rings, vacuum devices, intracavernosal injections and medication.

Medication
- Oral: sildenafil 50–100 mg taken on an empty stomach 40–60 min before intercourse enhances erections in 80% of patients, whether the cause is psychogenic or neurological.[214] Beware danger of interaction with cardiac nitrates (*BNF* section 7.4.5).
- Recent developments include two new phosphodiesterase type-5 inhibitors: tadalafil and vardenafil; both have fewer ocular side-effects than sildenafil.[215]
- Intraurethral: MUSE (prostaglandin E$_1$) 125–1000 mg inserted 10 min before intercourse produces erections in 40–50% of patients[216] (*BNF* section 7.4.5).
- Intracavernosal: prostaglandin E$_1$ 5–20 mg injected 10 min before intercourse produces erections in 80–90% of patients,[217] but long-term acceptability is low.

These medications are less effective in predominantly vasculogenic cases. See current NHS Executive guidelines for prescription of the above, either privately or on the NHS.

Premature ejaculation

Essential information for patient and partner
Persistent or recurrent onset of ejaculation and orgasm with minimal sexual stimulation before, on or shortly after penetration and before the person wishes it. Most young men learn to delay orgasm with sexual experience and ageing, but some continue to ejaculate prematurely. Premature ejaculation is typically seen in young men and is present from their first attempts at intercourse. When onset occurs later in life, it is often caused by a decreased frequency of sexual activity, intense performance anxiety with a new partner, or loss of ejaculatory control related to erectile dysfunction. It may also occur in men who have stopped regular use of alcohol.

Control of ejaculation is possible and can enhance sexual pleasure for both partners.

General advice and management to patient and partner
Reassure the patient that ejaculation can be delayed by learning new approaches during masturbatory training (eg the squeeze or stop–start technique). This, and other exercises, are set out in self-help books (see Resources below).

Medication
In some cases, delay can also be achieved with clomipramine or SSRI medication (paroxetine, sertraline) or clomipramine, but relapse is very common on cessation. Local anaesthetic sprays, if used cautiously, can delay ejaculation. Durex Performa is a new condom coated with a small amount of anaesthetic cream.

Orgasmic dysfunction or retarded ejaculation

Essential information for patient and partner
Persistent or recurrent delay in/absence of orgasm, following the normal excitement phase. The man typically feels aroused at the beginning, but thrusting gradually becomes a chore and less pleasurable.

This is a more difficult condition to treat; however, if ejaculation can be brought about in some way (eg through masturbation) the prognosis is better. Can be secondary to medication (eg antidepressants) or regular alcohol use.

General management and advice to patient and partner
Consider the patient's age and whether stimulation is adequate in focus, intensity and duration. Recommend exercises, such as self-pleasuring and penile stimulation with body oil, use of vibrator or masturbation close to the point of orgasm, plus use of sexual fantasy, followed by vaginal penetration shortly before ejaculatory 'point of no return'. Continue practice, and on repeated attempts try to penetrate progressively sooner.

Lack or loss of sexual desire

Essential information for patient and partner
The level of sexual desire varies widely between individuals. It may merely represent different expectations. Lack or loss of sexual desire has many causes, including stress and relationship problems, physical and psychiatric illnesses, bereavement or other losses, medication (SSRIs) and, rarely, hormonal deficiencies. Men with low/absent sexual desire typically do not usually initiate sexual activity or may only engage in it reluctantly when it is initiated by his partner.

General management and advice to patient and partner
Encourage stress reduction, balanced assertiveness and co-operation between partners and fostering intimacy through increased communication and shared pleasurable activities. 'Sensate focus' may be helpful in re-introducing structured but 'safe', non-performance-related sexual activity. Educational leaflets, books or videos might be helpful.

Referral
Patients can refer themselves to:

- Relate
- BASRT (British Association for Sexual and Relationship Therapy)-registered psychosexual therapist
- family planning clinics
- genito-urinary medicine clinics.

Consider referral if patient and doctor are unable to enter into a programme of treatment or if primary care treatment has failed:

- to a urologist for erectile dysfunction, if unresponsive to medication and counselling
- to a psychosexual specialist, if problem is predominantly psychogenic.

Resources for patients and partners

Relate 0845 1304 010/4561 310 (helpline)
Website: http://www.relate.org.uk
Counselling for adults with relationship difficulties, whether married or not.

BASRT (British Association for Sexual and Relationship Therapy) 020 8543 2707
Email: info@basrt.org.uk; website: http://www.basrt.org.uk
Registered therapists are multidisciplinary and work in the NHS as well as privately.

The Impotence Association 020 8767 7791 (helpline)
Email: theia@btinternet.com; website: http://www.impotence.org.uk

Brook Advisory Centres 020 7617 8000 (24-hour helpline)
Free counselling and confidential advice on contraception and sexual matters for young people (under 25).

AVERT http://www.avert.org.uk
Includes useful gay and young people's sections, which give basic information about homosexuality and sexual health.

Lovelife http://www.lovelife.uk.com
Designed for 16–24 year olds. Includes a list of GUM and family planning clinics around the country.

Impotence: A Guide for Men of All Ages by W Dinsmore and P Kell. RSM Press, 2002

Embarrassing Problems: Straight-Talking Good Advice by M Stern. Health Press Ltd, 1998
Men and Sex by B Zilbergeld. Fontana, 1980
Self-help exercises for erectile dysfunction and premature ejaculation.

Sexual Happiness by M Yaffe and E Fenwick. Dorling Kindersley, 1986

Sleep problems — F51
(Clinical term: Non-organic sleep disorders Eu51)

Insomnia

Presenting complaints

- Difficulty falling asleep.
- Recurrent waking during the night.
- Feeling unrefreshed (ie easily exhausted or fatigued) by sleep.
- Falling asleep at inappropriate times during the day.

Insomnia is associated with the following:

- complaints of poor memory and concentration
- irritability
- prone to accidents at work
- underperformance at work, or educational problems in young people
- psychosocial difficulties
- psychomotor impairment
- reduced quality of life
- more frequent use of health services owing to general ill health
- chronic dependence on hypnotic medication and sometimes alcohol as a (ineffective) means of 'sleeping' better.

Differential diagnosis
It is essential that the cause of insomnia be identified rather than attempting to treat the problem symptomatically, as treatment depends on cause.

- *Transient insomnia* (of several day's duration; commonplace) might result from worry about an anticipated event, upset related to a family dispute, unfamiliar sleeping environment, brief illness, withdrawal from hypnotic drugs.
- *Short-term insomnia* (lasting several weeks) might result from longer illness and worries about being ill, financial problems or difficulties at work, bereavement (may become prolonged if not resolved), psychiatric disorder with fluctuating course.
- *Chronic insomnia* (lasting months or years) may result from:
  — persistent psychological problems, especially stress
  — poor sleep hygiene, eg sleeping environment not conducive to sleep (including snoring or restless bed partner), excessive intake of caffeine or overuse of nicotine or alcohol, especially at night
  — physical disorders that disturb sleep (eg painful conditions, respiratory disorders)
  — psychiatric disorders, including '**Depression — F32#**', '**Generalized anxiety — F41.1**', psychotic states
  — medication, including some bronchodilators, decongestants, antidepressants and stimulants
  — other sleep disorders, including Restless legs syndrome
  — conditioned insomnia where original cause no longer applies but bed has become associated with being awake.

Assessment should include a full sleep history from patient (also the bed partner, family, etc., if possible), examination of mental state and review of medical, psychiatric and family histories. Screening sleep questionnaires and a sleep diary can be valuable.

Essential information for patient and family
- Temporary sleep problems are common and do not require treatment.

- People vary in the amount of sleep they need.
- If insomnia lasts more than a few days, advice should be sought and the cause identified (most causes are treatable).
- Generally avoid self-medication with over-the-counter or someone else's medication; using alcohol to sleep better; taking sleeping pills for more than a few days (and preferably not at all); lying awake in bed for long periods.

General management and advice to patient and family[218–220]
- Encourage the patient to practise good sleep hygiene:
  — Keep to regular hours for going to bed and getting up in the morning, including at weekends.
  — Make plans or think about problems before retiring to bed.
  — Keep a pen and pad next to the bed for writing down troublesome thoughts, which can then be reviewed.
  — Avoid caffeine and alcohol in the evenings.
  — Avoid daytime naps.
- Daytime exercise can help the patient to sleep regularly, but evening exercise might contribute to insomnia.
- Behavioural treatment is safer and more effective than medication (eg cognitive therapy, stimulus control, sleep restriction, relaxation) (R: 1–2).
- Self-help leaflets, books and groups may be useful (R: 9).
- Sleep diaries are often useful in assessment and monitoring of progress (R: 9).

Medication
- Address underlying psychosocial, psychiatric or physical conditions.
- Make changes to medication, as appropriate.
- A brief, time-limited use of hypnotic medication may sometimes be useful.
- Hypnotic medication may be used occasionally. Risk of dependence increases significantly after 14 days of use.
- Melatonin is only justified for jetlag.

Referral
Most cases will be dealt with in primary care.

Depending on likely cause of insomnia, referral might be appropriate to general medicine, neurology or psychiatry.

Referral for behavioural interventions may be useful where locally available.

Refer to a sleep disorders clinic, if available, if diagnosis is uncertain or treatment has failed.

Excessive daytime sleepiness (EDS)

Presenting complaints
- Prolonged overnight sleep.
- Falling asleep during the day.
- Feeling constantly tired, exhausted or fatigued.
- Poor memory and concentration.
- Irritability or depression.
- Automatic behaviour in a sleepy state.
- Periods of sleepiness, alternating with normal periods.

Excessive daytime sleepiness is associated with the following:

- Poor occupational or school performance.
- Increased accident rate (including road traffic accidents).
- Impaired marital relationships and social activities.
- Misdiagnosis as laziness, depression, intellectual decline.

Differential diagnosis
It is important to distinguish between sleepiness and fatigue without prominent sleepiness, which may be caused by physical disorders (eg anaemia) or primary psychiatric disorder.

- Chronic lack of sleep.
- Circadian rhythm sleep disorder, including irregular sleep–wake schedule or shift work.
- Disrupted (poor quality) sleep caused by obstructive sleep apnoea (common); caffeine, alcohol or nicotine excess, or other non-prescribed drugs (including withdrawal phase).
- Increased sleep tendency, eg narcolepsy (characterized by sleep attacks and cataplexy), over-sedation by medication.

Assessment should include sleep histories and a general review. Sleep questionnaires, sleep diary or actigraphy can be valuable. Polysomnography is often needed, including respiratory measures. Other specific interventions may be appropriate (eg a toxicology screen).

Essential information for patient and family
- Medical advice should be sought for sleepiness affecting everyday functioning.
- Underlying condition can usually be treated, if correctly diagnosed.
- Do not use stimulant drugs to stay awake.
- Avoid driving or other potentially hazardous activities until sleepiness is corrected.

General management and advice to patient and family
As for insomnia, above.

Chronotherapy (retiming of sleep phase) may be appropriate for circadian rhythm sleep disorders.

Medication
- Stimulant drugs are appropriate for narcolepsy.
- Continuous positive airway pressure is appropriate for obstructive sleep apnoea.

Referral
Drug treatment should be reserved for specialist recommendation.

Parasomnias

Presenting complaints
Some parasomnias (recurrent episodes of disturbed behaviour, experiences or physiological change occurring exclusively or predominantly in relation to sleep) are subtle; others are dramatic and frightening to experience or witness.

Diagnostic features
- Primary parasomnias:
  - pre-sleep period or sleep onset: sleep starts (sudden jerk or sensation often alarming); rhythmic movements, eg headbanging, rocking
  - early in the night in light non-rapid eye movement (NREM) sleep: teeth grinding, periodic limb movements (repetitive jerky movements)
  - early in the night in deep NREM sleep: confusional arousals (mainly in young children), sleepwalking, sleep (night) terrors
  - later in the night in REM (ie dreaming) sleep: nightmares, REM sleep behaviour disorder (in which dreams are acted out)
  - on waking: sleep paralysis
  - at various times during sleep: sleep talking, sleep-related eating disorders.
- Secondary parasomnias:

— physical: nocturnal epilepsy, awakenings associated with sleep-related breathing difficulties
— psychiatric: panic attacks, post-traumatic stress disorder, pseudoparasomnias (when the person is actually awake).

Differential diagnosis

The various parasomnias are often confused with each other, and all dramatic parasomnias can mistakenly be called 'nightmares' or 'night terrors'.
Assessment:

- Requires precise description of subjective and objective changes from start to finish of parasomnia, together with timing and circumstances in which they occur
- Audio-visual recording is very valuable
- Polysomnography with audio-visual recording is required in complicated cases
- A family history may be instructive, eg sleepwalking/sleep terrors
- A physical and psychiatric review is important.

Essential information for patient and family

- Many parasomnias of childhood improve spontaneously but protection may be necessary in the meantime (eg in sleepwalking).
- It is important to have the correct diagnosis.
- It should not be assumed that something is psychiatrically wrong with the person.

General management and advice to patient and family[221]

- Ensure the correct diagnosis on which treatment depends.
- Good sleep hygiene generally helps.

Referral

- Most common parasomnias should be identifiable in primary care, if assessed thoroughly.
- Refer to a sleep disorder clinic in complicated cases or uncertainty about type of parasomnia or its significance.

Special considerations in children and adolescents

Parental factors feature prominently in the cause, management and prognosis of children's sleep problems.

- Children and adolescents have the same basic sleep problems as adults but the underlying causes differ in certain ways; for example sleeplessness is often the result of parenting practices where the child has failed to acquire good sleep habits or has developed unsatisfactory ones.
- The clinical manifestations of basically the same disorder can be different in young and adult patients; for example obstructive sleep apnoea in children is usually caused by large tonsils and adenoids. It is not particularly limited to being overweight, and instead of sleepiness, it may result in overactivity and learning and behaviour problems.
- Medication plays even less of a role in treatment. Behavioural approaches are particularly important, although they require effective involvement of parents.
- Prognosis is better than in adults, where the condition may have become well established and complicated by the long-term consequences of the sleep disturbance.

Resources for patients and families

Resource leaflets: 1–2 *Learning to relax*, and 9 *Overcoming sleep problems* (includes *Sleep diary*).

British Sleep Society
Email: Martin.King@papworth_tr.anglex.nhs.uk; website: http://www.british-sleep-society.org.uk

UKAN (Narcolepsy Association UK) 020 7721 8904
Email: infor@narcolepsy.org.uk; website: http://www.narcolepsy.org.uk
Provides help for those suffering from narcolepsy.

British Snoring and Sleep Apnoea Association 0800 0851 097
Email: info@britishsnoring.demon.co.uk; website: http://www.britishsnoring.com
Leaflets available from the Royal College of Psychiatrists
(http://www.rcpsych.ac.uk): *Sleeping Well*, *Tiredness*.

Coping with Sleep Problems and *Coping with Children's Sleep Problems*. The Royal College of Psychiatrists. Talking Life, 1A Grosvenor Rd, Hoylake, Wirral CH47 3BS; tel: 0151 632 0662; website: http://www.talkinglife.co.uk.
Advice, information and strategies on tape for coping with insomnia (sleeplessness) and other disorders that lead to excessive daytime sleepiness. They present practical strategies to help parents cope with the sleep difficulties of their babies and young children.

Understanding Sleep Disorders in Adults by G Stores. Family Doctor Publications/ British Medical Association, 2003
A guide for the general public to sleep disorders in adults.

Solve Your Child's Sleep Problems by R Ferber. Dorling Kindersley, 1986.

Smoking cessation — F17.1

(Clinical term: Smoking cessation Eu137)

Smoking cessation interventions are highly cost-effective when compared with the long-term cost of illness and illness burden that is smoking related. Practitioners need to be positive and optimistic about the benefits of quitting smoking.

Some practitioners may wish to organize their practices systematically to screen and address smoking with all smokers at least once a year.

It is important to have available additional treatment resources for those who come asking for help to stop smoking.

Co-existing conditions

It is worthwhile using this opportunity to discuss alcohol and other lifestyle issues alongside smoking.

Essential information for patient and family

- Up to half of all current smokers will die of a smoking-related disease.
- Tobacco dependence is responsible for one in every five deaths in the UK, one-third of all cancers, over 80% of all chronic obstructive pulmonary disease (COPD) deaths and one-sixth of all ischaemic heart disease deaths. No single avoidable cause of disease accounts for more deaths, hospital admissions or GP consultations. Tobacco dependence shortens the lives of affected smokers by an average of 16 years.[222]
- Smoking cessation before middle age results in a 90% reduction in risk of lung cancer and a return to baseline risk of coronary heart disease within 10 years of stopping. Key improvements in mental and physical health will accrue more quickly.
- Smoking cessation treatments are demonstrably effective in that they double or more than double the chances that a person will stop and stay stopped for a defined period of time.

General management and advice to patient and family

- Doctors should raise the subject of smoking in a sensitive way in the context of an established rapport.
- The doctor should base their approach on an assessment of the patient's current readiness to change.[223] This will enable them to focus on what is most useful to the patient. For example, if a patient has already decided to attempt to quit, helping him/her implement the decision is more useful than rehearsing reasons for quitting; however, if the patient is not convinced of the reasons for quitting, then this should be addressed, rather than ways of trying to quit.
- Smokers should be offered support and encouragement to aid their attempt to quit.[224]
- Simple advice increases the chances of someone stopping by approximately one-third. If GPs identify smokers and advise cessation, an extra 2% of smokers will stop.[225]
- Opportunistically advise smokers to stop during routine consultations, giving advice on and/or prescribing effective medications to help them and referring them to specialist cessation services.[224–227]
- Aim to advise most smokers to stop, and record having done so, at least once a year.[226]
- Face-to-face behavioural intervention is the use of simple interventions that are motivational or provide strategies to assist in maintaining behavioural change. This is substantially more work-intensive than brief advice. It should be offered when time and skill resources are not available for more intensive interventions. Brief advice should still be tailored to a patient's readiness to change.

- Self-help materials describe the cessation process and the feelings associated with cessation, and recommend a range of coping strategies.
- Telephone counselling can be incorporated into the cessation phase but is also useful for relapse prevention in the first 12 months after stopping.

Medication

- Nicotine replacement therapy (NRT) and bupropion are recommended for smokers who have expressed a desire to quit and who feel they need pharmacological help in quitting, or who have had multiple previous failed attempts.[224]
- NRTs include gum, patches or sprays, and these work to enhance the impact of face-to-face behavioural interventions; there is little scientific basis for matching individual smokers to particular forms of NRT.[225,228]
- Bupropion can be used in combination with other interventions.
- Cautions and contraindications should be taken into account when prescribing these medications. Potential negative effects should be discussed with patients.

Referral

Specialist referral should be considered where locally available for people who have previously attempted to quit but continue to smoke and are motivated to try again.

Resources for patients and families

NHS Smoking Helpline 0800 169 0169 (7am–11pm daily; senior advisors [counsellors] 10am–11pm)
Website: http://www.givingupsmoking.co.uk

NHS Pregnancy Smoking Helpline 0800 169 9169 (12noon–9pm, daily)

Quit Line Smoking Helpline 0800 00 22 00 (9am–9pm, daily)

Action on Smoking and Health http://www.ash.org

Stroke and transient ischaemic attack — I60–I64, G45

(Clinical term: Stroke and cerebrovascular accident unspecified G66)

Presenting complaints

- Usually sudden-onset focal symptoms and signs, eg left or right hemiparesis/hemisensory deficit, ataxia, dysphasia or hemianopia. The evolution may be stuttering over a few days or, rarely, longer.
- Dysarthria is very common but not of localizing value, because it may occur with hemisphere or brainstem lesions.
- Some patients complain of headache at the time of stroke or leading up to it.

Transient ischaemic attacks (TIAs) have been arbitrarily defined as manifesting symptoms lasting less than 24 hours, and stroke more than 24 hours. However, it is the pathophysiology — and not the timing — that is important. The symptoms of a TIA should mimic a stroke. Isolated vertigo or amnesia is unlikely to be caused by transient ischaemia or stroke. Transient monocular blindness is common in TIA associated with ipsilateral carotid atheroma, but very rare in completed stroke.

Diagnostic features

Stroke is a clinical syndrome usually taken to mean 'sudden-onset focal symptoms or signs secondary to vascular disease'. There are no pathogonomic features. Physical signs usually reflect a lesion within a single vascular territory — hence the majority of patients present with hemiparesis. It is not possible to distinguish infarction (90% of cases) from haemorrhage (10%) clinically; therefore neuroimaging is essential.

With ischaemic stroke within the carotid or basilar circulation, occlusion of a small penetrating vessel (lacunar infarction) will usually result in one of the following:

- pure motor hemiparesis
- pure hemisensory deficit
- motor/sensory deficit
- ataxic hemiparesis
- dysarthria — Clumsy hand syndrome.

Cortical signs imply larger-vessel disease (eg middle cerebral artery occlusion):

- dysphasia in the dominant hemisphere
- neglect syndrome in either the dominant or more frequently non-dominant hemisphere
- hemianopia in either.

In large-vessel occlusion, these cortical signs are usually seen in conjunction with hemiplegia, but may be isolated (eg isolated acute hemianopia or dysphasia are very likely to be due to stroke).

Haemorrhage mimics any of the ischaemic stroke syndromes and there are no definite discerning features.

The vast majority of patients have underlying vascular risk factors. Hypertension is the single most important of these; others include ageing, diabetes and smoking. Hypercholesterolaemia may be present. Atrial fibrillation and carotid stenosis are also very important and need specific identification.

Differential diagnosis

Stroke is a syndrome and not a diagnosis; within the umbrella of 'stroke', the following distinctions are usually made:

- Infarct or haemorrhage
- Small-vessel disease, large-vessel disease or embolism from the heart
- Profile of risk factors leading to the above.

Although most strokes are the result of atherosclerosis or heart disease, rare causes of 'secondary' stroke need to be considered if the history is appropriate, for example:

- bacterial endocarditis
- meningitis
- dissection of carotid or vertebral artery
- venous sinus thrombosis.

In addition, 'mimics' of stroke that may also present with sudden-onset focal signs and need to be excluded by neuroimaging, for example:

- subdural haematoma
- intracranial tumour
- inflammatory lesions of the brain.

Essential information for patient and family
- Stroke is the result of a localized area of brain damage due to occlusion or rupture of a blood vessel.
- Predicting prognosis at the outset is difficult.
- Hospital treatment focuses first on preventing secondary brain damage and then planning a goal-orientated rehabilitation programme.
- Rehabilitation units focus on the needs of the individual patient.
- Attention will need to be paid to the environment of a person who has complex impairments.
- Secondary prevention lowers the risk of future stroke greatly but does not eliminate it; treating and monitoring hypertension is paramount in this regard.
- Depression is common following stroke.

General management and advice to patient and family
- Immediate diagnosis, treatment and rehabilitation are fundamental for improved outcomes.
- Vascular risk factors need aggressive management. Although treatment of hypertension should include lifestyle measures, this is rarely enough for secondary prevention. A similar approach is needed for lipids with diet, but the evidence is for drug treatments.
- Smoking and excessive alcohol are serious risk factors that patients need careful detoxification from with the help of formal programmes and drug treatments.
- Risk factors need long-term control — it does not matter if the blood pressure is a bit high one day; it is the long-term reduction that is beneficial.
- With risk factor control, the incidence of further stroke is approximately halved, but remains at 2–10% per year.
- Driving should cease for at least one month following stroke or TIA. Other than for LGV/PCV licences, there is no need to inform the DVLA unless there is residual neurological deficit.[3] Hemianopia contraindicates driving, and patients will need a formal ophthalmic assessment if in doubt — this can become a cause of much doctor/patient disharmony.

Medication[229,230]
Prompt treatment improves prognosis. Virtually all patients with stroke will need vascular risk factor control using medication.

- *Antihypertensives*: Hypertension remains the most important risk factor for haemorrhage and infarction.
  — It should not generally be treated immediately after stroke. Only malignant hypertension is treated acutely.

— Secondary prevention usually begins at about two weeks following stroke, aiming for a blood pressure <140/80 mmHg at all times.

— After TIA, if there is no immediate access to specialist assessment, antihypertensive medication can be started.

— The optimal first-line medication is a long-acting angiotensin-converting enzyme (ACE) inhibitor combined with a diuretic. However, it is likely that the most important action is to lower the blood pressure, with no definite evidence of a class-specific effect.[231]

— Lowering so-called 'normal' blood pressure after stroke may also be beneficial.[231]

- *Antiplatelet treatment*: This is usually given to all those with ischaemic stroke, both acutely and for secondary prevention. There is no definite evidence that giving aspirin acutely is detrimental to those with intracranial haemorrhage;[232] however, most defer until the results of neuroimaging. There are three main strategies for antiplatelet use in secondary prevention:

— aspirin alone (75 mg od)

— aspirin combined with slow-release persantin (Asasantin Retard 200 mg bd)

— clopidogrel (75 mg od)

Aspirin alone is first line, with clopidogrel usually reserved for those with aspirin intolerance and increasingly in those who have a further vascular event while taking aspirin (so-called 'aspirin failures'). Combination aspirin with persantin may be of greater benefit than aspirin alone,[233] but use of this combination first line is variable, some preferring to add persantin in the event of 'aspirin failure'. Persantin alone is rarely used. Clopidogrel as monotherapy or combined with aspirin is being used increasingly in high-risk patients and those with concurrent ischaemic heart disease[234] (*BNF* section 2.9).

- *Statins*: Beneficial in secondary and primary prevention, whatever the level of blood cholesterol. The current practice is to start a statin in almost everyone following an ischaemic stroke or TIA.[235]

- *Others*: Warfarin is reserved for patients with atrial fibrillation and some other cardiac conditions.

Antiplatelet treatment and statins are not monitored beyond ensuring normalization of cholesterol levels, if raised. Treatment of hypertension needs long-term and sometimes intensive short-term monitoring and titration. Patients after stroke need medication in addition to lifestyle measures. Patients need to understand that this triple approach is additive and that the reduction in risk afforded is long term and not from day to day.

Referral

- Ideally, all patients with stroke or TIA should be referred for specialist investigation and opinion.

- Patients with acute stroke should be admitted without delay to a hospital with an acute stroke unit because:

— intravenous thrombolytic therapy is effective when given within three hours in selected patients

— correction and control of abnormal physiological parameters (hyperglycaemia, hyperpyrexia, hypoxia, hypotension, dehydration) may improve outcome

— admission to a stroke unit reduces mortality and poor outcome

— multidisciplinary rehabilitation improves outcome.

- Patients with TIAs and mild strokes should have access to a rapid diagnostic and management service aimed at identifying the pathophysiology of the attack and correcting risk factors.

- Patients with multiple TIAs should be admitted urgently to hospital for further investigation.

- After investigation, the vast majority of vascular risk factor control can take place in a primary care setting, and the patient can be referred for further advice if deterioration occurs.

- Severe/uncontrolled hypertension should be managed by an appropriate specialist (eg a stroke physician, clinical pharmacologist or renal physician).
- A thorough knowledge of local community and inpatient rehabilitation services is necessary to optimize patient care and ensure appropriate placement and ongoing care.

Resources for patients and families

Stroke Association 0845 3003 3100 (helpline)
Email: stroke@stroke.org.uk; website: http://www.stroke.org.uk
Provides a comprehensive series of information leaflets, including *Stroke — Questions and Answers, Sex After Stroke, Cognitive Problems After Stroke, Stroke: a Carers Guide*, and many others.

Different Strokes http://www.differentstrokes.co.uk
Provides free services to younger stroke survivors throughout the UK.

My Year Off by Robert McCrum. New York; Broadway Books 1999
A personal account of recovery after stroke.

Unexplained somatic complaints — F45

(Clinical term: Somatoform disorders Eu45)

Presenting complaints
- Any physical symptom may be present.
- Symptoms may vary widely across cultures.
- Complaints may be single or multiple and may change over time.

Diagnostic features
- Physical symptoms that persist and remain unexplained following adequate examination, investigations and explanation by the doctor.
- Commonly, there are frequent medical visits in spite of negative investigations.
- Symptoms of depression and anxiety are common. The likelihood of psychiatric disorder (anxiety or depression) increases with increasing number of unexplained somatic symptoms.[236]

Some patients may be primarily concerned with obtaining relief from physical symptoms. Others may be worried about having a physical illness and be unable to believe that no physical condition is present (hypochondriasis).

Differential diagnosis
- **'Alcohol misuse — F10'.**
- **'Drug use disorders — F11#'** (eg seeking narcotics for relief of pain).
- If low or sad mood is prominent, see **'Depression — F32#'**.
- **'Generalized anxiety — F41.1'**, if anxiety symptoms are prominent.
- **'Panic disorder — F41.0'** (misinterpretation of the somatic signs associated with panic).
- **'Chronic mixed anxiety and depression — F41.2'.**
- **'Acute psychotic disorders — F23'** (if strange beliefs about symptoms are present [eg belief that organs are decaying]).
- An organic cause. Take a multiaxial approach. Although it is important not to overinvestigate, it is important to keep the physical side under review, because an organic problem may emerge.

Essential information for patient and family
- Stress often produces or exacerbates physical symptoms.
- Focus should be on managing the symptoms, not on discovering their cause.
- A cure might not always be possible; the goal should be to live the best life possible, even if symptoms continue.

General management and advice to patient and family[237] (R: 10)
- Acknowledge that the patient's physical symptoms are real to the patient.
- Ask about the patient's beliefs (what is causing the symptoms?) and fears (what do they fear might happen?).
- Be explicit early on about considering psychological issues. The exclusion of illness and exploration of emotional aspects should happen in parallel. Investigations should have a clear indication. It might be helpful to say to the patient, 'I think this result is going to be normal'.
- Avoid blanket reassurance; offer appropriate explanation (eg not all headaches indicate a brain tumour). Advise patients not to focus on medical worries.
- Discuss emotional stresses that were present when the symptoms arose.
- Explain the links between stress and physical symptoms, and how a vicious cycle can develop. For example, 'Stress can cause a tightening of the muscles in the gut. This

can lead to the development of abdominal pain or worsening of existing pain. The pain aggravates the tightening of the gut muscles'. A diagram may be helpful.

- Relaxation methods can help relieve symptoms related to tension (eg headache, neck or back pain) (R: 1–2).
- Encourage exercise and enjoyable activities. The patient need not wait until all symptoms are gone before returning to normal routines.
- Treat associated depression, anxiety, drug or alcohol problems.
- For patients with more chronic complaints, time-limited appointments that are regularly scheduled can prevent more frequent, urgent visits.[238]
- Structured problem-solving methods might help patients to manage current life problems or stresses that contribute to symptoms[133] (R: 1–1).
- Help the patient to:
  — identify the problem
  — list as many solutions as possible
  — list the pros and cons of each possible solution. (The patient should do this perhaps between appointments.)
  — support the patient in choosing their preferred approach
  — help the patient to work out the steps necessary to achieve the plan
  — set a date to review the plan. Identify and reinforce things that are working.

Medication

Avoid unnecessary diagnostic testing or prescription of new medication for each new symptom. Rationalize polypharmacy.

Where depression is also present, an antidepressant may be indicated. (See **'Depression — F32#'**.)

Even in the absence of clinical depression, a therapeutic trial of antidepressant medication may be helpful.[239]

Referral

- Patients are best managed in primary healthcare settings. Consistency of approach within the practice is essential. Seeing the same person is helpful. Consider referral to a partner for a second opinion. Documenting discussions with colleagues can reduce stress by sharing responsibility within the primary care team.
- Non-urgent referral to secondary mental health services is advised on the grounds of functional disability, especially if the patient is unable to work, and duration of symptoms, ie if the patient has had the symptoms for a long time.
- Cognitive behaviour therapy or interpersonal therapy, if available, might help some patients, though willingness of patients to participate is sometimes poor.[240–242]
- Refer to a liaison psychiatrist, if available, for those who persist in their belief that they have a physical cause for their symptoms, despite good evidence to the contrary.
- Avoid multiple referrals to medical specialists. Documented discussions with appropriate medical specialists may be helpful from time to time as, in some cases, underlying physical illness eventually emerges.
- After each specialist referral, the GP should review with the patient's understanding of his/her illness in the light of the specialist consultation. (The more doctors a patient sees, the greater the likelihood of apparent inconsistencies, which commonly serves to increase the patient's distress as well as their uncertainty about the reliability of the account offered by doctors and others.)

Resources for patients and families

Resources leaflets: 10 *Unexplained physical symptoms*, 1–2 *Learning to relax* and 1–1 *Problem solving*.

Depression Alliance http://www.depressionalliance.org
England: 020 8768 0123
Wales: 029 2069 2891 (10am–4pm, Monday–Friday)
Scotland: 0131 467 3050
Provides information and self-help groups.

CHILD & ADOLESCENT DISORDERS

Attention-deficit/hyperactivity disorder (ADHD) (most popular term for hyperkinetic disorder — F90)*

(Clinical term: Attention deficit disorder Eu97)

Presenting complaints

Most commonly presents in childhood as a result of complaints by parents or teachers about problems in behaviour and for learning.

Diagnostic features

All of the following:

- Six of nine features of inattention: careless with detail; fails to sustain attention; appears not to listen; does not finish instructed tasks; poor self-organization; avoids tasks requiring sustained mental effort; loses things; easily distracted; seems forgetful.
- Three of five features of hyperactivity: fidgets; leaves seat when should be seated; runs/climbs excessively and inappropriately; noisy in play; persistent motor activity unmodified by social context.
- One of four features of impulsivity: blurts out answers before question completed; fails to wait turn or queue; interrupts others' conversation or games; talks excessively for social context.
- Pattern of behaviour pervasive across at least two types of situation; information about school behaviour is therefore very valuable.
- Onset no later than age 7.
- Causing significant distress or impaired functioning.
- Not better explained by another psychiatric disorder.

Excitability, impatience and defiant angry outbursts are common, but as these have many other causes, they do not establish the diagnosis by themselves.

Differential diagnosis and co-existing conditions

- Normal boisterousness or dreaminess.
- **'Conduct or oppositional disorders — F91'.**
- **'Learning disability (mental retardation) — F70'.**
- Disinhibited attachment disorder.
- **'Depressive — F32#'**, especially in adolescent boys.
- **'Emotional disorders with onset specific to childhood — F93'.**
- Hearing impairment and epileptic seizures should be asked about.

Co-morbidity is common:

- developmental disorders (of reading, motor co-ordination, speech and language)
- antisocial behaviour
- illicit substance use
- emotional and mood disorders
- tic disorders and Tourette's syndrome
- autistic spectrum disorder.

*ADHD is a term taken from DSM-IV. In its US definition, it is a much broader category.

Essential information for patient and family

- It is essentially a syndrome with various causes, predominantly genetic but including low birth weight, serious early neglect, and fetal alcohol exposure.
- It is not directly a result of upbringing, but a child's behaviour may make it difficult for parents to be positive and supportive.
- Manifestations at school may differ from the picture at home.
- Recognizing co-morbidity can avoid some of the arguments that may otherwise arise about diagnosis.

General management and advice to patient and family[243,244]

- Treat as a chronic disorder.
- If you suspect a child has the condition, refer.
- Maintain consistency and structure: routines, stated expectations of behaviour, family rules.[245] Allowing the child to race around in an ungoverned way in an attempt to diminish hyperactivity will not work. In contrast, structured exercise might be helpful, particularly in improving sleep.
- Ensure the child has adequate sleep.
- Establish constructive communication with school to:
  — ensure teachers are informed
  — detect special educational needs
  — monitor progress (particularly if child is on medication).
- Keep confrontations to a minimum.
- Make a positive effort to have enjoyable interactions with child: *play* and *praise*.
- Positive interactions should outweigh negative interactions. This should be the basis for any disciplinary intervention; for example the 1–2–3 rule:
  1. Instruct the child to do something or desist
  2. Threat that if not complied with, the child will go to time out
  3. Time out — child placed out of communicative contact for one minute per year of age.
- Set realistic expectations, short-term goals, and praise success.
- Some children will become more excitable and active with certain foods. These vary from child to child, and parents will usually have identified them. Colouring and preservative exclusion can often be helpful, but radical exclusion diets should only be used under supervision from a paediatric dietician.
- There have been anecdotal reports of helpful change with some dietary additives, for example fish oils, evening primrose oil, zinc, with no evidence of harmful effects; some can be prescribed.

Medication

- Medication should always be considered in severe cases; this should follow a specialist assessment.
- Stimulant medication (methylphenidate, dexamphetamine) is the most effective means of controlling core symptoms.[246,247] It should only be initiated at specialist secondary care level (the paediatrician or child and adolescent psychiatrist). Primary care has an important role in supporting treatment and families. Shared care protocols vary, but primary care tasks typically include the following:
  — repeat prescriptions
  — checking height and weight and entering these on a growth chart
  — adjusting doses within narrow limits
  — reporting and managing adverse effects
  — encouraging child's positive view of treatment (not as coercion).
- Specialists are responsible for clear monitoring, supervision and dosage recommendation.
- Stimulant drugs are controlled and need to be prescribed in the doctor's writing, using words and figures to describe dosage and numbers of tablets to be prescribed. They do not, however, lead to dependence in children for whom they are prescribed.

- Extended-release preparations are often preferred to avoid the necessity of drugs being given at school.
- Second-line drugs include imipramine, bupropion, atomoxetine, risperidone and melatonin. At the time of writing, these are not necessarily licensed but may still be appropriate under specialist supervision.

Referral

ADHD should be considered in any child with hyperactive behaviour or inattentiveness reported by teachers. The diagnosis can be difficult in young children and where there is co-morbidity. Many localities have a specialist ADHD clinic; otherwise, there may be a choice between a paediatric clinic and Child and Adolescent Mental Health Services.

Resources for patients and families

ADDISS (The Attention Deficit Disorder Information and Support Service) 020 8906 9068
Website: http://www.addiss.co.uk
Advice, support, local self-help groups, conferences and literature.

CHADD (Children and Adults with ADHD) http://www.chadd.org
This is an American support group and a good source of information for parents.
The Mental Health Foundation produces the information booklet *All About ADHD*.
Publications, The Mental Health Foundation, 7th Floor, 83 Victoria Street, London SW1H 0HW; tel: 020 7802 0304; website: http://www.mentalhealth.org.uk
Leaflets are available from the Royal College of Psychiatrists
(http://www.rcpsych.ac.uk): *Attention Deficit Disorder and Hyperactivity*

Autism spectrum disorders (most popular term for pervasive developmental disorders — F84.0)

Includes disintegrative disorder, Asperger syndrome, Rett syndrome and pervasive developmental disorder not otherwise specified. These disorders have a range of severity.

(Clinical term: Childhood autism Eu84.0)

Presenting complaints

Children present in childhood with difficulties in socializing, communication and behaviour. Communication difficulties are often the first cause for concern.

Diagnostic features

Abnormal or impaired development is evident before the age of three in at least one of the following three areas:

- development of selective social attachments or of reciprocal social interaction
- receptive or expressive language, as used in social communication
- functional or symbolic play.

Difficulties are sometimes apparent from birth, or may follow a year or two of apparently normal development. Asperger syndrome might not be recognized until after a child starts school.

- Social difficulties:
  — These will depend on the age of the child, his/her developmental level and the severity of the disorder.
  — Children with autism have difficulties in interacting reciprocally with others; they may ignore other people or be relatively insensitive to their needs, thoughts or feelings.
  — Their use of non-verbal communication (eye contact, facial expression, body posture and gestures) in social situations is limited and they find it difficult to share enjoyment with others. Often, their best social interactions are with adults, and they usually show difficulties in interacting with same-age peers and in forming friendships.
  — The social difficulties of children with Asperger syndrome are similar but often more subtle: they may miss the unspoken rules of social interaction and fail to 'read' social situations.
- Communication difficulties:
  — Nearly all affected children are delayed in their acquisition of language (with some never acquiring useful speech) and usually there is little attempt to communicate using other means (gesture or mime).
  — Young children may show little interest in the speech of others.
  — Early language may consist of immediate repetitions of what is heard and spontaneous communication may be stereotyped or unusual.
  — About 30% of children with autism present with a loss/plateauing of language and/or other skills, most commonly in the second year of life.
  — Children with Asperger syndrome lack any clinically significant general delay in language or cognitive development. They may be early talkers but their language may be formal or somewhat stereotyped and, like children with autism, they show conversational difficulties.
  — Make believe and social play are usually deficient.
- Behaviour difficulties:

— Children with autism or Asperger syndrome show a tendency to routinized behaviour, resistance to change and sometimes have unusually intense interests. Some may insist on specific non-functional routines or rituals and be upset by minor environmental changes. Others might be unduly preoccupied with objects, activities or intellectual interests, which are sometimes unusual in quality, for example part objects or non-functional elements of play materials (eg wheels or wrappings).

— Interrupting these activities and interests can lead to distress.

— They may show stereotyped and repetitive motor mannerisms, for example hand or finger flapping or twisting, or whole body movements.

— Behaviours that are not specific to autism, such as tantrums or self-injury, can often be particularly problematic when children are young.

Boys are affected three to four times more commonly than girls.

Differential diagnosis and co-existing conditions

• The behaviours are not better explained by another psychiatric disorder (notably **'Attention-deficit/hyperactivity disorder — F90'**) or specific developmental disorder of receptive language, deafness or **'Learning disability — F70'.**

• It is important to exclude identifiable causes, particularly chromosomal abnormalities, the fragile X syndrome and tuberous sclerosis.
Some three-quarters of children with core autism have a performance IQ below the normal range.

• One-third of children with autism develop epilepsy, often in adolescence or early adult life. The possibility of epilepsy should be carefully investigated.

Essential information for patients and families

• Obtaining a correct diagnosis can be an important step in managing a child's developmental problems and planning for the future. Previously inexplicable behaviours may be seen to be part of a pattern of difficulties.

• Your child will need ongoing support and will benefit from the involvement of a wide network of professionals.

• Individuals with autism or Asperger syndrome often make significant developmental gains well into adult life, but they do not grow out of their difficulties.

• Playing to the individual's strengths and minimizing situations that require sophisticated social skills are important aspects of maximizing an individual's functioning and satisfaction.

• Some will need life-long supervision and care, while others can achieve greater levels of independence.

• Advice and support can be provided through your local National Autistic Society group.

General management and advice to patients and families

• The child's educational placement is a crucial element in ensuring the child's potential is maximized.

• The optimal provision should be decided on an individual basis following a full assessment, and taking into account the severity of the child's difficulties, their overall level of intelligence and their language abilities.

• Children may be best placed in a specialist school for children with autism or in a unit for children with autism or communication difficulties within a mainstream or special school. Higher functioning children may benefit from education in mainstream school, although they usually need additional help and support.

• Affected children generally need explicit teaching about social conventions and guidance and feedback on appropriate ways of interacting with others. Break times and lunch times can be particularly difficult for children in mainstream schools, who are vulnerable to bullying.

- At home, parents should complement the behavioural and teaching strategies of teachers, speech therapists and other professionals. However, the behaviour of children with autism can vary substantially across different environments and parents might need advice and help to deal with particularly problematic behaviours at home, for example sleep problems, feeding difficulties with rigid adherence to certain foods, difficulty with change in routines. There is evidence that parents can manage these behaviours successfully using parent training approaches.[248]

Medication

There is only a limited role for medication in the management of children with autism, although it can sometimes be a useful adjunct to behavioural treatments of sleep and behaviour difficulties.

Those who develop epilepsy may require anticonvulsant medication.

Liaison and referral

There should be liaison with Education Services, including Educational psychology and any specialist autism teaching support teams. Community paediatricians and speech therapists will also be involved in most cases. Clinical psychologists and child psychiatrists can provide parents with expert advice on the management of behavioural problems. Social Services can, depending on need, provide help in the home and advice on attendance and disability allowances. Respite care can be an important component of the management of children with autism.

Resources for patients and families

The National Autistic Society (Office: 020 7833 2299; Helpline: 020 7903 3555) Email: nas@nas.org.uk; website: http://www.oneworld.org/autism_uk Information service, national diagnostic and assessment service, supported employment scheme, local groups and other services.

The Mental Health Foundation produces the information booklet *All About Autistic Spectrum Disorders*. Publications, The Mental Health Foundation, 7th Floor, 83 Victoria Street, London SW1H 0HW; tel: 020 7802 0304; website: http://www.mentalhealth.org.uk

Why Does Chris Do That? by Tony Atwood. The National Autistic Society, 1993 (revised reprint 2002); website: http://www.oneworld.org/autism_uk

The Autistic Spectrum: A Guide for Parents and Professionals by Judith Gould. Constable and Robinson, 1996 (paperback published 2002)

It Can Get Better... Dealing with Common Behaviour Problems in Young Autistic Children by Paul Dickinson and Liz Hannah. The National Autistic Society, 1998; website: http://www.oneworld.org/autism_uk

Asperger Syndrome: A Guide for Parents and Professionals by Tony Atwood. Jessica Kingsley Publishers, 1998

Bereavement and loss in childhood — Z63.4*

(Clinical term: Grief reaction E2900)

Presentation

Reaction of children over the age of 10 to the death of a parent or other close family member is similar to that of adults.

- Adolescents may develop a depressive disorder and may self-medicate with alcohol or non-prescribed drugs. If depressed, they need assessment for suicidality (see **'Deliberate self-harm in children and adolescents'**).
- Children of normal intelligence who have reached the age of five to seven are capable of comprehending a concept of death that includes the ideas of irreversibility, non-functionality (dead people cannot move, breathe, eat, see, hear, feel) and universality.
- Children may not express grief directly but indirectly through play and behaviour. Anger may predominate. They might believe their parent will return, and seem indifferent or unfeeling to others.
- They are capable of expressing grief and taking part in community mourning rituals but will often need help and encouragement to do so.
- If the death was violent and witnessed by the child, such as in an accident, or where there was also a perceived threat to their own life, post-traumatic stress symptoms are likely to interfere with the normal grief process.
- Children younger than four are unable to understand the reasons for their parent's disappearance and may attribute it to their own 'bad' behaviour.
- They may react to loss by predominantly somatic symptoms or a mixture of somatic and behavioural symptoms. These are usually non-specific and include sleeping and eating problems, complaints of abdominal pain and headache, as well as an increase in oppositional or withdrawn behaviour.
- Separation anxiety is likely to be present, which may present as **'School refusal'**.
- Children will also be affected by the grief reaction of their surviving parent, which rarely may lead to neglect.

Essential information for carers and family

- Bereavement in childhood is a risk factor for later difficulties (separation anxiety disorder, anxiety, depression or other emotional disorders during childhood and adolescence, and depressive disorder in adult life). The risk can be reduced by good early management and therapeutic intervention, if indicated (see below).
- Multiple losses such as moving house or school or repeat changes of carer should be avoided. If unavoidable, try to prepare the child, and enable them to keep contact with previous attachment figures for a time after any move.
- Children over five, if well supported, might benefit by seeing the dead parent, because this helps them to understand about the non-functionality of death. (They do not benefit from seeing a mutilated or unrecognizable parent.)
- They also are helped by attending the funeral, providing they wish to, and the surviving parent agrees.
- Agencies such as Cruse Bereavement Care offer bereavement support and counselling and publish book lists and pamphlets for children and adolescents.
- Family therapy has been shown to improve children's functioning after bereavement.

*The current ICD-10 classification does not distinguish between adults and children/adolescents.

This might be available from the local Child and Adolescent Mental Health Service (CAMHS), and other agencies.

General management and advice to patient, family and carers[249,250]

- If attending a parent with a terminal illness, consider with the family when and what to tell the child and who should do it.
- Explain directly to the child what is happening or has happened to their parent or other family member and answer questions they may have. Reassure them that they will be looked after.
- Anticipate that young children may have distorted or immature thinking, eg they might think it was their fault or that their parent/family member will return soon.
- Ascertain child's worries about the health of the remaining parent and any siblings, and reassure.
- Encourage participation in the funeral, as appropriate.
- Encourage the family to talk about the dead person, share their sorrow together and remember good times. They should help children keep mementos of the dead person, perhaps in a memory box.
- Discourage families from giving explanations to the child that are developmentally inappropriate; for example, discourage the explanation that 'Mummy has gone to heaven'. If a religious explanation is desired, it is better to say, 'Mummy's soul has gone to be with God in heaven. Her body doesn't work any more and has to be buried or cremated'.
- Advise the family to maintain child's normal routines as far as possible (eg school, nursery).
- Reassure the family that most bereaved children recover from the loss with good support; children are resilient.
- Ensure that the child's school is aware of their bereavement and is supportive.
- Anticipate anniversary reactions — the first Christmas, birthday and anniversary of the death. Monitor the child's progress for the next year.
- Bereavement support or counselling for child and family (perhaps including family therapy) should be considered in each case as a preventive intervention.
- Some charities run groups and/or camps for bereaved children (eg Winston's Wish in Gloucestershire), again as a preventive intervention.
- If the bereavement was a violent, traumatic one, watch for post-traumatic stress symptoms (flashbacks, high arousal, avoidance) and arrange appropriate referral if these persist. Traumatic bereavement giving rise to PTSD is best treated early with cognitive behavioural therapy.

Medication

There is rarely a place for medication with children.

Referral

- Refer to voluntary agency for bereavement counselling for child and parent. Cruse Bereavement Care or the Child Bereavement Network can give details of local services.
- Refer to CAMHS if the child or adolescent is showing symptoms or signs of continuing dysfunction (eg school refusal, continuing separation anxiety, persistent somatic or other behavioural problems, parasuicidal behaviour, PTSD).
- If health services were involved with the person who died (eg a hospice), these can be very helpful.
- If family therapy is indicated, CAMHS, some Social Services departments or training institutes might be the appropriate source.

Resources for patients and families

Cruse Bereavement Care 020 8939 9530, Youthline 0808 808 1677
Website: http://www.crusebereavementcare.org.uk
Voluntary bereavement care with 150 branches throughout the UK. Offers support, training, direct telephone help to children and young people (of 12–18 years) through the Youthline; publications, help in finding local counselling. The website has a useful guide to 'Helping children'.

Child Bereavement Trust 01494 446 648.
Website: http://www.childbereavement.org.uk/
Offers training for counselling bereaved children and advice on where to obtain help in UK. The website has advice sheets for parents and young people and a list of useful resources, including videos for young people.

Child Bereavement Network 0115 911 8070
Website: http://www.ncb.org.uk/cbn/index.htm
This site has an online directory of accessible specialist bereavement support services throughout the UK.

Winston's Wish 0845 203 0405
Website: http://www.winstonswish.org.uk
This is an organization supporting bereaved children and young people, and offering guidance and information to anyone concerned about a child after bereavement.

SAMM (Support after Murder and Manslaughter) 020 7735 3838
Email: enquiries@samm.org.uk; website: http://www.samm.org.uk
A helpline and useful publications, including some for carers.

SOBS (Survivors of Bereavement by Suicide) 0870 241 3337 (9am–9pm, daily)
Website: http://www.uk-sobs.org.uk
This site offers emotional and practical support to those affected by suicide. Provides a factsheet entitled *Understanding Childhood Bereavement*.

Institute of Family Therapy 020 7391 9150
Website: http://www.instituteoffamilytherapy.org.uk
Offers family therapy and training in family therapy.

BACP (British Association for Counselling and Psychotherapy) 0870 443 5252
Email: bacp@bacp.co.uk; website: http://www.counselling.co.uk
Will advise on sources of individual counselling and family therapy in the UK. A leaflet is available from the Royal College of Psychiatrists (http://www.rcpsych.ac.uk): *Death in the Family — Helping Children to Cope*

When Someone Very Special Dies and *When Something Terrible Happens* (traumatic bereavement) by M Heegaard. Cruse Bereavement Care, 126 Sheen Road, Richmond, Surrey TW9 1UR; tel: 020 8939 9530.
Work books for children.

Beyond the Rough Rock. Supporting a Child who has been Bereaved Through Suicide by D Crossley and J Stokes, 2002. Winston's Wish, The Clara Burgess Centre, Gloucestershire Hospital, Great Western Road, Gloucester GL1 3NN; tel: 0845 203 0405.
Book to help children.

Bullying

(Clinical term: Bullying 13ZF.)

Bullying is defined as the intentional, unprovoked abuse of power by one or more children to inflict pain or cause distress to another child on repeated occasions. It occurs in social groups with clear power relationships and low supervision, to some extent in all schools, and often without apparent provocation.

Presenting complaints

Bullying can have a major impact on the physical and mental health of victims, as well as on their education. It is perceived as stressful by those who experience it.[251]
Victims of bullying may present with a variety of psychosomatic symptoms or mental health problems, including the following:

- sleeping difficulties
- bed wetting
- feeling sad
- headaches
- stomach aches
- irritability, poor concentration
- depression, suicidal ideation, deliberate self-harm
- somatic symptoms
- anxiety
- social dysfunction.

Health professionals seeing school children who present with any of these should consider bullying as a possible contributory factor.
There is some evidence to suggest that bullying can have long-term mental health effects.[252,253] Former victims of bullying are more likely than non-victimized peers to:

- be depressed
- be anxious
- be lonely
- have low self-esteem
- feel less comfortable with the opposite sex.

Diagnostic features

Compared with other children, 'passive victims' of bullying tend to:

- be cautious
- be sensitive
- be quiet
- be more anxious and insecure
- have fewer friends
- feel unhappy and lonely
- have low self-esteem
- have a negative view of themselves and their situation
- look upon themselves as failures
- feel stupid, ashamed and unattractive.

A smaller group — 'proactive victims' — is characterized by a combination of anxious and aggressive reaction patterns. These children have concentration difficulties, may be overactive and often behave in ways that cause irritation and tension around them. Their behaviour frequently provokes other children, who retaliate in a negative fashion.

Although any child can be bullied, it is more likely to occur to the following vulnerable children. Those who:

- are shy or lacking in close friends at school
- come from an overprotective family environment or a family experiencing crisis or distress
- come from a different racial or ethnic group from the majority
- differ in some obvious respect from the majority, eg by stammering, having a physical disability or being of short stature
- have special educational needs
- provoke their peers by their inappropriate behaviour
- have Asperger syndrome or other autistic spectrum disorder.

Essential information for patient and family
- Bullying is more common in boys and in the youngest pupils in a school.
- The commonest type of bullying is general name-calling, followed by being physically hit, being threatened and having rumours spread about the bullied individual.
- Research suggests an incidence of about one in five for being bullied (with higher figures for children who attend remedial classes or who are of Asian origin) and up to one in ten for bullying others.

General management and advice to patient and family
- Encourage the child to tell their parents and teacher. Reassure them they were right to tell and that the adults will try to work together to keep them safe.
- In the first instance, bullying should be dealt with by approaching the school directly to inform it of the problem. Consider involving a school or practice counsellor.[254]
- Encourage parents to raise the issue with school, possibly against the child's wishes, if the problem persists.
- Bullying interventions in schools include:
  — the setting up of whole-school policies
  — curriculum-based strategies
  — intervening in bullying situations by working directly with pupils involved in bully/victim problems
  — setting up school tribunals or 'bully courts'
  — assertiveness training for victims
  — making changes to playgrounds
  — peer-led interventions (eg peer counselling)
  — working with lunch time supervisors.
- Being bullied is one of the stressors most strongly associated with suicidal behaviour in adolescents. Both bullies and victims are at increased risk of suicide.[255] Bullies need help too (see 'Conduct disorder — F91#').

Liaison and referral
Bullying by fellow pupils is a primary responsibility of the school; every school should have an anti-bullying policy.

Referral to a specialist Child and Adolescent Mental Health Service is advised if the child or adolescent:

- is severely depressed
- has suicidal thoughts
- is self-harming
- shows social withdrawal
- refuses to eat
- is severely anxious or has insomnia
- is developing school refusal.

Resources for patients and families

Anti-Bullying Campaign 020 7378 1446
Provides help if a child is being bullied or if a child is a bully.

Childwatch 01482 325 552
Website: http://www.childwatch.org.uk
Advice for children on bullying and abuse that occurs at home and at school.

ChildLine 0800 1111 (24-hour helpline)
Website: http://www.childline.org.uk
Telephone service for all children and young people providing confidential counselling, support and advice on any issue. Parents can also write to ChildLine.

Kidscape 020 7730 3300
Website: http://www.kidscape.org.uk/childrenteens/childrenteensindex.shtml
This is a charity set up to protect children from danger — whether from peers, adults they know or complete strangers.

NSPCC (National Society for the Prevention of Cruelty to Children)
0808 800 5000 (helpline)
Website: http://www.nspcc.org.uk/html/home/needadvice/bullying.htm
Charity specializing in child protection and the prevention of cruelty to children.

Bullying Online http://www.bullying.co.uk
Gives help and advice for parents and pupils in dealing with school bullying.

The Bullying Project http://www.bullying.org
Provides online mentoring support programmes, as well as educational resources.
A leaflet is available from the Royal College of Psychiatrists
(http://www.rcpsych.ac.uk): The emotional cost of bullying

Tackling Bullying: Listening to the Views of Children and Young People. Summary Report by Christine Oliver and Mano Candappa of the Thomas Coram Research Unit, Department for Education and Skills, 2003. Available from ChildLine, 45 Folgate Street, London E1 6GL; Tel: 020 7650 3200; Website:
http://www.dfes.gov.uk/bullying/

Child abuse and neglect — Z61.4, Z61.5, Z61.6*

(Clinical term: Child abuse ZV612)

Presenting complaints

Abuse is not usually presented as the problem. Instead, children present with complaints that are the sequelae of abuse or neglect. Most of these are psychological or behavioural; some are physical.

Recognition and diagnostic features

Four forms of maltreatment are recognized:

- neglect — the persistent failure to meet a child's physical and psychological needs by lack of supervision or provision (N)
- physical abuse and non-accidental injury (which includes fabricated or induced illness) (PA)
- sexual abuse (CSA)
- emotional abuse (EA).

Different forms may lead to different sequelae, but there is often co-occurrence of more than one form. All forms include some element of emotional maltreatment, but emotional abuse may occur on its own.

Children with disabilities are particularly vulnerable. Children of all ages may experience abuse and neglect.

- Physical neglect and emotional abuse often continue from early childhood
- Physical abuse in infancy may cause serious injury and occasionally death or lasting disability. Later in childhood, it is associated more with inappropriate and harsh punishment.
- Sexual abuse is more common in adolescence and in girls, although young boys are also abused.

Child abuse and neglect are recognized by:

- ill-treatment that the child receives (including both omission and commission). Neglect and emotional abuse are observable forms of ill treatment
- harm arising from the abuse or neglect.

During routine or unrelated medical examinations, children may be found to have signs of the results of child abuse and neglect. Occasionally, an injured child may be brought for treatment.

Signs of physical harm:

- Multiple superficial injuries of varying ages, for which no reasonable explanation is given — for example, bruises (which may resemble the shape of the article used to inflict the bruise), abrasions, cuts or cigarette burns (PA).
- Fractures — rib, metaphyseal and spiral fracture; skull in non-ambulant children (PA).
- Retinal and subdural haemorrhages in non-ambulant children (PA).
- Failure to thrive and short stature (EA; N).
- Poisoning, asphyxiation (PA — induced illness).

*This is the coding for sexual and physical abuse; neglect and emotional abuse are not specifically coded under the current ICD-10 classification.

- Delayed or no immunizations (N).
- Untreated medical conditions (N).
- Sexually transmitted diseases (CSA).

Indicators of psychological harm:

- **'Depression — F32#'** (CSA).
- Anxiety (recent onset) (EA; CSA).
- Low self-esteem (PA; EA; CSA).
- **'Post-traumatic stress disorder — F43.1'**(CSA).
- **'Conduct or oppositional-defiant disorder — F91'** (PA; EA).
- Sexualized behaviour inappropriate to age and stage of development (CSA).
- **'Deliberate self-harm'** (CSA).
- **'Substance misuse — F10, F11#'** (CSA).
- Educational underachievement (N; EA).
- Social isolation (EA).

Recognition of sexual abuse ultimately relies most strongly on the child's verbal disclosures or descriptions. The reliability and credibility of a child's descriptions are often closely scrutinized and challenged, despite the fact that false allegations are rare. Most cases of child sexual abuse have no physical signs and, when found, are rarely conclusive proof of abuse, being regarded as (only) compatible with the child's account of sexual abuse.

Differential diagnosis

Child abuse and neglect is often disputed or denied by the parents or alleged abusers. There may well be a delay in presentation of the child to a doctor, and the history/explanation might be inconsistent, changing and not compatible with the injury or child's development.

Some forms of ill-treatment are readily observable:

- Neglect with lack of supervision, leading to accidents or lack of hygiene and provision of basic care
- Emotional abuse, including frequent negativity towards, and excessive punishment of, the child.

What may be in dispute is the extent to which these forms of parent–child interaction are actually harming the child and qualify for the term 'abuse'.

None of the list of possible presentations is caused exclusively by child abuse or neglect, although some patterns of physical injury (eg certain fractures, bruises, retinal and subdural haemorrhages, genital and perianal signs) are strongly suggestive or typical of abuse. They require immediate intervention to safeguard the child, and expert validation.

It is important to exclude likely alternative explanations for the child's difficulties. Mental ill-health of the parent or suspected abuser, or their substance abuse or domestic violence are risk factors for child abuse and neglect. However, not all troubled adults are responsible for child abuse and neglect.

Essential information for patient and family

- Everyone, particularly those in a professional role, has a responsibility to report any concerns.
- Professionals must work together in partnership with the family to protect the child(ren); there may be a need to override confidentiality in the interests of interdisciplinary communication.
- The child is not responsible for the abuse.
- Child protection procedures and the statutory centrality of Social Services should be explained.

General management and advice to patient and family[256]

- *Sharing information and reporting:*
  - Follow local area child protection committee (ACPC) guidelines
  - If in doubt about possible child abuse and neglect, discuss with health visitor and named or designated doctor in the primary care team
  - If suspicious or likely child abuse and neglect, report to Social Services.
- *Immediate treatment:*
  - Few children require immediate medical or psychiatric treatment. Exceptions are those who have been seriously injured, infected with a sexually-transmitted disease, are pregnant, or those acutely traumatized by the abuse.
- *Multidisciplinary response:*
  - The first step is to determine whether the child and other children in the family need immediate protection. The closer the relationship between the non-abusing caregiver(s) and the (suspected) abuser, the more precarious the position of the child. The term 'close' includes love, fear or dependency.
  - This requires a multidisciplinary assessment, led by Social Services usually in collaboration with other agencies — health, police, voluntary organizations (eg the NSPCC).
  - A strategy discussion may be followed by a Child Protection Conference (CPC). It is important that the GP attends the CPC or sends a report of salient information about the child and family
  - ensuring protection may require an emergency protection order and placing of the child's name on the Child Protection Register with a protection plan and sometimes through court proceedings.
- *Supporting the child and family:*
  - Acknowledge the crisis and distress that investigation and intervention cause to the child and family.
  - Acknowledge that there may be conflicting interests between the needs of the child and those of the parents.
  - Explain that in law (Children Act 1989, see page 217) the child's welfare is paramount.
  - Facilitate meaningful contact for the child with trusted and familiar persons who are supportive of the child's needs.
  - Support the child who discloses abuse not to feel responsible for the abuse or guilty about disclosing it. Beyond the needs of the medical history taking, do not question the child about the concern and do not make unrealistic promises.
  - Actively support the non-abusing parent(s), who is often very distressed and who may feel torn between the abuser and child.
  - Help the parents to accept that acknowledging responsibility for the maltreatment is a difficult, painful but necessary process in order to achieve positive change for the child and family.
- *Treatment:*
  - The GP must ensure treatment is provided for children whose names are not on the Child Protection Register and for whom there is therefore no protection plan.
  - A comprehensive treatment plan includes help for the child, the non-abusing caregiver(s), siblings and the abuser.
  - Parents may require parenting work and considerable social support. Such help often needs to be maintained for long periods, as change may not be sustained after a short but intensive course of intervention.
  - Many abused children require educational remediation for their associated educational underachievement.
  - Treatment for the child depends on the nature of the maltreatment and the sequelae; there is no unitary post-abuse syndrome, not even following specific forms such as sexual abuse. Treatment needs to be based on an individual's needs at any given time and may be given in groups or individually.

— Group therapy is not appropriate where a case is subject to a criminal inquiry that may result in criminal court proceedings.[257]
— Cognitive behavioural therapy is effective for PTSD and sexualized behaviour.
— Treatment should be given for **'Depressive disorder — F32#'**, **'Substance misuse — F10, F11#'** and **'Deliberate self-harm'** which often develop in adolescence .
— As well as emotional and behavioural difficulties, some maltreated children undergo social disruption as part of the necessary protection process. They experience considerable difficulties arising from separations and impermanence and require active support through this process.
— Some children require more intensive psychotherapy for the effects of the abuse.

Liaison and referral

Treating agencies include social services, family centres, child and adolescent mental health services, adult mental health and substance misuse services, and voluntary agencies (eg the NSPCC).

Resources for patients and family

NSPCC (National Society for the Protection of Children) 0808 800 5000 (24-hour child protection helpline)
Email: help@nspcc.org.uk; website: http://www.nspcc.org.uk
This is a charity specializing in child protection and the prevention of cruelty to children.

ChildLine 0800 1111 (24-hour helpline)
Website: http://www.childline.org.uk
A telephone service for all children and young people providing confidential counselling, support and advice on any issue. Parents can also write to ChildLine.

Like it is
Email: likeitis@stopes.org.uk; website: http://www.likeitis.org.uk
Sex education for young people.

Youth2Youth 020 8896 3675
Email: help@youth2youth.co.uk; website: http://www.youth2youth.co.uk
Telephone, email and online chat line run by young people for young people.

Ask Brook 020 7284 6040
Email: admin@brookcentres.org.uk; website: http://www.brook.org.uk
Provides free and confidential sexual health advice and contraception to young people up to the age of 25
Leaflets are available from the Royal College of Psychiatrists
(http://www.rcpsych.ac.uk): *Domestic Violence: It's Effects on Children*, and *Child Abuse and Neglect: the Emotional Effects*
A leaflet is available from the Royal College of General Practitioners
(http://www.rcgp.org.uk): *Domestic Violence in Families with Children*

Conduct disorder (including oppositional-defiant disorder) — F91#

(Clinical term: Conduct disorders Eu91)

All children are defiant at times and it is a normal part of adolescence to do the opposite of what one is told. Oppositional-defiant disorder mainly applies to children whose functioning at home and at school is impaired by constant conflict with adults and other children. Conduct disorder mainly applies to adolescents whose behaviour goes to antisocial extremes; many are excluded from school or in trouble with the law.

Presenting complaints
- In younger children: marked tantrums, defiance, fighting and bullying.
- In older children and adolescents: serious law-breaking, such as stealing, damage to property, assault.
- Can be confined only to school or only to home.

Diagnostic features
- A pattern of repetitive, persistent and excessive antisocial, aggressive or defiant behaviour lasting six months or more.
- These features must be out of keeping with the child's development level, norms of peer group behaviour, and cultural context (eg isolated tantrums in a three-year-old should not be regarded as abnormal).
- In younger children (say, three to eight year-olds), the behaviours are characteristic of the *oppositional-defiant type* of conduct disorder: angry outbursts, loss of temper, refusal to obey commands and rules, destructiveness, hitting, but without the presence of serious law-breaking.
- In older children and adolescents (say, nine to 18 year olds), the behaviours are characteristic of *conduct disorder per se*: vandalism, cruelty to people and animals, bullying, lying, stealing outside the home, truancy, drug and alcohol misuse, and criminal acts, plus all the features of the oppositional-defiant type.

Differential diagnosis and co-existing conditions
Co-existent disorders are common and do not rule out the diagnosis; they are easily missed so should be carefully checked for the following:

- **'Attention-deficit/hyperactivity disorder — F90'.**
- Hyperactivity.
- **'Depressive disorder — F32#'.**
- Specific reading retardation (dyslexia).
- Generalized **'Learning disability (mental retardation) — F70'.**
- **'Autism spectrum disorders — F84'.**
- Adjustment reaction (this follows a clear stressor, such as parental divorce, bereavement, trauma, abuse, or change of caregiver).

Parenting problems are commonly associated and include a lack of positive joint activities with the child, insufficient praise, inconsistent discipline, harsh punishments, hostility, rejection or emotional abuse, sexual abuse, and poor monitoring of the whereabouts of older children.

Essential information for patients and family
- The child is likely to be temperamentally different from their siblings, and cannot easily control their actions.
- Antisocial behaviour is learned and can be corrected (unlearned).

- The long-term prognosis is not good without intervention (they do not 'grow out of it') but is good with appropriate management, especially parent behavioural management training.[258–260]

General management and advice to patient and family

- Promote daily play and positive joint activities between parent and child for at least 10 minutes per day, despite both sides' initial reluctance.
- Encourage praise and rewards for specific, agreed desired behaviours. If appropriate, monitor with a chart. Negotiate rewards with the child and change target behaviours every two to six weeks and rewards more often.
- Set clear house rules and give short specific commands about the desired behaviour, not prohibitions about undesired behaviour (eg 'Please walk slowly', rather than 'Don't run').
- Provide consistent and calm consequences for misbehaviour. Many unwanted behaviours can be ignored, and will then stop (but may increase when this technique is first tried). Distracting the child from an unwanted behaviour is likely to be more effective than saying, 'Don't do it'. If neither ignoring nor distraction is appropriate, 'time out' (to avoid the unwanted behaviour receiving positive reinforcement) may be effective. This can involve leaving the child alone to calm down or sending them to a quiet, boring 'time out' room (or other space in the house) for no more than one minute per year of age, and 10 minutes maximum. Avoid getting into arguments or explanations with the child, as this merely provides additional attention for the misbehaviour.
- Reorganize the child's day to prevent trouble. Examples include asking a neighbour to look after the child while going to the supermarket, ensuring that activities are available for long car journeys, and arranging activities in separate rooms for siblings who are prone to fight.
- Monitor the whereabouts of teenagers. Telephone the parents of friends whom they say they are visiting.
- Liaise with school and suggest similar principles are applied. Parents should put pressure on the child's school to look hard for specific learning difficulties such as dyslexia.

Medication

No drugs are effective. Methylphenidate is effective for co-morbid hyperkinetic disorder and may reduce conduct problems in children with both problems (see **'Attention-deficit/hyperactivity disorder — F90'**).

Liaison and referral

- If problems are mainly or exclusively at school, parents should request that the school involves educational services, such as the Educational Psychology Service (for assessment of specific learning difficulty), the Educational Welfare Service (for attendance problems) or local behaviour support teams. Some schools employ school counsellors or specialized teachers who may be skilled in anger-management training.
- Referral to a local Child and Adolescent Mental Health Service (CAMHS) should be considered for cases that fail to improve, where the behaviour is leading to major impairment, or where co-existing problems such as hyperkinetic disorder or autism spectrum disorder are suspected.
- For adolescents with law-breaking behaviour (delinquency), youth-offending teams can often provide an intensive intervention package for the duration of the court's involvement. This may include parenting groups for behavioural management training.
- For preschool children, health visitors are often trained to educate parents in behavioural management techniques. Local parent support agencies such as Sure

Start may be able to provide more intensive input.
- Social Services must be involved in cases of suspected abuse (of any sort), when a young person's behaviour is beyond the control of parents, and with adopted children. They may not have the resources to help in more straightforward cases.

Resources for parents and carers
National Family and Parenting Institute 020 7424 3460
Email: info@nfpi.org; website: http://www.nfpi.org
Details of the most studied form of parent managements training can be found at http://www.incredibleyears.com
A leaflet is available from the Royal College of Psychiatrists (http://www.rcpsych.ac.uk): *Behavioural Problems and Conduct Disorder*

Deliberate self-harm in children and adolescents — X60–X84

(Clinical term: self-harm in children and adolescents U2…)

Presenting complaints

Deliberate self-harm in children and adolescents usually presents with a deliberate overdose of tablets or cutting. It occasionally presents with other methods of self-harm, such as attempted hanging, strangulation, burning or running in front of a car.

Assessment

The diagnosis of deliberate self-harm in primary care settings is usually straightforward. However, some children and adolescents who have harmed themselves may try to conceal their true intent, claiming for instance that an overdose was accidental. Many others will conceal self-harm from parents and the practitioner.

Assessment is directed to four main issues:

- assessment and management of the current episode
- identification and management of associated problems
- identification and promotion of the child and family's resources
- prevention of repetition.

Assessment and management of the current episode

- All children and adolescents who have taken an overdose should receive prompt medical attention.
- Suicidal intent should be assessed. Circumstances suggesting a high intent include the use of very dangerous methods, precautions to avoid discovery, and final acts such as leaving a note or giving possessions away.
- The triggers of the current episode should be identified. These include arguments with family members, disciplinary crises at home or school, rows with peers, and breaking up with a boyfriend or girlfriend.
- Cutting often occurs when the young person experiences strong feelings of tension, and the young person might report that cutting provides some temporary relief. Most young people who cut themselves have long-standing problems such as low self-esteem or substance abuse.

Identification and management of associated problems

- Self-harm in adolescents is associated with depression, drug or alcohol abuse, behavioural problems, and physical illness.
- There is often an association with family difficulties, including parental discord and violence, parental depression or substance abuse, role models of suicidal behaviour in the family, abuse of all kinds, and bereavement.
- Other associated problems include bullying at school, peer role models of self-harm, models of self-harm in the media, and educational difficulties.

Identification and promotion of the child and family's resources

- Factors in the child that protect them from self-harm, or from repetition of self-harm include being particularly good at something (eg a sport), positive peer relationships, good school attendance and academic achievement, and positive plans for the future.
- Family factors that reduce the risk of self-harm include a close relationship with at least one positive role model, parenting styles that encourage rather than punish, and clear methods for communication within the family.

Prevention of repetition
- This should begin with an assessment of the risk factors for frequent repetition or suicide — male gender, older age, use of dangerous methods, severe mental health problems (such as depression), high suicidal intent during the index episode of self-harm, and continuing suicidal intent.
- Factors suggesting there is continuing suicidal intent include a clear statement that the young person intends to harm themselves again (such a statement should always be taken seriously), depression, unresolved personal or family problems (particularly if these appeared to precipitate previous self-harm), hopelessness, clear suicidal plans, easy access to dangerous methods, and frequent previous attempts.
- Assessment of mental state and continuing suicidal intent will usually require that the young person be interviewed without the parent.
- There is no evidence that encouraging children and adolescents to talk with professionals about suicidal feelings and suicidal plans precipitates self-harm.
- The risk of repetition and suicide is not static, but changes over time, and may require regular assessment.

Essential information for patient and family
- Deliberate self-harm should always be taken seriously, even if the actual intent to die seems to have been low.
- Take whatever steps are necessary to prevent the young person gaining access to methods of harming themselves again (eg parents should clear old tablets out of the medicine cupboard, lock away essential medicines and hide sharp knives).
- Do not make the adolescent feel guilty or reject them because of the self-harming behaviour. This will simply make matters worse.
- Although many families want to draw a veil over the episode, it can often be important to talk about it. The young person needs to feel that their behaviour is being listened to and understood, not devalued or ridiculed.
- Parents should create an atmosphere for listening if the young person wants to talk; parents should be around, but not hover.
- Helplines, such as the Samaritans, and local emergency services are available 24 hours a day.

General management and advice to patient and family
- Assessment of suicidal thinking and planning is an important part of the mental-state examination of any young person who presents with emotional or behavioural difficulties.
- Underlying mental health problems, particularly depression and substance misuse, need to be assessed and managed.
- Risk of repetition should be reviewed regularly, particularly in patients who are at high risk of further self-harm.

Medication
Medication is not usually required by adolescents who self-harm, but if the young person has major depression then an SSRI can be prescribed.

Referral
- All children and adolescents who have taken an overdose should be referred to hospital for medical evaluation, admission and subsequent evaluation by a mental health professional.
- Urgent referral to secondary mental health services should be considered when there is a high risk of further self-harm or completed suicide. All children and adolescents who engage in serious methods of self-harm (eg attempted hanging), or who use methods suggesting high suicidal intent, should be referred.
- Consider referral for psychological therapies, as appropriate.

Resources for patients and families

Self Harm Alliance 01242 578 820 (Helpline 6pm–7pm, Tuesday, Sunday; 11am–1pm, Thursday)
Email: selfharmalliance@aol.com; website: http://www.selfharmalliance.org
Helpline, produces monthly newsletters, provides postal and email support and offers an advocacy service.

ChildLine 0800 1111 (24-hour helpline)
Website: http://www.childline.org.uk
Telephone service for all children and young people providing confidential counselling, support and advice on any issue. Parents can also write to ChildLine.

Change our Minds http://www.changeourminds.com
A website run by the Samaritans, targeted at a younger audience.

Self Injury and Related Issues (SIARI)
Email: jan@siari.uk; website: http://www.siari.co.uk
Forum for self-harmers.

Suicide Information and Education Centre (Canada) http://www.suicideinfo.ca
Library, resources and specific youth links.
A leaflet is available from the Royal College of Psychiatrists
(http://www.rcpsych.ac.uk): *Fact Sheet 30: Deliberate Self Harm in Young People.*

Depressive disorder in adolescents — F32#*
(Clinical term: Depressive episode Eu32)

Depressive disorder in pre-adolescents is very rare and difficult to distinguish from the intense emotional reactions and misery that are common in small children. All cases of suspected depressive disorder in pre-adolescents should be referred. This guideline is concerned with depressive disorder in adolescents aged 11 and over.

Presenting complaints
Adolescents usually present with symptoms of depressive disorder such as depression, suicidality or sleep disturbance. Depressive disorder can also present with its complications (eg school refusal) or with co-morbid problems (eg behavioural difficulties). Adolescents frequently present with physical symptoms, such as headaches or abdominal pain. Irritability can also be a symptom of depression.

Diagnostic features
Depression is diagnosed using the same criteria as in adults:

- Low or sad mood is present most days.
- Loss of interest or pleasure is present most days.

As well as several of the following associated symptoms:

- Hopelessness
- Poor concentration
- Poor or excessive sleep for developmental stage
- Weight loss (or failure to gain weight normally) or excessive weight gain
- Suicidal thoughts or acts
- Low self-esteem
- Loss of energy
- Agitation or slowing of movement or speech.

To qualify for a diagnosis of depressive disorder, these symptoms should lead to significant suffering or impairment and should persist for at least one month.

Several factors increase the risk of depression, and their presence should alert the practitioner to the possibility of this diagnosis. These include being in care, recent bereavement, family breakdown, and adolescents with shy personalities who have peer relationship problems.

Differential diagnosis and co-existing conditions
- **Anxiety disorder** (Depressive disorder should only be diagnosed if the symptoms are clearly prominent and not part of an anxiety disorder).
- Normal adolescent emotionality (Depressive disorder should only be diagnosed if there is social impairment, or there are serious symptoms such as a suicide attempt).
- **'Conduct disorder — F91#'** (Depressive disorder should only be diagnosed if the symptoms are clearly prominent and not part of the behavioural disorder).
- **'Drug use — F11#'** (diagnose depression as secondary if it occurs only in conjunction with heavy substance abuse [eg misuse of marijuana]).
- **'Bipolar disorder — F31'** (in referred samples, about 1 in 20 adolescents with severe depression go on to develop bipolar disorder; the risk is higher if there are features of psychotic depression and a family history of bipolar disorder).

*The current ICD-10 classification does not distinguish between adults and adolescents.   177

Some medications used by adolescents, eg preparations for acne, oral contraceptives and corticosteroids, can be associated with depression.

A wide range of problems can occur in conjunction with depression, which makes the diagnosis more difficult. Symptoms of general or separation anxiety (fear of being away from a major attachment figure) are frequently present. Other co-morbidities include behavioural problems, substance misuse, school attendance problems and family difficulties.

Essential information for patient and family
- The adolescent is not making the symptoms up. What looks like laziness or crossness can be symptoms of depression.
- Depression can affect relationships within the family and the ability to do school work or to go to school.
- Effective treatments are available for depression, and there is a good chance of recovery.

General management and advice to patient and family[261]
- Identify current life problems or stresses and try to reduce them.
- Try to keep the adolescent active by planning enjoyable activities with them.
- If the depression is not severe, encourage the adolescent to go to school.
- Encourage the adolescent to take exercise, to get to bed early and to eat a balanced diet.
- If the adolescent has made a suicidal attempt, the parent should be encouraged to secure medication and sharp objects. Offer the patient and family an emergency telephone number (see **'Deliberate self-harm'**).
- Involve both patient and family in discussing the advantages and disadvantages of psychological and physical treatments. Many adolescents and families are worried about taking antidepressant medication, so respect this decision and continue to monitor.
- Individual psychological treatments, such as cognitive behavioural therapy and interpersonal therapy, are the treatment of first choice, if available.
- Family therapy has not been found to be effective, but might be indicated if family problems are obviously contributing to the adolescent's depression.
- Response to the initial treatment usually occurs within eight weeks. If it has not, consider a second line of treatment.

Medication[261]
- In general, medication is not the first-line treatment.
- Consider antidepressants, however, if the depression is so severe that psychological treatment is unlikely to work by itself, if non-medical treatments have failed or are not available.
- Tricyclic antidepressants should be avoided — there is little evidence they are effective in adolescent depression and they are dangerous in overdose.
- SSRIs are the first-line antidepressants.
- Start with half the adult dose and increase slowly, as adherence is particularly poor in this age group and perceived side-effects are the most common reason for not taking medication.
- Explain that the medication must be taken every day, that improvement in symptoms takes three to four weeks, and that there may be some mild side-effects but that these usually fade within two weeks.

Referral
Referral may be necessary if structured psychological therapies are not available in primary care.

Referral to a Child and Adolescent Mental Health Service is advised:

- in an emergency, when there is a high risk of self-harm, psychotic symptoms, or refusal to drink
- if depression persists despite initial treatment in primary care
- if the depression occurs in the context of complex family or social difficulties
- if the cause of the depression is likely to include abuse
- if the depression is co-morbid with severe behavioural disorder or substance abuse.

Resources for patients and families

Young Minds Trust 020 7336 8445
Parent information service: 0800 018 2138; website:
http://www.youngminds.org.uk
Aims to improve the mental health of all children and young people. Produces a range of leaflets for parents and young people.

Change our Minds http://www.changeourminds.com
A website run by the Samaritans targeted at a younger audience.
A leaflet is available from the Royal College of Psychiatrists
(http://www.rcpsych.ac.uk): *Depression in Children and Young People*

So Young, So Sad, So Listen by P Graham and C Hughes. Gaskell Press, 1995.
A book discussing childhood depression.

Eating disorders in children and adolescents — F50*

(F98.2 refers only to infants and early childhood)
(Clinical term: Eating disorders Eu50)

Presenting complaints

- The family may ask for help because of the patient's loss of weight, refusal to eat, vomiting or amenorrhea. The family unit is often under considerable stress by the time help is sought.
- Patients may present with symptoms of binge-eating and purging or laxative abuse.

Diagnostic features

Eating disorders are much more common in girls than in boys.

Anorexia nervosa

Common features are as follows:

- Weight loss or failure to gain weight during the period of pre-adolescent growth (10–14 years) in the absence of a causative physical illness.
- Determined food avoidance and strict dieting.
- Fear of fatness, drive for thinness.
- Denial of seriousness of low body weight.
- Preoccupation with body weight and calories.
- Presence of intensive fear of gaining weight and disturbance in body image depends on cognitive development. Younger children will often not verbalize such fears and distortion.
- Excessive efforts to control weight (strict dieting, excessive exercise). Self-induced vomiting and laxative abuse are less common than in adults.
- Amenorrhea in post-pubertal patients or delay of menarche in younger girls.

Bulimia nervosa

Bulimia nervosa is less common than anorexia nervosa, especially in children and young adolescents.

Food restriction is accompanied by episodes of binge-eating and purging (self-induced vomiting or other weight-control behaviours).

Many of the features are the same as in anorexia nervosa, in particular:

- extreme concern about weight and body shape
- overwhelming fear of fatness and food restriction
- low self-esteem, fluctuating or low mood.

Specific signs that may indicate the presence of bulimia nervosa are:

- unexplained weight loss or fluctuations
- a chaotic pattern of eating
- unexplained disappearances of large amounts of food at home
- refusal to eat with others or secretive behaviour around food
- 'puffy' cheeks due to the enlargement of salivary glands caused by frequent vomiting
- sore throat and erosion of tooth enamel from vomiting

---

*The current ICD-10 classification does not distinguish between adults and children and adolescents.

- Russell's sign — abrasions to back of hand or knuckles caused by repeated, self-induced vomiting
- disappearing to the lavatory immediately after meals
- evidence of laxative abuse.

Differential diagnosis
- 'Depressive disorder — F32#' (often occurs along with bulimia or anorexia).
- Physical illness (eg tuberculosis, acquired immune deficiency disease, endocrine disorders, inflammatory bowel disease and hyperthyroidism) may cause weight loss, but it can usually be distinguished by the lack of a distorted body image and a desire to put on weight.
- Food refusal — refusal of food which does not involve preoccupation with body shape or weight and which is best viewed as oppositional behavioural difficulties that often resolve with time.
- Selective eating — children consume an extremely narrow range of food, but are generally of appropriate height and weight, indicating that their energy intake is probably sufficient. Sometimes this occurs as part of Asperger syndrome.
- Food avoidance emotional disorder — this term is applied to emotional disorders in which food avoidance is prominent, eg certain cases of depression, obsessive-compulsive disorder or school refusal, but which do not fulfil the diagnostic criteria for anorexia nervosa.
- Functional dysphagia — a rare condition in which the history is of a traumatic episode of choking or difficulty swallowing, followed by food avoidance, which is usually selective and which may lead to weight loss.
- Pervasive refusal syndrome — profound and pervasive refusal to eat, drink, walk, talk, or engage in any form of self-care.

Routine laboratory investigations should include serum electrolytes, liver enzymes, full blood count, renal function, glucose tolerance, full protein and albumin.

Essential information for patient and family
- In children and adolescents, some eating disorders (anorexia nervosa and pervasive refusal syndrome) represent potentially life-threatening conditions that impede physical, emotional and behavioural growth and development.
- If treated soon after onset, child and adolescent eating disorders have a relatively good prognosis; however, if not treated they may become chronic conditions by adulthood.
- In severe cases of pre-pubertal anorexia nervosa, the medical consequences may be irreversible. For example, growth retardation; delayed puberty may result in sterility and incomplete development of secondary sex characteristics; and impaired acquisition of peak bone mass during the second decade of life may result in osteoporosis in adulthood.

General management and advice to patients and families[262]
Eating disorders are serious conditions with a high lifetime mortality, mainly from suicide.

The GP can undertake early simple steps to treat an eating disorder with the help of the practice nurse, counsellor and/or dietician.

Anorexia nervosa
- Family involvement is essential for any intervention with children and adolescents.[263]
- The patient, parents and other family members need information and education about the disorder.
- Expect denial from the patient. Encourage and empower parents to be in charge concerning the child's health, eating and safety. Emphasis should be placed on empowering parents as controllers of the patient's food intake.

- Weigh the patient weekly and chart their weight. Set manageable goals in agreement with the patient and their family; for example, aim for a 0.5 kg weight increase per week. For patients who are denying the illness, setting the task of gaining weight can often be usefully presented as 'diagnostic' — someone who is not suffering from an eating disorder should be able to gain weight relatively easily.
- Older adolescents might benefit from individual support.

Bulimia nervosa
- Family involvement and providing information and education are equally important as they are in anorexia nervosa.[263]
- Older adolescents might benefit from individual support and the use of appropriate self-help literature.

Medication
- Antidepressant medication (eg fluoxetine up to 60 mg daily) usually helps to reduce the frequency of bingeing and vomiting in some patients with bulimia nervosa, but it is not a cure (*BNF* 4.3.3).
- No psychoactive medication has proven effective with anorexia nervosa. Antidepressant medication may be beneficial for children and adolescents with concurrent depressive disorder.

Liaison and referral
Young people with eating disorders are at risk of other mental health problems, including suicide; therefore, liaison with the Child and Adolescent Mental Health Service (CAMHS) is always recommended.

Anorexia nervosa
- If there is lack of a rapid improvement in eating patterns and weight, refer to the CAMHS or to the more specialist Children and Adolescent Eating Disorder Service, if locally available. Intensive treatments of early-onset anorexia nervosa can prevent many of the more severe consequences from occurring. In addition, evidence indicates that treatment outcomes are more favourable when eating disorders are treated soon after their onset.
- Refer for urgent assessment if there has been rapid weight loss or the body mass index (BMI) of the patient is low. The BMI cut-offs need to be adjusted for growth. Specialist intervention might prevent the need for inpatient treatment, even in individuals who are seriously underweight.

Bulimia nervosa
- Consider referral to CAMHS or a specialist Eating Disorder Service if there is a lack of progress in primary care or if more specific treatments (eg cognitive behavioural therapy or family therapy) are not available.

Resources for patients and families
Eating Disorders Association (EDA) 0845 634 7650 (Youthline [for under 19s] 4.00pm–6.30pm, weekdays)
Email: info@edauk.com; website: http://www.edauk.com
Self-help support groups for sufferers, their relatives and friends. Assists in putting people in touch with sources of help in their own area.
Leaflets are available from the Royal College of Psychiatrists
(http://www.rcpsych.ac.uk): *Anorexia and Bulimia, Changing Minds: Anorexia and Bulimia, Understanding Eating Disorders in Young People and Worries about Weight.*

Emotional disorders with onset specific to childhood — F93

(Clinical term: Emotional disorders with onset specific to childhood Eu93)

Children may experience a number of different emotional disorders. This guideline concerns anxiety disorders and symptoms that are specific to childhood, and is intended for use with children aged 10 years and younger. For anxious adolescents and adult-type emotional disorders that may also be seen in childhood (including obsessive-compulsive disorder and post-traumatic stress disorder), see adult guidelines.

Presenting complaints

Anxiety symptoms in childhood can take a number of forms. Most children experiencing anxiety difficulties will demonstrate behavioural, cognitive or somatic features.

Behavioural features

- Avoidance of feared activities, eg reluctance to go to school or to go swimming; feared objects, eg animals.
- Clinginess or reluctance to separate from trusted adults. This can include refusal to sleep alone.
- Withdrawal. This can take the form of shyness in the presence of strangers or large groups of people. In some cases, a more general withdrawal from people and situations is seen, and in severe cases, children may become mute.
- Tantrums/tearfulness/other outward displays of distress, when asked to engage in a feared activity or to separate from a parent.
- General irritability.

Cognitive features

Many children, especially those of school age, will be able to report cognitive symptoms of anxiety. In particular, they (or more often their parents) report that they worry about feared catastrophes. These worries are often unrealistic, but the child may not recognize this.

Somatic features

Many anxious children report a range of somatic symptoms, including:

- palpitations
- stomach aches, headaches, other aches and pains with no obvious organic cause
- breathlessness
- difficultly getting to sleep
- nausea
- feeling wobbly or 'jelly legs'
- 'butterflies'.

Some may present their anxiety in an entirely physical form, although with further sensitive questioning, evidence of behavioural and cognitive symptoms of anxiety is usually also present.

Differential diagnosis and co-existing conditions

- **'Depressive disorder — F32#'** often co-exists with anxiety and can be very difficult to distinguish in this age group. Marked sleep disturbance, disturbed appetite, dysphoric mood, or tearfulness in the absence of direct anxiety provocation could indicate that a child is depressed.

183

- **'Obsessive-compulsive disorder (OCD) — F42'**, indicated by the presence of marked rituals or compulsive behaviours. Most children have phases of ritualized behaviour, which can usually be distinguished from OCD by the degree of distress caused if a ritual is interrupted, and the number of rituals present at any one stage.
- **'Post-traumatic stress disorder — F43.1'** if the onset of anxiety was preceded by an extremely distressing experience.
- Maltreatment — children who have experienced physical, emotional or sexual abuse are at high risk of developing emotional difficulties; this possibility should always be borne in mind. Concern should be raised when anxiety onset occurs over a short period subsequent to relatively normal development and when no other explanation (eg change of school/family circumstances) is apparent.
- Physical illness — it is important to exclude an organic cause for emotional difficulties, particularly where the child presents with mostly physical symptoms. When physical symptoms occur only in specific situations (eg severe headaches on weekdays, but symptom free at weekends and during school holidays), this is a good indication that they might be anxiety-related. It is then usually safe to conclude that symptoms have a psychological origin.
- Normal behaviour — it is often difficult to diagnose anxiety disorder in young children, because a moderate level of anxiety is normative at certain developmental stages. For example, most toddlers show some anxiety when separated from their primary caregiver; a large minority of pre-school and infant school-aged children will express fears of the dark, animals, monsters/ghosts and the like. These worries should not, on their own, raise too much concern, unless they are causing marked distress for the parent or child, or they interfere with the child's ability to engage in developmentally important activities (eg a child who is unable to sleep in their own bed because they are afraid of the dark).

General management and advice to parents and carers

GPs wishing to manage a case themselves should attempt to determine the factors that might be maintaining or causing the anxiety. Multiple factors should be investigated:

- Is an external problem causing the child to be anxious, for example bullying at school or academic difficulties? This should be addressed in the first instance.
- Is the parent anxious? Anxious children very often have an anxious parent. It is thought that children can learn to be anxious from their parents. Advise parents to minimize their own displays of fear or worry when the child is present. A referral to adult mental health services might also be appropriate.
- Does the parent allow the child to avoid feared activities?
  - Gently explain that the child needs to learn to cope with their fear, and should not be allowed to avoid feared activities.
  - Expose a child with a severe phobia to their fear in a number of graded steps; do not suddenly force them to cope with their fear unsupported. If the practitioner does not feel confident in helping the family to develop this 'hierarchy', a referral to specialist services should be made.
  - Encourage parents to display a calm and confident appearance when their child is being exposed to their fear. If they appear upset at their child's distress, the child will pick this up and will then become more distressed.
- How are brave behaviours being encouraged in the family? Encourage parents to praise and give small rewards for displaying brave behaviour. For example, a shy child might be told, 'If you go into the shop and ask the lady for some sweets, I will give you the money to pay for them'. If the child does not approach the assistant, do not provide sweets on that occasion. School-age children respond well to star charts. The rules for using star charts for brave behaviour are as follows:
  - only focus on one or two behaviours at a time
  - have one star chart per behaviour

— negotiate rules for the star chart, for example 'sleeping in own bed for one night = one star; four stars = trip to the swimming pool'

— ignore mistakes and failures — do not ever mark them on the star chart. Simply carry on awarding stars when they are earned.

- Does the parent have good basic parenting skills? Are they consistent and gentle in their use of discipline, or do they shout a lot, or use smacking? Do they use praise and reward to encourage desirable behaviour? There is evidence that many parents of anxious children have impaired parenting skills. If basic advice on these issues is not adequate to change parenting practice (and it is often very difficult for parents to change), attendance at a parenting class may be helpful. Most communities now have access to parenting classes.
- Does the child have a relatively healthy lifestyle? In particular, parents should be encouraged to:
  — monitor their child's caffeine intake
  — make sure that their child eats regularly
  — establish regular daily routines for their child.

The practitioner should also do the following:

- Reassure parents that anxiety often passes, and by following the advice given above, there is a strong likelihood of a good outcome.
- Educate parents about their child's anxiety. It is often helpful to explain the fight/flight response and its role in causing distressing physical symptoms. Parents often fail to push their child to expose to their fear, because the physical symptoms that this elicits are so worrying. Strongly emphasize that these symptoms are *not harmful* to the child.

Medication
Medication is not advised for this age group.

Referral
Referral to specialist mental health services should be considered in the following circumstances:

- When the child has multiple symptoms of anxiety; for example, he/she is very afraid of dogs and distressed by separation from parents.
- When anxiety threatens to interfere with education; for example, the child is very reluctant to go to school, and the parent is not managing to maintain full attendance.
- When symptoms are threatening the achievement of other developmentally important goals; for example, a shy child who is reluctant to mix with other children.
- When the child or parent is very distressed by the symptom(s).
- Where there are co-morbid behaviour problems.
- Where there is felt to be risk of significant harm to the child or other person. Refer to specialist services as an emergency.

Catching anxiety problems early may have long-term benefits. Therefore, where good mental health services are available, the GP should consider referring all cases of anxiety to specialist services, no matter how minor.

Resources for patients and families

Child Anxiety Network (CAN)
www.childhoodanxietynetwork.org
A US-based resource for parents, teachers and health workers regarding childhood anxiety disorders.

Helping your Anxious Child: A Step by Step Guide for Parents by RM Rapee, S Spence, V Cobham and Wignall. New Harbinger Publications, 2000.
A self-help book for parents.

School refusal

Presentation

The commonest ages of presentation are at five and 11 (because of school transitions), and 14–15 (because of accumulating social and academic pressures).

- The child is reluctant to leave home and attend school. There are often physical complaints, such as abdominal pain, headache, sore throat, often with no signs of physical illness. The symptoms are typically worse on weekday mornings and absent at weekends and holidays. Some children complain of anxiety symptoms that include a racing heart, shaking, sweating, difficulty breathing, butterflies in the tummy or nausea, pins and needles. All symptoms are likely to be interpreted as signs of physical illness; the clue is that they subside during school holidays or on Friday evenings, or are present only in the morning. Attempts by the parents to insist on attendance result in heightened distress, or temper outbursts.
- The child may express fears about the school environment (usually bullying, social ostracism or difficulty with school work), or they may be fearful about leaving the home because of worries such as family illness, death or disability, or maternal depression with threats of self-harm. Often, the child cannot voice these fears, and then they can only be guessed at.
- There is often a history of separation difficulties on first starting school.
- Background family factors include ineffectual organization and discipline, often with an absent or uninvolved father, emotional over-involvement with the child, with excessive anxiety about physical symptoms, and difficulties seeking or using help from teachers when school problems first emerge.
- There may be an underlying depressive disorder or generalized anxiety. School refusal can be an expression of a particular fear or phobia or a manifestation of generalized anxiety. Pointers to this can include social withdrawal or avoidance. In depressive disorder, symptoms such as loss of interest and enjoyment may pre-date the school attendance problem. Some children with an anxiety disorder show no symptoms so long as they are off school.

Differential diagnosis

Truancy is the wilful avoidance of school without parental knowledge and is less likely to present in primary care. In contrast, the whereabouts of school refusers are usually known to parents. Some children have features of both these conditions.

A third possibility is that parents might wilfully keep their child away from school for reasons of their own. Genuine illness such as asthma or migraine may be combined with a school refusal picture. This can be due to the main caregiver having a specific reason to be anxious, such as having had a relative who died from asthma, or from a brain tumour.

Essential information for parents and carers

- The outcome is best in younger children and those who have been out of school for a short time.
- A change of school is usually unhelpful because the problems tend to recur in the new setting.
- Parents need to work together and agree a firm and consistent approach to their child's difficulties.
- It is crucially important for there to be good communication with the school.

General management and advice to parents and carers

- Provide a rapid consultation to exclude physical illness and give reassurance about fitness for school.
- Explore with the child and parents the source of the child's anxieties about attending school/leaving home, and deal with these as far as possible.
- Exclude an underlying depression that might need treatment or referral.

The following steps will enable many children to return to school successfully:

- Establish parental agreement for the goal of the child's return to school.
- Encourage the parents to make close links with a key member of the school staff, to work out and support school return plans and deal with issues such as bullying or academic difficulties.
- The child's return to school may need to be in small steps with consolidation of success at each stage.
- The plans usually involve parents taking the child to school until confidence is restored, and the father's involvement in this is often crucial to success.
- Encourage parents to take a firm and consistent line over keeping to the school return plans. There may be an upsurge of distress from their child to start with, which needs to be managed calmly, and praise given when the child succeeds.
- Once the child is back in school, they may experience a recurrence of some anxiety about returning to school after holidays or illnesses. Prompt action is needed to ensure the attendance problem does not recur.

Medication

- In general, school refusal should be managed without medication.
- A depressive disorder might require antidepressants.
- Co-existent physical illness such as migraine may require its own dietary or pharmacological treatment.

Liaison and referral

- If parents feel the child is too ill to attend school, and will not accept the reassurance of the primary care team, referral to a paediatrician for reassurance can be helpful.
- Referral to the Educational Social Worker (Educational Welfare Officer) will be needed for children with persistent school attendance problems. It is their role to link with the school and other sources of help as necessary. Sometimes, parents are threatened with court proceedings; an early approach by the parent to this service can make this less likely.
- Parents can ask the school to refer their child to an educational psychologist or special needs teacher within the school to look for possible undetected academic difficulties.
- The local Child and Adolescent Mental Health Services (CAMHS) might be needed to assess the child's level of depression or anxiety, or to help parents establish authority and control.
- In some areas, a local tutorial unit may provide a valuable halfway house between school and the social isolation of staying at home that is more acceptable to the young person than returning to a large school.
- Home tutors can play a useful role with persistent school refusers by helping them to make the transition between home and school, or between home and tutorial unit, then tutorial unit and school.

Resources for parents

Advisory Centre for Education (ACE) 0808 800 5793 (general advice line)
Website: http://www.ace-ed.org.uk
Independent advice centre for parents, offering free advice on many topics including exclusion from school, bullying, special educational needs and school admission appeals.

Young Minds Parent information line 0800 018 2138
Website: http://www.youngminds.org.uk
Produces books and leaflets about young people's mental health and offers seminars and training.
A leaflet is available from the Royal College of Psychiatrists (http://www.rcpsych.ac.uk): *Factsheet 9: Children Who Do Not Go To School.*

Substance misuse in young people — F10, F11#*

(Clinical term: Mental and behavioural disorders due to use of alcohol Eu10, Mental and behavioural disorders due to use of opioids Eu11)

Substance misuse in young people should be considered in the context of 'normal' adolescent risk-taking and experimentation: 65% of young people (aged under 18) will experiment with illegal drugs; 96% of this experimentation is with cannabis and only 4% go on to regular abuse and long-term problems. Polydrug use is common as part of the 'club scene' in older adolescents, so a variety of substances — legal and illegal — are used on a sporadic basis.

Presenting complaints

Presentation is often at the instigation of others (parents, teachers, social services, criminal justice), often precipitated by physical, psychological or social 'events'. Young people's advisory services may suggest GP consultation to a young person where they feel significant medical problems may arise.

Diagnostic features

May be divided into physical, psychological and social features but the patient will usually present with a mixture of these.

- Physical:
  — respiratory symptoms caused by smoking
  — peri-oral and peri-nasal lesions caused by inhalation or snorting
  — physical injuries incurred during intoxication
  — agitation after polydrug or prolonged use
  — needle tracks, thrombosis or abscesses owing to intravenous use
  — withdrawal syndromes.
- Psychological:
  — mood changes: depression on withdrawal of stimulants, irritability as part of withdrawal syndrome
  — acute mental disorders, psychosis, confusion, etc.
  — deliberate self-harm or suicide attempt.
- Social:
  — deteriorating educational performance
  — family conflict
  — crime: petty associated with intoxication; theft to provide funds; 'dealing' as part of more serious association with drug culture.

Substance *misuse* is defined as use that is medically, legally or socially unacceptable (therefore potentially subject to changing levels of acceptability). This might apply to 'legal' substances such as tobacco in a young person over 16 if there is potential physical or social harm caused by its use.

Risk factors for substance misuse include the following:

- Living in an area of high 'usage'
- 'Social' factors. For example, parental conflict, separation, divorce; physical or sexual abuse; neglect; poor monitoring or supervision; family history of substance misuse

---

*The current ICD-10 classification code does not distinguish between adults and children and adolescents, nor does the clinical term code.

- 'Psychological' factors, such as psychological distress, psychiatric disorder, conduct and emotional disorder
- 'Exclusion' factors, such as unemployment, truancy and criminal activities.

Harmful use is a subclassification of misuse, where actual physical or psychological harm ensues (for example blood-borne virus infections with needle use; overdose and death with solvent use; cardiovascular disease (embolus etc); injuries during intoxication; and social exclusion). Not all misuse leads to harm but the risk of this is significant, even at first use of some substances.

Dependence is diagnosed if at least three of the following criteria have been present in the preceding 12 months:

- narrowing of the substance repertoire
- persistent substance use, despite evidence of its harmful consequences
- difficulties in controlling the use of the substance
- neglect of interests and an increased amount of time taken to obtain the substance or recover from its effects
- evidence of tolerance such that higher doses are required to achieve the same effect
- compulsion: a strong desire to take the substance
- a withdrawal syndrome when substance use ceases or is reduced. The young person might also report the use of substances to relieve the withdrawal symptoms.

Differential diagnosis

Substance misuse may be a 'symptom' of an underlying psychological problem.

- **'Deliberate self-harm'** — intoxication or overdose may not be accidental; an underlying suicidal intent should be suspected because substance use is strongly linked to suicide.
- Affective disorder.
- Anxiety disorder.
- **'Eating disorders — F50'.**
- **'Psychotic disorder — F20#'.**
- **'Personality disorders — F60-69'.**
- **'Attention-deficit/hyperactivity disorder — F90'.**
- Acute or chronic confusional state.

Essential information for patient and family

- Although substance misuse in young people is very common and often 'on–off', it is occasionally fatal and should be taken seriously.
- Substance misuse in young people can be a 'symptom' of an underlying psychological problem that itself requires treatment.
- If identified early, there is less likelihood of progression to a more severe condition, as well as social, psychological and physical consequences.
- Even if the problem has progressed, there is benefit in reducing or stopping and in social 'interventions'.
- Engagement and retention in treatment and family support are key, even if the long-term goal of abstinence cannot be immediately achieved.
- Voluntary organizations and drug services and agencies provide valuable support and are often the most appropriate source of help.

General management and advice to patient and family

- Confidentiality and access to services for young people need specific consideration. Local services will have well-formulated policies on confidentiality about which the primary care team needs to be aware.
- Instil positive expectations of success and offer support and encouragement.
- Assess motivation for psychological change.
- Give advice on cessation and harm reduction (eg 'safe levels' of drinking).

- Confirmatory urine/saliva analysis, information (from professionals, family and friends), regular monitoring and review of compliance represent satisfactory co-operation with agreed treatment options and plan.
- Discuss a *referral* plan with the young person and family and obtain their support for it, within the confines of medical confidentiality and consent.
- Management options include counselling, motivational enhancement, cognitive behavioural therapy, family therapy and group therapy. The choice depends on the nature and extent of the problem and which approach appears most appropriate and suitable for a particular young person and their family.

Medication

A diagnosis of definite clinical dependence is necessary for prescribing. Only exceptionally should GPs prescribe — with specialist advice, support and supervision. Almost all medications are not licensed for patients under 18.

Referral

Community drug and alcohol services for young people are usually the initial source of help.

Early referral for specialist assessment or admission may be necessary for the following:

- severe physical illness
- co-morbid severe mental illness
- abuse of multiple substances
- frequent relapses of substance misuse
- unstable social circumstances, living alone, homelessness.

Resources for patients and families

DrugScope 020 7928 1211
Email: services@drugscope.org.uk; website: http://www.drugscope.org.uk

ChildLine 0800 1111 (24-hour helpline)
Website: http://www.childline.org.uk
Telephone service for all children and young people providing confidential counselling, support and advice on any issue. Parents can also write to ChildLine.

Drinkline National Alcohol Helpline 0800 917 8282 (11am–7pm, Monday–Friday)
Website: http://www.wrecked.co.uk
For young people. Provides confidential information, help and advice about drinking.

HIT http://www.hit.org.uk
Leaflets are available from the Royal College of Psychiatrists (http://www.rcpsych.ac.uk): Factsheet 34: Mental Health and Growing Up, Second Edition: *Drug and Alcohol Misuse*, and Factsheet 35 (for parents and teachers): Mental Health and Growing Up, Second Edition: *Alcohol and Drugs — What Parents Need to Know*.

Unexplained medical symptoms — F45.0, including chronic fatigue — G93.3*†

Presenting complaints
- Recurrent physical complaints unexplained by a medical disorder.
- Common symptoms are abdominal pains, headaches, muscle and joint pains.
- Less commonly seen is an inability to control or lack of sensitivity in parts of the body, sensory deficits, sudden and unexpected spasmodic movements resembling epileptic seizures.
- Fatigue is commonly associated with other unexplained symptoms or sometimes it can be the main presenting symptom.

Diagnostic features
- There are recurrent, persistent, medically and psychiatrically unexplained physical symptoms.
- There are often several simultaneous physical symptoms.
- There may be marked sleep and appetite changes.
- Children with chronic fatigue are tired, easily fatigued and exhibit a poor response to rest.
- There is impairment resulting from symptoms, most noticeably school absence.
- There are frequently associated mood or behavioural changes or full co-morbid psychiatric (often emotional [anxiety, depressive]) disorders.
- Pain and chronic fatigue can last for months or years.
- Sudden loss of movement may have a more acute course.
- It often follows a trigger illness (eg an episode of diarrhoea and vomiting leading to recurrent abdominal pains; trauma in loss of movement; a 'flu'-type infection or Epstein–Barr virus infection in chronic fatigue).
- There may be parental concern about the symptoms and medical consultations.
- Any child who has missed 15 school days in a month should have the cause assessed.

Differential diagnosis
- A full history and physical examination are necessary. Referral to specialist paediatric services will be required when indicated medically, in protracted cases and in severely impaired children.
- Investigations are as for adult guidelines, to exclude an explanatory medical disorder. For example, investigations for chronic fatigue should include full blood count, CRP (or ESR), thyroid function tests, urea and electrolytes, blood sugar and liver function tests, tests for glandular fever (link to EBV). If clinically indicated, screening for gluten-sensitive enteropathy or autoimmune disease might be helpful.
- School phobia (phobic anxiety disorder).
- 'Generalized anxiety —F41.1' and/or 'Panic disorder — F41.0'.
- 'Depressive disorder — F32#'.
- 'Eating disorders — F50'.

Essential information for patient and family

---

*The current ICD-10 classification does not distinguish between adults and adolescents.
†See page 45 for discussion of coding of chronic fatigue. [cross-reference to adult CFS guideline]

- Recurrent unexplained physical symptoms (eg headaches, abdominal pains and fatigue) are very frequent in children and adolescents (about 10% in the general population). Severely incapacitating problems are far less common.
- Few children develop explanatory physical illness at a later stage.
- Encouraging maintenance of or gradual resumption of normal activities is helpful.

General management and advice to patient and family

- The fact that the symptoms are not an indication of medical illness does not mean that they are not real or only 'in the child's mind'.
- Explore carefully what the child and parents think about what the symptoms mean and give detailed explanations about what illness the child does NOT have.
- Enquire about any perceived stresses to the child in school (working too hard, putting themselves under pressure, preoccupied with criticism from teachers or unsympathetic pupils, occasionally bulling) and at home (discord, separations, other stresses).
- Help the child and family look for solutions for the above (including relief of school pressure), as this can help towards recovery.
- Understand parental concerns about the child.
- Support the development of a regular sleep routine and dietary advice, when appropriate.
- Encourage reduction of attention (verbal and non-verbal) to physical symptoms and an increase in joint pleasant and enjoyable activities.
- Relaxation exercises can be helpful with symptoms such as headaches.
- Emphasize the importance of gradual re-integration to school (total or gradually increasing). Some sort of educational support is often indicated, and home tuition may be appropriate; if so, it is usually short term.
- Encourage parents to bring the child to the surgery if in doubt about symptoms, rather than missing school.

Medication

- SSRIs are suitable, if there is associated depression or incapacitating anxiety.
- The usual pain-relieving agents can be helpful sometimes.

Liaison and referral

- Liaison with school and/or educational department is often helpful.
- Community therapists (eg physiotherapists or local pain services) might be helpful in some cases.
- Refer to paediatric services when further medication investigations and opinion are required, and in protracted or incapacitating cases.
- Refer to Child and Adolescent Mental Health Services, ideally liaison psychiatric services if available, if there is suspected:
  — co-morbid psychiatric disorders
  — suicidal risk
  — no improvement despite the above measures.

Resources for patient and family

Association of Young People with ME (AYME) 01908 373 300
Email: info@ayme.org.uk; website: http://www.ayme.org.uk
Gives support and advice to young people with ME.

Chronic Fatigue Syndrome: A Clinical Perspective. A Sonkey and MJJ Thompson
University of Southampton, distributed by Oxford Education Resources Ltd., PO
Box 106, Kidlington, Oxford OX5 1JY; website: http://www.oer.co.uk.
Video. Young people affected by Chronic fatigue syndrome and their parents
describe the condition. Specialists explain what causes the condition, and why it can
be so difficult to diagnose. The successful multidisciplinary regime adopted by
Southampton is described; this combines a steady controlled increase in physical
and mental activity, a structured daily timetable and a graded exercise programme,
with (as appropriate) medication, cognitive behavioural therapy and family therapy.

LEARNING DISABILITY

Learning disability — F70

(Also referred to as 'mental retardation' in ICD-10. Clinical term: Mild mental retardation Eu70)

Presenting complaints

At birth:

- Unusual faces (dysmorphia)
- Poor thriving, eg Down syndrome.

In children:

- Delay in usual development (eg sitting up, walking, speaking and toilet training)
- Difficulty managing school work as well as other children, because of learning disabilities
- Behavioural problems, especially overactive behaviour and poor socialization
- Often, these children are the target of stigma and bullying, because of their different appearance, abilities and behaviour.

In adolescents:

- Difficulties with peers, leading to reduced social opportunities and isolation
- Inappropriate sexual behaviour
- Difficulties in making the transition to adulthood, especially in terms of forming relationships and developing independence.

In adults:

- Difficulties in everyday functioning, requiring extra support (eg cooking and cleaning), with consequent increased costs of living
- Problems with normal social development and establishing an independent life in adulthood (eg finding work, marriage and child-rearing)
- Inappropriate sexual behaviour and other antisocial behaviour.

Diagnostic features

- Slow or incomplete mental development resulting in:
  — learning difficulties
  — social adjustment problems (which are present from early in life).
- The range of severity includes:
  — severe learning disability (usually identified before two years of age. The individual requires help with daily tasks throughout life and is capable of only simple speech)
  — moderate learning disability (usually identified between ages three and five. The individual is able to do simple work with support, and needs guidance or support in daily activities)
  — mild or borderline learning disability (usually identified during school years. The individual is limited in school work, but is able to live alone and maintain some form of paid employment).

Differential diagnosis and co-existing conditions

Learning disability is associated with an increased prevalence of many other disorders. The most common include the following:

- 'Epilepsy — G40, G41' (25% people with learning disability and 50% of those with severe learning disability).
- Hypothyroidism (people with Down syndrome).
- Physical disabilities and dysmorphia (30%).

- Incontinence (10%).
- Hearing impairments (40%).
- Visual impairments (40%).
- **'Autism spectrum disorders — F84'** (10% individuals with learning disability and 30% of those with moderate to severe learning disability).
- Psychiatric and behavioural disorders (at least 35%).
- **'Dementia — F00#'** (people with Down syndrome and those over 50).

Diagnosis of these conditions can be made harder by unusual presentations of the illness; for example, irritability (which might present as agitation or even aggression) may be an indication of pain or emotional distress.

The following may also interfere with performance at school:

- sensory problems (eg deafness)
- specific learning difficulties (eg dyslexia)
- attention-deficit/hyperactivity disorder
- motor disorders (eg cerebral palsy)
- autism in children of normal intellectual ability.

Malnutrition, extreme social deprivation, or chronic medical illness can cause developmental delays. Most causes of learning disabilities cannot be cured. The more common, treatable causes of learning disability include hypothyroidism, lead poisoning, and some inborn errors of metabolism (eg phenylketonuria).

Essential information for patient and family

- Early training can help a person with learning disability towards self-care and independence.
- People with learning disability are capable of loving relationships and have the same needs as any other person for love, security, play, friendship, clear boundaries and limits on behaviour.
- The person's intellect and skills must be accurately assessed, so that key learning needs are determined and they are helped to attain the appropriate level of independence, and use appropriate support services where necessary. The functional assessment should match the realistic social expectations.
- Sudden changes in behaviour may indicate physical illness and the need for medical examination.

General management and advice to patient and family

- Reward effort. Allow disabled children and adults to function at the highest level of their ability in school, work and within the family.
- Teach the same set of social rules as to other children.
- Advise families that learning and practising skills will be helpful, but that 'miracle cures' do not exist. It is usually impossible to predict, at diagnosis, how a child with learning disability will function as an adult. However, with careful long-term follow-up, it does become clearer what an individual may attain, in terms of independence and need for support.
- Families may feel conflicting emotions — intense love, disappointment, anger, great loss — and may take time and continuing support to adjust to being the parent of a child with learning disability and to deal with the different life stages and transitions (eg leaving school, employment, social life and sexuality, death of parents). It may be helpful to talk things through with someone who has the same experiences (see Resources below). Preparing a transition plan that involves the young person, their family and relevant services is good practice for when they leave school, whether or not the child has a statement of special educational need.
- Inform families that people with learning disability frequently under-report illness. Arranging regular health screening can be useful actively to seek out treatable sensory disorders, depression, obesity, skin infections, diabetes and other conditions.

It is valuable to review healthcare at times of transition (eg school leaving) and of family illness. Creating a health action plan is one recommended way to be proactive in maintaining health.[264]

- Primary-care teams should make a regular slot (eg every six months) to review patients with learning disability, and keep a recall register. There is evidence that these patients have health needs that are only detected by this kind of proactive contact.
- Encourage the patient to see the same doctor and nurse at every planned appointment, if possible, in order to build trust and reduce problems in communication.
- Invite a carer to come too; carers who know the patient well are invaluable as informants.
- Allow extra time for the appointment so that communication and examination can occur at a pace that suits both staff and patient.
- Use additional user-friendly literature to prepare the patient for examinations such as well-woman checks (see Resources below).

Medication

- Except in the case of certain physical or psychiatric disorders, medical treatment cannot improve cognitive function.
- Careful treatment of psychiatric problems can substantially improve functioning, by promoting improved concentration and learning. It is helpful to review social networks and social support in addition to other treatment.
- Learning disability can occur with other disorders that require medical treatment (eg seizures, cerebral palsy and psychiatric illness such as depression).
- A good rule regarding psychiatric medication is to 'start low' (dose) and 'go slow' (increasing dose) to avoid polypharmacy.
- Unnecessary medication should be avoided, and medication reviewed regularly, because side-effects and idiosyncratic reactions are common. People with learning disability underreport side-effects; therefore, consideration should be given to proactive checks (eg blood levels of anticonvulsants).

Referral

Referral to a community paediatric team or learning disability services (depending on local arrangement) is advised when the learning disability is first identified, to help plan for education and specialist care. Psychiatrists specializing in learning disability may be skilled in investigating and treating epilepsy as well as psychiatric illness. Referral for specialist support is also indicated:

- where there are significant changes in behaviour, which persist for longer than one month
- where there is significant weight change, which persists for longer than one month, to exclude emotional or psychiatric disorder
- following the death of a carer or close relative, because there is increased risk of pathological grief.

For further information about learning disability, see *Once a Day* NHS Executive guidelines for primary healthcare teams, March 1999. Department of Health, PO Box 410, Wetherby LS23 7LN.

Resources for patients and families

Association for Spina Bifida and Hydrocephalus (ASBAH) 01733 555 988
(9am–5pm Monday–Friday)
Website: http://www.asbah.org

Downs Syndrome Association 020 8682 4001 (10am–4pm, Tuesday–Thursday)
Email: info@downs-syndrome.org.uk; website: http://www.downs-syndrome.org.uk.
Information and support for people with Down syndrome and their families.

Mencap http://www.mencap.org.uk
England and Wales: 020 7696 5593 (information line)
Northern Ireland: 0345 636 227 (family advisory service line)
Information and support for people with a learning disability and their families in
the UK. Provides residential, employment, further education and leisure and
holiday services.

Scope 0800 626216 (helpline)
Website: http://www.scope.org.uk
Information, emotional support and support groups for people with cerebral palsy
and their families. Only some people with cerebral palsy have learning disability in
addition to their physical disabilities.

Contact a Family 0808 808 3555 (helpline 10am–4pm, Monday–Friday)
Website: http://www.cafamily.org.uk
Works across the UK to support families caring for children with any disability. It is
particularly useful where there is a rare condition.

Circles Network 01788 816 671
Website: http://www.circlesnetwork.org.uk
Provides information on setting up circles of friends and circles of support to help
people with a learning disability have a more interesting social life.

I CAN 0870 010 4066
Email: info@ican.org.uk; website: http://www.ican.org.uk
National educational charity for children and young people with speech and
language difficulties.

**Association to Aid the Sexual and Personal Relationships of People with a
Disability (SPOD)** 020 7607 8851
Website: http://www.spod-uk.org
An online resource exploring the issues of personal and sexual relationships of
people with a disability
Benefits Enquiry Line 0800 882 200
For information about Social Security benefits for disabled people.

The Family Fund 0845 130 45 42
Website: http://www.familyfundtrust.org.uk
An independent organization helping families caring for a child with severe
disabilities. They may help pay one-off costs such as holidays and washing
machines.
Leaflets are available from the Royal College of Psychiatrists
(http://www.rcpsych.ac.uk): *Depression in People with Learning Disability* and
Patient's Rights and Monies
Leaflets are available from the Mental Health Foundation, tel: 020 7802 0300;
website: http://www.mentalhealth.org.uk: *Learning Disabilities and the Family: the
Young Child with Learning Disabilities*, and *Learning Disabilities and the Family: the
Teenager with a Severe Learning Disability*.

Books Beyond Words is a series of picture-books for adolescents and adults who cannot read. They can be used by parents, carers, GPs, nurses and others to help communication about important topics. Titles include *Feeling Blue,* about depression, *Going to the Doctor, Going to the Hospital, Going to Outpatients, Keeping Healthy Down Below, When Dad Died, Making Friends.* The Royal College of Psychiatrists, 17 Belgrave Square, London SW1X 8PG; tel: 020 7235 2351; website: www.rcpsych.ac.uk/publications/index.htm

The Foundation for People with Learning Disabilities produces the information booklets *Get Moving* (for people with learning disabilities who are thinking about leaving home), *Leaving Home, Moving On* (to help parents who are planning leaving home with their son or daughter), *Learning Disabilities and The Family: The Young Child, Learning Disabilities and The Family: The Teenager.* Publications, The Mental Health Foundation, 7th Floor, 83 Victoria Street, London SW1H 0HW, tel: 020 7802 0301; Email: fpld@fpld.org.uk; website: http://www.learningdisabilities.org.uk

Assessment under the Mental Health Act England and Wales 1983: a basic guide for General Practitioners

Introduction

General Practitioners can be involved in Mental Health Act assessments in a variety of settings:

- Home — the patient may be causing serious concern to family or neighbours.
- Hospital — the patient may have already been admitted informally, or even admitted for treatment for a physical illness and is now needing to be detained under an emergency, assessment or treatment section of the Act as they meet the criteria for mental disorder under the Act and are unwilling to accept treatment as an informal patient.
- Police station — the patient may have been taken to a police station following arrest for an offence or as a place of safety after being found in a public place exhibiting symptoms of mental disorder (section 136 of the Act).

Use of the Mental Health Act 1983

The Mental Health Act 1983 makes statutory provision for the compulsory assessment, care and treatment in hospital of patients with a mental disorder as defined in section 1 of the Act. The patient may be in the community or in hospital at the time of assessment.

Mental disorder comprises mental illness, mental impairment, severe mental impairment and psychopathic disorder. In the Act, mental illness is not defined but is a matter for clinical judgement.

The most common civil sections of the Act under which patients are compulsorily admitted to a hospital are:

- section 2: admission to hospital for up to 28 days for assessment
- section 3: admission to hospital for up to six months for treatment
- section 4: admission on an emergency basis for up to 72 hours.

Criteria for detention under the Mental Health Act 1983

Compulsory admission for assessment and/or treatment can only occur when:

- the patient is suffering from mental disorder within the meaning of section 1 of the Act
- the mental disorder is sufficiently serious to need further assessment and/or medical treatment in hospital
- the patient needs to be compulsorily admitted under the Act in the interests of his or her own health or safety, and/or for the protection of other people.

When assessments under the Act may be needed

GPs are frequently approached in the first instance by a relative or other carer of a patient, worried about the mental health of a patient. Following his/her own assessment it is normal practice for the GP to request a domiciliary visit by a consultant psychiatrist where this is warranted.

If, following an examination by the consultant psychiatrist, a patient needs admission to hospital and it appears that informal admission is not appropriate, an Approved Social Worker (ASW) should be contacted to make arrangements for the patient to be formally assessed for admission to hospital under the Act.

The Act allows the compulsory admission of a patient who is very distressed or ill (for example, actively psychotic or manic) solely in order to improve their health, even if they are not thought to be at immediate risk of harming themselves or others.

There will be situations where an emergency admission is required and it may not be possible or practicable for a consultant psychiatrist to examine a patient before a request for a compulsory admission to hospital is made. In these situations the GP should approach the ASW directly.

Where the patient is thought to need hospital admission but is unwilling to be admitted to hospital as an informal patient the ASW will make the arrangements for the patient to be formally assessed for admission under the Act. The ASW will usually ask the GP to carry out a medical examination and, if appropriate, provide a written medical recommendation for detention of the patient under the Act.

A patient may also, in some circumstances, be detained by the police under section 136 of the Act to enable him/her to be examined by a registered medical practitioner and interviewed by an ASW. Where this occurs the patient's GP, where known, will usually be contacted.

The Act cannot be used for the compulsory treatment of addictions unless the criteria for detention under the Act are also met.

The Medical Recommendations

The recommendations required for the purposes of an application for admission to hospital under the Act have to be provided by two doctors ('registered medical practitioners') who have personally examined the patient either jointly or separately. In the case of an application for an 'emergency admission' under section 4, however, only one medical recommendation is required. This recommendation may also be provided by a GP.

GPs may apply to become 'section 12 approved'. The local Strategic Health Authority should be able to provide further information.

First medical recommendation: Every application must be supported by a recommendation from a practitioner approved under section 12(2) of the Act 'as having special experience in the diagnosis or treatment of mental disorder'. Health Service Guideline (HSG) (96)3, available from the Department of Health sets out criteria for approval under section 12(2) of the Act. In the wake of devolution of powers to Strategic Health Authorities with effect from 1 April 2002, revised guidance was issued (December 2002) to recognize the new structure and impact. The revised guidance indicated that the regional and approval arrangements that existed prior to 1 April 2002 would effectively continue to operate as before. (Both publications are available on the Department of Health website at www.doh.gov.uk.)

Second medical recommendation: In accordance with section 12(2) of the Act the second recommendation shall, if practicable, be provided by a doctor with previous acquaintance' with the patient unless the doctor making the first medical recommendation has previous acquaintance with the patient. GPs are often best placed to undertake this role, and do not need to be specially approved under the Act to do so. Where there is no obvious person to provide the second medical recommendation, for example, because the patient is not registered with a GP or is not known to local mental health services, another section 12 approved doctor is usually asked to assess the patient. In cases where this is not practicable any registered medical practitioner may provide the second recommendation as long as they do not work in the same hospital as the doctor providing the first recommendation.

How to arrange a Mental Health Act assessment

A Mental Health Assessment is activated by telephoning the Duty ASW. Other arrangements may be in place depending upon local policy.

Where a GP does not have a telephone number for the ASW service it should be possible to contact the duty ASW both during and out of normal office hours by ringing the general telephone number for the social services authority or local council.

He or she will need the following information:

- name
- date of birth
- address
- reason for assessment
- previous history, including name of key worker, next of kin (if known) and past history of violence or self harm (if known).

He or she will need enough information to decide if there is the possibility of an admission under the Mental Health Act 1983 and to decide that the full assessment process is warranted.

Management of the patient should be discussed with the duty ASW (or the duty consultant, depending on local policy).

The ASW will then take responsibility for co-ordinating the assessment, bringing relevant papers, ensuring the process complies with the law and arranging for the transport of the patient.

Before the assessment

Information is an important component of the assessment. If you can access your records, check for previous history and response to treatment, risk of neglect, violence or self-harm, and any known contact names. If there is a relative or informant, ask about the recent situation, its duration, whether there is any support, whether there have been threats or violence and if the patient is known to carry or have access to weapons. Liaise with the ASW about directions, access to premises, where to meet and the need for police attendance.

It is good practice if the medical assessments take place jointly with the ASW at the same agreed time because it is safer, communication is better and disruption of the patient is minimized. Although if this is not possible, they are legally allowed to be 5 days apart. In all cases, the two doctors must discuss their decision.

If the patient is suffering from the short-term effect of drugs, alcohol or sedative medication, discussion should take place about deferring the assessment until a more productive interview can take place.

If access to home is denied, section 135 (warrant to search for and remove patients) may need to be used. This warrant is obtained from a Magistrates' Court by an ASW.

During the assessment

Except in the case of emergencies, an application for assessment (section 2, 28 days) or treatment (section 3, 6 months) must be founded on two medical recommendations from:

- a medical practitioner approved under section 12 of the Act as having special experience in the diagnosis or treatment of mental disorder (usually a psychiatrist, often the duty consultant or specialist registrar)
- a doctor with prior knowledge of the patient (ideally the GP).

The GP and others in the primary care team often have prior knowledge of the patient, including access to records and an existing relationship with the patient and/or family. This facilitates the assessment. The psychiatrist may not know the patient but often contributes clinical experience and expertise. The ASW makes a more comprehensive assessment of the social aspects of the case and advises on the legal issues that may arise during the process. He or she sees that the patient is interviewed 'in a suitable manner', ie taking into account the guiding principles set out in Chapter 1 of the Code of Practice to the Mental Health Act 1983 (1999).

The patient is interviewed as comfortably as possible with the following questions in mind:

• Is there any possible evidence of mental illness?

• Is there a risk to the health or safety of the patient or a danger to others?

If the answer to both of these questions is yes:

• Will the patient consent to informal admission, and if so, is that realistic based on past experience or aspects of the current interview?
• Are there any community alternatives to admission? eg giving medication at home, CPN visits, crisis services, day hospitals.

All professionals strive to reach a consensus and if the doctors agree to make the medical recommendations for compulsory admission, the ASW makes the application to the admitting hospital managers.

Section 2 is appropriate if there is no previous history, the diagnosis is unclear or no treatment plan is in place.

Section 3 specifies the category of mental disorder and is mainly used for patients already known to the service. If the nearest relative objects to the detention, the application cannot proceed.

Arranging admission

If the decision of the team is to admit the patient, the level of security required should be considered. Arrangements for a bed are usually made by the psychiatrist and for appropriate transport by the ASW. The ASW usually accompanies the patient and delivers the section papers in person. He/she is responsible for securing the premises. The ASW informs the patient and nearest relative of the decision.

If the patient is not admitted

When the patient is not admitted to hospital, a package of follow-up care needs to be agreed with the patient and nearest relative, if appropriate. Arrangements may need to be made to contact mental health or social work teams during working hours to inform them of the assessment and/or to make a referral.

You are entitled to submit a claim form (usually held by the ASW).

This is not intended to be a comprehensive guide to the Mental Health Act 1983. The Code of Practice (1999 version) provides guidance to doctors, managers and staff of hospitals and registered mental nursing homes, and to ASWs on how they should proceed when undertaking duties under the Act.

The Department of Health published guidance to assist GPs in understanding the processes involved in undertaking mental health assessments under the Mental Health Act 1983 and to clarify their role in those processes. It can be accessed on the Department of Health's website on www.doh.gov.uk/mhact1983.htm.

Forms to be used in making medical recommendations for admission to hospital under the Mental Health Act 1983

• First and second medical recommendations must be made on the relevant statutory forms.
• There are different forms for separate and joint medical recommendations and care should be taken to ensure that the correct form is completed in each case. An incorrectly completed form may make an application for detention invalid.
• The second medical recommendation may be completed before the first but the medical examinations must be completed within five clear days of each other.
• The Code of Practice states that 'unless there are good reasons for undertaking separate assessments, assessments should be carried out jointly by the ASW and doctor(s)'. When this is not possible a doctor may undertake the examination, make the recommendation and, where clinically appropriate, leave the scene. However, he/she must make arrangements for the form to be given to the ASW or to the admitting hospital in those instances where the patient is already an in-patient. But 'it is essential that at least one of the doctors undertaking the medical assessment

discusses the patient with the applicant (ASW or nearest relative) and is desirable for both of them to do this'. (Code of Practice, para 2.3).

- Primary Care Trusts (under the umbrella of their respective Strategic Health Authorities) are required to maintain and provide lists of doctors approved under section 12 of the Mental Health Act 1983 as having special experience in the diagnosis or treatment of mental disorder.

Clean and sample copies of these forms are attached at Appendix 1 to the Department of Health's 'Guidance for GPs: Medical Examinations and Medical Recommendations under the Act'. It can be accessed at www.doh.gov.uk/mhact1983.htm.

Key action points for GPs in making assessments and recommendations for admission

These can be accessed at Appendix 2 of the above Guidance.

The role of the 'nearest relative'

The nearest relative has the power to:

- make an application for detention of the patient
- object to an application for the detention of a patient (an application can be made to the county court for the functions of the nearest relative to be transferred to the local Social Services authority or another person if relative objects unreasonably)
- apply to the Hospital Managers for the discharge of the patient (application must be made in writing giving 72 hours notice, patient must be discharged unless within the 72 hours, the RMO reports to Managers that patient is likely to be a danger to self or others)
- receive information about the detention and treatment of a patient.

Payment and claiming fees

Currently the fees payable are £162.70 for section 12 approved doctors and £50.45 for other registered practitioners excluding travel expenses.

Use of the Mental Health (Northern Ireland) Order 1986: a basic guide for general practitioners

The 1986 Mental Health (Northern Ireland) Order provides the legal framework in Northern Ireland for compulsory admission and treatment of patients suffering from mental illness. GPs can be involved in Mental Health Order assessments in different settings:

- *Community*: The patient may be causing serious concern to family or neighbours. An application can be made for compulsory hospital admission for seven days, renewable to 14 days for assessment (Article 4). In extreme circumstances, if access is denied, a warrant authorizing a police constable to secure access may need to be used (Article 129). This warrant is obtained by an approved social worker (ASW), other officer of the Health and Social Services Trust or a police constable from a Justice of the Peace. If the constable has to enter the premises, by force or otherwise, they must be accompanied by a medical practitioner (usually a GP) who will administer medical treatment, if required.
- *Hospital*: The patient may have been admitted informally and now wants to leave or is refusing treatment. An application for assessment involves the patient's own GP (or another practitioner who has previous knowledge of the patient) in attending hospital to give the medical recommendation. A doctor on the staff of the hospital in which it is intended that the assessment should be carried out cannot give the recommendation, except in a case of urgent necessity.

Use of the Mental Health Order

Compulsory admission for assessment of a patient can only occur when:

- they are suffering from a mental disorder of a nature or degree that warrants detention in hospital for assessment (or for assessment followed by medical treatment); and
- failure to detain the patient would create a substantial likelihood of serious physical harm to themselves or to other persons.

Criteria for likelihood of serious physical harm are evidence of one of the following:

- the patient has inflicted, or threatened or attempted to inflict, serious physical harm on themselves
- the patient's judgement is so affected that they are, or would soon be, unable to protect themselves against serious physical harm and that reasonable provision for their protection is not available in the community
- the patient has behaved violently towards other persons or so behaved themselves that other persons are placed in reasonable fear of serious physical harm to themselves.

Mental disorder comprises mental illness, mental handicap, severe mental handicap and severe mental impairment. In the Order, mental illness is defined as a 'state of mind which affects a person's thinking, perceiving, emotion or judgment to the extent that he requires care or medical treatment in his own interests or the interests of other persons'.

The Order cannot be used for the compulsory treatment of addictions, personality disorders or sexual deviancy, unless the above criteria are also met.

How to arrange a Mental Health Order assessment

An application for compulsory admission needs to be made by either the nearest relative (on form 1) or an ASW (form 2), supported by a medical recommendation (form 3), usually the patient's own GP or, if not, a doctor who knows the patient personally and is not (except of urgent necessity) on the staff of the receiving hospital. Guidance on who is considered the 'nearest relative' under the Order can be found on the back of form 1. See www.n-i.nhs.uk

A Mental Health Order assessment is activated by telephoning the duty ASW. An ASW might be essential (in order to make the application) or highly desirable in order to support and advise the relative making the application. The ASW also assesses the social aspects of the case and provides a social report. Telephone them with the following information: name, date of birth, address, reason for assessment, previous history, including name of key worker, next of kin (if known), and past history of violence of self-harm (if known).

They will need enough information to decide if there is the possibility of an admission under the Mental Health Order and that the full assessment process is warranted.

If you want to discuss the management of the patient, either telephone the duty ASW or the duty consultant.

Before the assessment
Information is an important component of the assessment.

- If you can access your records, check for previous history and response to treatment, risk of neglect, violence or self-harm, and any known contact names.
- If there is a relative or informant, ask about the recent situation, its duration, whether there is any support, whether there have been threats or violence and if the patient is known to carry or have access to weapons.
- Contact the duty ASW. An ASW might be essential (in order to make the application) or desirable in order to support and advise the relative who is making the application. Liaise with the ASW about directions, access to premises, where to meet, and the need for police attendance.
- Where no ASW is involved, liaise with the nearest relative or other informant about directions, access to premises, and the need for police attendance. Bring forms 1 and 3 with you (available from the Health and Social Services Trust). Arrange police attendance, if necessary.
- It is good practice (because it is safer, communication is better and disruption of the patient is minimized) for the professionals involved in the application for admission to be present at the same time (although it might be helpful for each to interview the patient separately). Everyone involved should be aware of the need to provide mutual support. In any case, the applicant — whether relative or ASW — must have seen the patient within two days of signing the application and the doctor must examine the patient not less than two days before signing the application.

If the patient is suffering from the short-term effect of drugs, alcohol or sedative medication, discussion should take place about deferring the assessment until a more productive interview can take place.

During the assessment
The team necessary to make an application for compulsory admission is either:

- the nearest relative and a doctor (patient's own GP or doctor who knows the patient personally); or
- an ASW and the patient's own GP or a doctor who knows the patient personally.

Where the nearest relative makes the application, advise them that they can ask for an ASW to consider making the application in their stead (because sometimes making such an application can be detrimental to family relationships).

Where an ASW makes the application, they must consult the nearest relative, unless this causes unreasonable delay. If the nearest relative objects to the application, the ASW must consult another ASW. Where no ASW is involved, a social worker (not necessarily an approved one) must interview the patient as soon as is practicable and provide a social report to the registered medical officer in the receiving hospital.

The patient is interviewed as comfortably as possible, with the following questions in mind:

- Is there any possible evidence of mental illness?
- Is there a substantial risk of serious physical harm to the patient or others?

If the answer to both of these questions is yes:

- Will the patient consent to informal admission? And if so, is that realistic, based on past experience or aspects of the current interview?
- Are there any community alternatives to admission (such as giving medication at home, community mental health nurse visits, crisis services, day hospitals)?

The relatives and, if practicable, other significant informants, are interviewed to find out their views of the patient's needs and whether and in what ways the patient's behaviour is different from their normal behaviour.

All parties strive to reach a *consensus*, and if the doctor agrees to make the medical recommendation for compulsory admission, the social worker or the nearest relative makes the application to the admitting hospital managers.

The doctor's recommendation must be made on form 3 and must include the following information: the grounds, including a clinical description of the mental condition of the patient, for the opinion that the detention is warranted; the evidence for the opinion that failure to detain the patient would create a substantial likelihood of serious physical harm. Examples of what might be considered in assessing the likelihood of serious physical harm include uncontrolled overactivity likely to lead to exhaustion, gross and protracted neglect of diet which would lead to malnutrition, gross neglect of hygiene and personal safety which would create a hazard to the patient or others, disinhibited behaviour likely to lead to serious physical harm to the patient, their family or other persons. A diagnosis of the specific form of mental disorder is not required

Arranging admission

If the decision of the team is to admit the patient, the level of security required should be considered.

If an ASW is involved, arrangements for a bed are usually made by the doctor and by the ASW for appropriate transport, unless an ambulance is required, in which case the doctor arranges this. The ASW usually accompanies the patient and delivers the application papers in person. They are responsible for securing the premises. The ASW informs the patient and nearest relative of the decision.

If no ASW is involved, liaise with the receiving hospital about arrangements for the patient's admission, transport to hospital and the patient's need for care during removal, including medical and nursing escorts if required. Ensure the premises are secured and inform the patient of the decision. The nearest relative may accompany the patient and deliver the application papers.

The patient must be admitted to hospital within two days from the date on which the medical recommendation was signed; otherwise, the authority to detain them expires.

If the patient is not admitted

When the patient is not admitted to hospital, a package of follow-up care needs to be agreed with the patient and nearest relative, if appropriate. Arrangements may need to be made to contact mental health or social work teams during working hours to inform them of the assessment and/or to make a referral.

This is not intended to be a comprehensive guide to the Mental Health Order. Consultation of the Code of Practice, the Guide and the Mental Health Order is recommended.

Use of the Mental Health (Scotland) Act 1984: a basic guide for general practitioners

The 1984 Mental Health (Scotland) Act provides the legal framework in Scotland for compulsory admission and treatment of patients suffering from mental disorder. A new Act — the Mental Health (Care and Treatment) (Scotland) Act 2003 — has been passed by the Scottish Parliament and is expected to come into effect after October 2004 (see below). Until it does, the 1984 Act remains in force.

GPs can be involved in using the Mental Health Act in a variety of circumstances:

- *Emergency recommendation for detention (Section 24)*: This is used where admission is urgently required and use of Section 18 would introduce undesirable delay. Admission under Section 24 allows for a period of 72 hours of assessment. Any doctor can legally make the recommendation, but the consent of a mental health officer (MHO; a social worker with special training) or a near relative must be obtained, wherever practicable.
- *Non-emergency admission for up to six months (Section 18)*: This is used where admission is required less urgently (eg where the patient's mental state deteriorates over time). In practice, this is mainly used for patients known to the service. An application is required from a MHO (or occasionally the nearest relative) and recommendations from a Section-20-approved doctor (usually a psychiatrist, and, where the patient is known to the service, the patient's own consultant psychiatrist) and the GP or another doctor with previous knowledge of the patient.
- *Power of Entry (Section 117)*: This might need to be where a patient with possible mental disorder in the community refuses assessment and help. For example, the patient may be behaving eccentrically, live in very poor conditions, be ill-treated or neglected by others, or alone and unable to care for themselves. This warrant is obtained by a MHO from a Justice of the Peace. It allows a police officer, accompanied by a doctor, to force entry. The person may then be removed to a place of safety, with a view to assessment for admission under Section 24.
- *Treatment of a patient who is on leave of absence*: A detained patient may be allowed out of hospital on 'leave of absence' for up to one year. GPs must only prescribe psychiatric medications that are consistent with the agreed treatment plan, set out on form 9 (where the patient is consenting to treatment) or form 10 (where the patient is not consenting to treatment) – see www.show.scot.nhs.uk. GPs should expect to be told of the conditions of the leave of absence, of the circumstances in which the patient is likely to be recalled to hospital, and the arrangements in relation to treatment.

Use of the Mental Health Act

Compulsory admission can only occur when:

- there is a mental disorder; and
- the patient requires hospital admission in the interest of the health or safety of the patient or the protection of others; and
- such admission cannot be achieved without compulsory measures.

The Act allows the compulsory admission of a patient who is very distressed or ill (eg actively psychotic or manic) solely in order to improve their health, even if they are not thought to be at immediate risk of harming themselves or others.

Mental disorder comprises mental illness, mental impairment, severe mental impairment and persistent disorder manifested only by persistent abnormally aggressive or seriously irresponsible conduct. In the Act, mental illness is not defined but is a matter for clinical judgement, but it excludes those for reasons only of promiscuity or other 'immoral' conduct, sexual deviancy, or dependence on alcohol or drugs (although psychiatric symptoms secondary to drug and alcohol abuse — for example drug-induced paranoid psychosis and Korsakoff psychosis — are included). Mental disorder manifested only by mental impairment or only by abnormally aggressive or seriously irresponsible conduct might be grounds for detention under Section 18 only where treatment in hospital is likely to alleviate or prevent a deterioration in the patient's condition.

Before the assessment

Information is an important component of the assessment, including information about domestic, employment and social factors, as well as a person's mental state.

- If you can access your records, check for previous history and response to treatment, risk of neglect, violence or self-harm, and any known contact names.
- If there is a relative or informant, ask about the recent situation, its duration, whether there is any support, whether there have been threats or violence and if the patient is known to carry or have access to weapons.
- Contact the duty MHO. For Section 24, involvement of an MHO is desirable. For Section 18, involvement of an MHO is essential. They will need the following information: name, date of birth, address, reason for assessment, previous history, including name of key worker, next of kin (if known), and past history of violence or self-harm (if known). They will need enough information to decide if there is the possibility of an admission under the Mental Health Act.
- Liaise with the MHO about directions, access to premises, where to meet and the need for police attendance. It is good practice (because it is safer, communication is better and disruption of the patient is minimized) if the medical assessment(s) take place jointly with the MHO at the same agreed time. For Section 24, only one medical recommendation is needed; for Section 18, two are required. They can be provided up to five days apart.
- If the patient is suffering from the short-term effect of drugs, alcohol or sedative medication, discussion should take place about deferring the assessment until a more productive interview can take place.
- Take copies of form A (the emergency detention form) with you. If no copies are available, take practice-headed notepaper, if possible.
- If you want to discuss the management of the patient, either telephone the duty MHO or the duty consultant.

During the assessment

The patient is interviewed as comfortably as possible with the following questions in mind:

- Is there any possible evidence of mental disorder?
- Is there a risk to the health or safety of the patient or a danger to others?

If the answer to both of these questions is yes:

- Will the patient consent to informal admission? And if so, is that realistic based on past experience or aspects of the current interview?
- Are there any community alternatives to admission, eg giving medication at home, community mental health nurse visits, crisis services, day hospitals?

For Section 24:

- Seek the consent of the MHO or a near relative. A list of who is considered a 'relative' under the Act can be found on form A. Being involved in the compulsory admission of a relative to hospital can sometimes damage family relationships; therefore, if practicable, advise the relative that there is an alternative (ie an MHO can perform the consent role). If it is not practicable to seek consent from either an

MHO or a near relative, a single doctor's recommendation is sufficient, but the reason for failure to seek consent must be explained on the recommendation form. If the relative and MHO refuse consent, compulsory admission cannot go ahead.

- Complete the recommendation on form A (or on practice-headed notepaper). Include the following: full details of your qualifications; a declaration that you have examined the patient at the time of the application; that the patient is subject to a mental disorder; that treatment is necessary in the interests of the health or safety of the patient or the protection of others; state the reasons why detention is urgently necessary and use of section 18 is precluded; whose consent has been obtained or reasons why it has not been possible to obtain the consent of an MHO or a near relative. The documentation must be completed on the same day as the patient examination.

For Section 18:
The MHO will normally take responsibility for co-ordinating the assessment, bringing relevant papers and ensuring the process complies with the law.
The team needed for a Section 18 (six months for treatment) is:

- a Section-20-approved doctor. Where the patient is known to the service, this doctor should be the patient's own consultant psychiatrist.
- The nearest relative or a MHO (the MHO makes a more comprehensive assessment of the social aspects of the case and advises on the legal issues that may arise during the process).
- A doctor with prior knowledge of the patient (ideally the GP).

All professionals strive to reach a consensus and if the two doctors agree to make the medical recommendations for compulsory admission, the MHO makes the application to the Sheriff within seven days. The MHO must make the application even if the two doctors disagree with the medical recommendations. The Sheriff may call a hearing, which may involve the attendance of the GP to court.

Arranging admission
If the decision of the team is to admit the patient, the level of security required should be considered.

Discuss with the MHO how the patient is to be managed, including who is to accompany the patient and deliver the section papers, who will secure the premises and who will inform the patient and relative of the decision. Liaise with the receiving hospital to ensure a bed is available, to discuss arrangements for the patient's admission, transport to hospital and patient's need for care during removal, including medical and nursing escorts if required.

Emergency detention is not a 'treatment order' and the patient cannot therefore be forced to accept any form of treatment. However, in emergency circumstances, medication can be given under the common law principle of necessity to control acute symptomatology or behavioural disturbance where risk to life and safety are involved.

If the patient is not admitted
When the patient is not admitted to hospital, a package of follow-up care needs to be agreed with the patient and nearest relative, if appropriate. Arrangements may need to be made to contact mental health or social work teams during working hours to inform them of the assessment and/or to make a referral.

This is not intended to be a comprehensive guide to the Mental Health Act. Reference should be made to the relevant Code of Practice, which is available from the Stationery Office, see www.hmso.gov.uk

The Mental Health (Care and Treatment) (Scotland) Act 2003
As noted above, mental health law in Scotland is in the process of being reformed. This new Act has been passed by the Scottish Parliament and is expected to be brought into

force on a staged basis from October 2004. Sections relating to civil compulsion are expected to come into force from April 2005.

The new Act retains the current three-pronged structure of civil compulsion:

- 72-hour (emergency detention)
- 28-day (short-term detention)
- longer-term (through what are called 'Compulsory Treatment Orders').

However, the criteria for compulsion are more clearly spelt out, as are the procedures that must be followed. More detail on these procedures will be provided in a Code of Practice on the new Act, which will be published in advance of the Act being brought into effect. A draft of the Code of Practice will be published for consultation during 2004.

For more information on the new Act and on its implementation, contact the Mental Health Division of the Scottish Executive Health Department, St Andrew's House, Edinburgh EH1 3DG; http://www.scotland.gov.uk/health/mentalhealthlaw.

The Children Act 1989

The Children Act 1989 is the relevant statute that relates to the welfare of children. Its key elements are as follows:

- *The paramountcy principle*: This states that the welfare of children is at all times paramount and overrides all other considerations.
- *The welfare checklist*: This refers to a list of factors that are used to ensure that any decision made by the statutory agencies is done so with the child's best interests in mind. These factors include:
  — the child's physical, emotional and educational needs
  — the perceived effect (positive or otherwise) of changing their environment
  — the child's wishes and views, wherever possible
  — the capability of the child's parents to meet their needs.
- *The no delay/no order principle*: No delay should occur in making decisions about a child's future, and courts should not make an order unless it is absolutely in the child's best interests to do so.

Implications for GPs
- Although GPs provide care for people of all ages, their primary responsibility lies with the child.
- GPs who encounter children in need of protection should discuss their concerns either with social services or with named paediatricians who have a special interest in child protection.
- Sharing of information is a focal point of the child protection process. The Child Protection Case Conference represents the principle venue whereby this happens. Although attendance at conferences might not always be possible, it is important that the views of GPs are represented at conferences by means of a written report.
- All health professionals who have concerns regarding the welfare of children must maintain accurate and contemporaneous clinical notes.
- GPs are uniquely placed to provide continuing support for vulnerable families.

Template chart for local resources — statutory services

It is important for clinicians in primary care to have ready access to information about local agencies that can help their patients. The following table contains a suggested template for a simple wall chart. Alternatively, the information can be available in computer consultations. You may find it helpful to fill in the names and telephone numbers of local agencies, plus the arrangements for referral (for example, what is considered to be an emergency and the standard time to appointment for an urgent referral), enlarge and copy the chart and put it on the walls of all consulting rooms. Set a date for re-checking the telephone numbers and up-dating the charts, and delegate this task to a specific person. This could be done on a primary-care organization or practice basis.

Local statutory services for mental health and learning disability

	Adults	Elderly	Child and adolescent	Learning disability
Inpatient services				
Community services		Old age psychiatrist Neurologist Community resource team Day care Chiropody Incontinence nurse Clinical psychology Counselling services Therapists, eg speech and language therapy	Child and Adolescent Mental Health Clinic	Learning disability psychiatric team Occupational therapist Learning disability nurse Child development centre Toy library Physiotherapy Speech therapy Day care
Social services	Adult mental health teams ASW services	Elderly teams Occupational therapist Elderly mental health services	Child care teams Child disability teams Post-adoption teams Foster-care support teams Leaving care teams	Adult learning disability social care team Residential care
Educational services			Educational psychology service Educational welfare service Behaviour support team	
Department of Social Security				
Agreed priority groups				
Referral arrangements:				
Emergency referrals (9am–5pm Mon–Fri)				
Emergency referrals (outside working hours)				
Urgent referrals				
Routine referrals				

Template chart for local resources – voluntary agencies

This is a suggested template for a simple wall chart. Alternatively, the information can be available in computer consultations. You may find it helpful to fill in the names and telephone numbers of local agencies under each heading, enlarge and copy the chart and put it on the walls of all consulting rooms. Set a date for re-checking the telephone numbers and updating the charts, and delegate this task to a specific person. This could be done on a primary-care organization or practice basis.

Non-statutory, voluntary services for mental health and learning disability		
Alcohol/drug support	**Carer support**	**Ethnic support**
Anxiety/stress	**Depression**	**Parents and children**
Learning disability	**Counselling**	**Suicidal thoughts and self harm**
Bereavement	**Elderly support**	**Relationships**
Welfare Citizens Advice Bureau Benefits Agency Debt Counselling	**Mental Illness** Mind Manic Depression Fellowship Rethink User support service	**Young people**

Resource directory

The following self-help, non-statutory and voluntary organizations are all national organizations, and the telephone numbers are head office numbers. Many of the agencies have networks of support groups across the country and they will be able to tell you the location of your nearest group. All encourage self-referral. You may wish to adapt this directory to include details of your local groups.

Alcohol misuse

Al-Anon Family Groups UK and Eire (local groups)
61 Great Dover Street, London SE1 4YF

Helpline: 020 7403 0888 (10am–10pm Daily)
Website: http://www.al-anon.org/

Understanding and support for families and friends of alcoholics whether still drinking or not.

Alateen
Helpline: 020 7403 0888 (10am–10pm Daily)
Website: http://www.al-anon.alateen.org/

For young people aged 12–20 affected by others' drinking.

Alcoholics Anonymous (local groups)
PO Box 1, Stonebow House, General Service Office, Stonebow, York YO1 7NJ

Administration: 01904 644 026
Helpline: 0845 769 7555 (24-hour)
Website: http://www.alcoholics-anonymous.org.uk

Helpline and support groups for men and women trying to achieve and maintain sobriety and help other alcoholics to get sober.

Drinkline National Alcohol Helpline
Freepost, PO Box 4000, Glasgow, G3 8XX

Helpline: 0800 917 8282 (9am–11pm, Tuesday–Thursday, Friday 9am–Monday 11pm)
Asian line (Hindu, Urdu, Gujerati, Pujabi): 0990 133 480 (1pm–8pm, Monday)

Confidential alcohol counselling and information service.

National Association for Children of Alcoholics
PO Box 64, Fishponds, Bristol, BS16 2UH

Office: 0117 924 8005
Helpline: 0800 358 3456 (10am–7pm, Monday–Friday)

Provides information and support to children of alcoholics.

Northern Ireland Community Addiction Service
40 Elmwood Avenue, Belfast BT9 6AZ

02890 664 434 (8.45am–5pm Monday–Thursday, 8.45am–4.30pm Friday)

Secular Organisations for Sobriety (SOS)
Office: 020 8698 9332

Helpline: 020 8698 9332/8291 5572

A non-religious self-help group.

Anxiety, obsessive-compulsive disorder, panic and phobias

First Steps to Freedom (local groups)
1 Taylor Close, Kennelworth, Warwickshire, CV8 2LW

Office: 01926 864 473
Helpline: 01926 851 608 (24-hour)
Email: info@firststeps.demon.co.uk; website: http://www.first-steps.org

Runs self-help groups.

The International Stress Management Association (ISMA) UK
PO Box 348, Waltham Cross, EN8 8ZL

Helpline: 07000 780 430
Email: stress@isma.org.uk; website: http://www.isma.org.uk

Promotes knowledge and best practice in the prevention and reduction of acute stress.

No Panic (local groups)
Brands Farm Way, Telford TF3 2JQ

Helpline: 0808 808 0545 (10am–10pm Daily, and a taped crisis message through the night) — gives numbers of volunteers for the day
Website: http://www.nopanic.org.uk
Email: ceo@nopanic.org.uk

Helpline, information booklets, local self-help groups (including telephone recovery groups) for people with anxiety, phobias, obsessions, panic.

OCD Action
Aberdeen Centre, 22–24 Highbury Grove, London N5 2EA

020 7226 4000 (9.30am–5pm, Tuesday, Wednesday; 11am–5pm, Thursday)
Email: info@ocdaction.org.uk; website: http://www.ocdaction.org.uk

Provides information, advice and support for people with Obsessive-compulsive disorder and related disorders such as body dysmorphic disorder and trichotillomania.

Social Anxiety UK (local groups)
Website: http://www.social-anxiety.org.uk

Information and support for sufferers of social anxiety and related problems. Has chat room and details of local meetings across the UK.

Stresswatch Scotland (local groups)
The Barn, 42 Barnweil Road, Kilmarnock KA1 4JF

Office: 01563 574 144
Helpline: 01563 528 910 (10am–1pm, Monday–Friday, excluding Wednesday)

Advice, information, materials on panic, anxiety, stress, phobias.

Triumph Over Phobia (TOP UK)(local groups)
PO Box1831, Bath BA2 4YW

Office: 01225 330 353
Email: triumphoverphobia@compuserve.com; website:
http://www.triumphoverphobia.com

Structured self-help groups for sufferers from phobias or Obsessive-compulsive
disorder. Produces self-help materials.

Attention-deficit/hyperactivity disorder and Autism

Attention Deficit Disorder Information and Support Service (ADDISS) (local groups)
10 Station Road, Mill Hill, London NW7 2JU

020 8906 9068
Website: http://www.addiss.co.uk

Advice, support, local self-help groups, conferences and literature.

The National Autistic Society (local groups)
393 City Road, London EC1V 1NG

Office: 020 7833 2299
Helpline: 020 7903 3555
Email: nas@nas.org.uk; website: http://www.nas.org.uk

Information service, national diagnostic and assessment service, supported
employment scheme, local groups and other services.

Autism Connect
Website: http://www.autismconnect.org

A website for anyone interested in autism, providing news, events, world maps, and
rapid access to other websites with information on autism.

Bereavement and loss

Childhood Bereavement Network
National Children's Bureau, 8 Wakley Street, London EC1V 7QE,

020 7843 6309
Website: http://www.ncb.org.uk/cbn/directory

Has an online directory of accessible specialist bereavement support services
throughout UK.

The Child Bereavement Trust
Ashton House, High Street, High Wycombe, Buckinghamshire HP14 3AG

Office: 01494 446 648
Information line and support for professionals only: 0845 357 1000
Email: enquiries@childbereavement.org.uk; website:
http://www.childbereavement.org.uk

Offers training for counselling bereaved children and advice on where to obtain help in
the UK. Website has advice sheets for parents and young people and list of useful
resources including videos for young people.

The Compassionate Friends
53 North Street, Bristol BS3 1EN

Helpline: 0117 953 9639 (10am–4pm and 6.30–10.30pm, open 365 days a year)
Email: info@tcf.org.uk; website: http://www.tcf.org.uk

Organization of bereaved parents offering friendship and understanding to others after the death of a child.

Cruse Bereavement Care (local groups)
Cruse House, 126 Sheen Road, Richmond, Surrey TW9 1UR

020 8939 9530
Helpline: 0870 167 1677 (9.30am–5.00pm, Monday–Friday)
Youthline (for those aged 12–18): 0808 808 1677
Email: info@crusebereavementcare.org.uk; website:
http://www.crusebereavementcare.org.uk

Offers support, information, training and direct telephone help to anyone who has been affected by a death. Over 150 branches throughout the UK.

The Foundation for the Study of Infant Deaths (FSID) (local groups)
Artillery House, 11–19 Artillery Row, London, SW1P 1RT

Administration: 0870 787 0885
Helpline: 0870 787 0554 (9–11am Monday–Friday; 6–11pm, Saturday and Sunday)
Email: fsid@sids.org.uk; website: http://www.sids.org.uk

National helpline, local parent groups and befrienders.

Papyrus
c/o The Administration, Rosendale GH, Union Road, Rawtenstall, Rosendale, Lancs BB4 6NE

01706 214 449

Self-help for parents of young people who have committed suicide.

SAMM (Support after Murder and Manslaughter)
Cranmer House, 39 Brixton Road, London SW9 6DZ

Helpline: 020 7735 3838 (9am–5pm Monday–Friday)
Email: samm@victimsupport.org.uk; website: http://www.samm.org.uk

Helpline and useful publications including some for carers.

SOBS (Survivors of Bereavement by Suicide) (Local groups)
Centre 88, Saner Street, Hull HU3 2TR

Administrator: 01482 610 728
Helpline: 0870 241 3337 (9am–9pm, 365 days of the year)
Email: sobs.support@care4free.net; website: http://www.uk-sobs.org.uk

Offers emotional and practical support to those affected by suicide.

Stillbirth and Neonatal Death Society (SANDS)
28 Portland Place, London W1B 1LY

Office: 020 7436 3715
Helpline: 020 7436 5881 (9.30am–4pm Monday–Friday, and answerphone outside normal hours)
Email: support@uk-sands.org; website: http://www.uk-sands.org

Provides support for parents and families whose baby is stillborn, or dies shortly after birth.

Winston's Wish
The Clara Burgess Centre, Gloucestershire Hospital, Great Western Road, Gloucester GL1 3NN

General enquiries: 01452 394 377
Family line: 0845 203 0405 (9am-5pm, Monday–Friday)
Email: info@winstonswish.org.uk; website: http://www.winstonswish.org.uk

Organization supporting bereaved children and young people, and offering guidance and information to anyone concerned about a child after bereavement.

Bipolar disorder (manic depression)

The Manic Depression Fellowship (MDF) (local groups)
England
Castle Works, 21 St George's Road, London SE1 6ES

Office: 020 7793 2600
Email: mdf@mdf.org.uk (information); smt@mdf.org.uk (self-management); groups@mdf.org.uk (self-help groups); website: http://www.mdf.org.uk

Scotland
Studio 1019, Mile End Mill, Abbey Mill Business Park, Seedhill Road, Paisley PA1 1TJ

0141 560 2050
Email: info@mdfscotland.co.uk; website: http://www.mdfscotland.co.uk

Wales
1 Palmyra Place, Newport, South Wales, NP20 4EJ

08456 340 080
Email: info@mdfwales.org.uk; website: http://www.manicdepressionwales.org.uk

Advice, support, local self-help groups and publications list for people with a manic depressive illness.

Carers

Carers UK
20–25 Glasshouse Yard, London EC1A 4JT

020 7490 8818
Helpline: 0808 808 7777 (10am–12noon and 2–4pm, Monday–Friday)
Email: info@ukcarers.org.uk; website: http://www.carersonline.org.uk

Formerly the National Carers Association. Provides information and advice on all aspects of care for both carers and professionals.

Counsel and Care
Twyman House, 16 Bonny Street, London NW1 9PG

020 7485 1566 (10am–1pm, Monday–Friday)
Website: http://www.counselandcare.org.uk

Advice and information on home and residential care for older people.

Crossroads Association (local groups)
10 Regent Place, Rugby CV21 2PN

0845 450 0350
Email: communications@crossroads.org.uk; website: http://www.crossroads.org.uk

There are regional centres throughout the UK, providing practical support and help for carers, including respite care, day centres, befriending and night care. There is a scheme for young carers also.

Children and adolescents (see also Parents and children)

Anti-Bullying Campaign
185 Tower Bridge Road, London SE1 2UF

020 7378 1446

Provides help if children are being bullied or if children are bullying.

Bullying Online
Website: http://www.bullying.co.uk

Gives help and advice for parents and pupils in dealing with school bullying.

The Bullying Project
Website: http://www.bullying.org

Provides online mentoring support programmes, as well as educational resources.

Change our Minds
Website: http://www.changeourminds.com

A website run by the Samaritans targeted at a younger audience.

ChildLine
45 Folgate Street, London E1 6GL

Office: 020 7650 3200
Helpline: 0800 1111 (24-hour, freephone)
Website: http://www.childline.org.uk

Telephone service for all children and young people providing confidential counselling, support and advice on any issue. Parents can also write to ChildLine.

Childwatch
19 Spring Bank, Hull, East Yorkshire HU3 1AF

01482 325 552
Website: http://www.childwatch.org.uk

Advice for children on bullying and abuse that occurs at home and at school.

Kidscape
2 Grosvenor Gardens, London SW1W 0DH

020 7730 3300
Website: http://www.kidscape.org.uk

This is a charity set up to protect children from danger — whether from peers, adults they know or complete strangers.

Like it is
Email: likeitis@stopes.org.uk; website: http://www.likeitis.org.uk

Sex education for young people.

NSPCC (National Society for the Prevention of Cruelty to Children)
Weston House, 42 Curtain Road, London EC2A 3NH

020 7825 2500
Helpline: 0808 800 5000
Website: http://www.nspcc.org.uk

A charity specializing in child protection and the prevention of cruelty to children.

Teenage Health Freak
Website: http://www.teenagehealthfreak.org

Aimed primarily at teenagers aged 11–16 years, provides teenage-friendly health information.

Youth in Mind
Website: http://www.youthinmind.net

Website helping stressed children, teenagers and those who care for them access information and services.

Young Minds Trust
102–108 Clerkenwell Road, London EC1M 5SA

020 7336 8445
Parent information service: 0800 018 2138
Website: http://www.youngminds.org.uk

Aims to improve the mental health of all children and young people. Produces a range of leaflets for parents and young people.

Youth2Youth
Helpline: 020 8896 3675 (6.30–9.30pm, Monday and Thursday)
Email: admin@youth2youth.co.uk; website: http://www.youth2youth.co.uk

Telephone, email and online chat line run by young people (16–21-years-old) for young people.

Chronic fatigue

Action for ME (AfME)
PO Box 1302, Wells, Somerset, BA5 1YE

01749 670799
Email: admin@afme.org.uk; website: http://www.afme.org.uk

A national charity campaigning for patients and a useful source of information

Association of Young People with ME
PO 605, Milton Keynes, Bucks, MK2 2XD

01908 373 300
Email: info@ayme.org.uk; website: http://www.ayme.org.uk

Gives support and advice to young people with ME.

Counselling and psychotherapy

BACP (British Association for Counselling and Psychotherapy)
BACP House, 35–37 Albert Street, Rugby CV21 2SG

0870 443 5252.
Website: http://www.counselling.co.uk

Provides advice on sources of individual counselling and family therapy in the UK.

British Association for Behavioural and Cognitive Psychotherapies
Globe Centre, PO Box 9, Accrington, BB5 2GD

01254 875 277
Email: babcp@babcp.com; website: http://www.babcp.org.uk

Provides a free directory of accredited cognitive behavioural practitioners.

The British Confederation of Psychotherapists
West Hill House, Swains Lane, London N6 6QS

020 8830 5173
Website: http://www.bcp.org.uk

Register of psychotherapists, including psychoanalysts, analytical psychologists, psychoanalytical psychotherapists and child psychotherapists.

The British Psychological Society
St Andrew's House, 48 Princess Road East, Leicester LE1 7DR

01162 549 568
Website: http://www.bps.org.uk

Produces a directory of chartered clinical psychologists.

Counsellors and Psychotherpists in Primary Care (CPC)
Queensway House, Queensway, Bognor Regis, West Sussex PO21 1QT

01243 870701
Email: cpc@cpc-online.co.uk; website: http://www.cpc-online.co.uk

Represents counsellors and psychotherapists working in the NHS as a self-regulating professional association.

Institute for Counselling and Personal Development Trust
Interpoint, 20–24 York Street, Belfast BT15 1AQ

02890 330 996
Email: diane@icpd.thegap.com

Offers counselling and psychotherapy (normally free), course for helpers and community training and development courses.

United Kingdom Council for Psychotherapy (UKCP)
167–169 Great Portland Street, London, W1W 5PF

020 7436 3002

Email: ukcp@psychotherapy.org.uk; website: http://www.psychotherapy.org.uk

Provides information on registered therapists and training organizations.

Debt (see also Welfare)

National Debtline
The Arch, 48–52 Floodgate Street, Birmingham B5 5SL

Freephone: 0808 808 4000
Website: http://www.nationaldebtline.co.uk

Dementia

Age Concern

England
Astral House, 1268 London Road, London SW16 4ER

Information line: 0800 009 966 (7am–7pm, daily)
Email: ace@ace.org.uk; website: http://www.ace.org.uk

Northern Ireland
02890 245 729
Email: info@ageconcernni.org

Wales
029 2037 1566
Email: enquiries@accymru.org.uk

Scotland
0131 220 3345
Email: enquiries@acscot.org.uk

Provides information and advice relating to older people.

Alzheimer's Society
Gordon House, 10 Greencoat Place, London, SW1P 1PH

020 7306 0606; helpline: 0845 300 0336
Email: helpline@alzheimers.org.uk; website: http://www.alzheimers.org.uk

Provides support to people with all forms of dementia, not just Alzheimer's, their family and friends, and supports research on education and training for primary care.

Help the Aged
Website: http://www.helptheaged.org.uk

England
207–221 Pentonville Road, London N1 9UZ

020 7278 1114
Email: info@helptheaged.org.uk;

Wales
12 Cathedral Road, Cardiff CF11 9LJ

02920 346 550
Email: infocymru@helptheaged.org.uk

Scotland
11 Granton Square, Edinburgh EH5 1HX

0131 551 6331
Email: infoscot@helptheaged.org.uk

Northern Ireland
Ascot House, 24–30 Shaftesbury Square, Belfast BT2 7DB

02890 230 666
Email: infoni@helptheaged.org.uk

Provides advice and support to older people

Depression

Aware Defeat Depression Ltd. (local groups)
22 Great James Street, Derry, Co Londonderry BT48 7DA

02871 260 602
Email: info@aware-ni.org; website: http://www.aware-ni.org

Provides information leaflets, lectures and runs support groups for sufferers and relatives.

Campaign Against Living Miserably (CALM)
Helpline: 0800 585 858

Helpline for 15–24-year-old men at the onset of depression, to give advice, guidance, referrals and counselling.

Depression Alliance (local groups)
Website: http://www.depressionalliance.org

England
35 Westminster Bridge Road, London SE1 7JB

020 8768 0123

Wales
11 Plas Melin, Westbourne Rd, Whitchurch, Cardiff CF14 2BT

029 2069 2891 (10am–4pm Monday–Friday)

Scotland
3 Grosvenor Gardens, Edinburgh EH12 5JU

0131 467 3050

Provides information and self-help groups.

SAD (Seasonal Affective Disorder) Association
PO Box 989, Steyning BN44 3HS

01903 814 942
Website: http://www.sada.org.uk

Information about seasonal affective disorder (SAD). Offers advice and support to members.

Domestic violence

Domestic Violence Unit or Community Safety Unit
Contact your local Police Force for details.

Everyman Project
40 Stockwell Road, Stockwell, London SW9 9ES

020 7737 6747
Website: http://www.changeweb.org.uk/new_page_22.htm

Counselling, support and advice to men who are violent or concerned about their violence, and anyone affected by that violence.

Kiran: Asian Women's Aid
020 8558 1986, Fax: 020 8532 8260
Email: kiranawa@btopenworld.com

Advice, support, refuge for Asian women, and women from other cultures (eg Turkey, Iran, Morocco and Malaysia).

Refuge
National Crisis Line: 0870 599 5443 (24-hour)

Offers support, information and referrals. Runs own refuges in London and South East.

Relate
Herbert Gray College, Little Church Street, Rugby, Warwickshire CV21 3AP

01788 573 241/0800 456 1310
Website: http://www.relate.org.uk

Counselling for adults with relationship difficulties, whether married or not.

Women's Aid Federation
PO Box 391, Bristol BS99 7WS

National Domestic Violence 24-hour helpline:

England: 08457 023 468

Wales: 029 2039 0874

Northern Ireland: 01232 249 041/358

Scotland: 0131 221 0401
Website: http://www.womensaid.org.uk

Support, advice, information and refuge referrals for women experiencing domestic violence.

Zero Tolerance
Helpline: 0800 028 3398
Website: www.domesticviolenceprevention.com

Support, advice and information for women experiencing domestic violence.

Drug misuse

ADFAM National

Waterbridge House, 32–36 Loman Street, London SE1 0EE

Helpline 020 7928 8900 (10am–5pm, Monday, Wednesday–Friday; 10am–6.45pm, Tuesday)
Website: http://www.adfam.org.uk

Confidential support and information for families and friends of drug users.

CITA (Council for Involuntary Tranquilliser Addiction)

Cavendish House, Brighton Road, Waterloo, Liverpool L22 5NG

Office: 0151 474 9626
Helpline 0151 949 0102 (10.00am–1.00pm, Monday–Friday: emergency weekend number available)

Offers advice on withdrawing from tranquilisers and help with anxiety and depression.

DrugScope

Waterbridge House, 32–36 Loman Street, London SE1 0EE

020 7928 1211
Email: services@drugscope.org.uk

Families Anonymous (local groups)

Unit 37, The Doddington and Rollo Community Association, Charlotte Despard Avenue, Battersea, London SW11 5JE

020 7498 4680 (1–5pm, Monday–Friday)
Email: office@famanon.org.uk; website: http://www.famanon.org.uk

Runs self-help groups in the UK for families and friends of those with a drug problem.

Narcotics Anonymous

020 7730 0009
Email: helpline@ukna.org; website: http://www.ukna.org

For leaflets, telephone the UK Service Officer: 020 7251 4007.
A network of recovering addicts supporting each other to live without drugs.

National Drugs Helpline/Talk to Frank

Helpline: 0800 776600 (24-hour)
Website: http://www.talktofrank.com

Provides free confidential advice, including information on local services.

Release

388 Old Street, London EC1V 9LT
Advice line: 020 7729 9904 (10am–5.30pm Monday–Friday)
Email: info@release.org.uk; website: http://www.release.org.uk

Advice, support and information to drug users and their friends and families on all aspects of drug use and drug-related legal problems.

Eating disorders

Anorexia Bulimia Careline (Northern Ireland)
84 University Street, Belfast BT7 1HE

Helpline: 02890 614 440

Centre for Eating Disorders (Scotland)
3 Sciennes Road, Edinburgh EH9 1LE

0131 668 3051

Psychotherapy for individuals, self help manuals and information packs.

Eating Disorders Association (local groups)
1st Floor, Wensum House, 103 Prince of Wales Road, Norwich NR1 1DW

Office: 01603 619 090
Helpline: 01603 621 414 (9am–6.30pm, Monday–Friday)
Youthline (for under 19s): 01603 765050 (4–6.30pm Mon-Fri)
Email: info@edauk.com; website: http://www.edauk.com

Self-help support groups for sufferers, their relatives and friends. Assists in putting people in touch with sources of help in their own area.

Ethnic minorities

Commission for Racial Equality (local groups)
St Dunstan's House, 201–211 Borough High Street, London SE1 1GZ

020 7939 0000
Email info@cre.gov.uk; website: http://www.cre.gov.uk

Provides help to individuals with cases of racial discrimination.

Jewish Association for the Mentally Ill (JAMI)
707 High Road, Finchley, London N12 0BT

020 8343 1111

Offers guidance, counselling and support to sufferers and carers. Runs a help and referral line.

NAFSIYAT
278 Seven Sisters Road, London N4 2HY

020 7686 8666

This is an intercultural therapy centre. Its own services are local but it might be able to provide information about counsellors from black and ethnic minority groups in other areas of the UK.

Refugee Council
3 Bondway, London SW8 1SJ

020 7820 3000
Website: http://www.refugeecouncil.org.uk

Gives practical support and advice to refugees. Provides information on mental health services to refugees and their advisers.

Refugee Support Centre
47 South Lambeth Road, London SW8 1RH

020 7820 3606

Provides counselling to refugees, asylum seekers; plus training and information to health and social care professionals on psycho-social needs of refugees.

Learning disability

Down Syndrome Association
155 Mitcham Road, London SW17 9PG

020 8682 4001 (10am–4pm, Tuesday–Thursday)
Email: info@downs-syndrome.org.uk; website: http://www.downs-syndrome.org.uk

Information and support for people with Down syndrome and their families.

Mencap

England and Wales
123 Golden Lane, London EC1Y 0RT

020 7454 0454
Information line: 020 7696 5593
Website: http://www.mencap.org.uk

Northern Ireland
Segal House, 4 Annadale Avenue, Belfast BT7 3JH

02890 691351
Family Advisory Service Line: 0345 636 227

Information and support for people with a learning disability and their families in the UK. It provides residential, employment, further education and leisure and holiday services.

Scope (local groups)
12 Park Crescent, London W1N 4EQ

020 7636 5020
Helpline: 0800 626 216
Website: http://www.scope.org.uk

Information, emotional support, and support groups for people with cerebral palsy and their families. Only some people with cerebral palsy have learning disabilities in addition to their physical disabilities.

Mental health and illness: general

Cause for Mental Health
2 Castle Village, Carrickfer, County Antrim BT38 7BH

01960 367 728
Helpline: 0845 603 0291

Mental Health Foundation
7th Floor, 83 Victoria Street, London SW1H 0HW

020 7802 0300
Email: mhf@mhf.org.uk; website: http://www.mentalhealth.org.uk

Free leaflets about mental illness and learning disabilities for the general public.

MIND
Granta House, 15–19 Broadway, Stratford, London E15 4BQ

Office: 020 8519 2122
MINDinfoLINE: 0845 766 0163
Email: info@mind.org.uk; website: http://www.mind.org.uk

Information service for matters relating to mental health.

Northern Ireland Association for Mental Health
Central Office, 80 University Street, Belfast BT7 1HE

02890 328 474

Provides services in the community for people with mental needs.

SANELine
Helpline: 08457 678 000 (12noon–2.00am Daily)
Website: http://www.sane.org.uk

Helpline offering information and advice on all aspects of mental health for those experiencing illness or their families or friends.

Scottish Association for Mental Health
Cumbrae House, 15 Carlton Court, Glasgow G59JP

0141 568 7000
Website: http://www.samh.org.uk

Mental Health Care
Website: www.mentalhealthcare.org.uk

Information about mental health and the latest research from the South London and Maudsley NHS Trust and the Institute of Psychiatry. Particularly suited to the carers, friends and family of anyone with mental illness. The site currently deals with schizophrenia and psychosis.

Neurological disorders and stroke

Epilepsy Action
New Anstey House, Gate Way Drive, Yeadon, Leeds LS19 7XY

Helpline: 0808 800 5050 (9am–4.30pm, Monday–Thursday; 9am–4pm, Friday)
Email: helpline@epilepsy.org.uk; website: http://www.epilepsy.org.uk

Epilepsy Action is the working name for British Epilepsy Association.

Epilepsy Bereaved
PO Box 112, Wantage, Oxon OX12 8XT

Bereavement Support Contact Line (24-hour answering service): 01235 772 852
Email: epilepsybereaved@dial.pipex.com

Epilepsy Youth in Europe
Website: http://www.eyie.org

Provides an opportunity for young people to discuss epilepsy and its effect on their lives.

The National Society for Epilepsy
Chesham Lane, Chalfont St Peter, Bucks SL9 0RJ

Office 01494 601 300
UK Epilepsy Helpline: 01494 601 400 (10am–4pm, Monday–Friday)
Website: http://www.epilepsynse.org.uk

Migraine Action Association
Unit 6, Oakley Hay Lodge Business Park, Great Folds Road, Great Oakley, Northants NN18 9AS

01536 461 333 (best time to phone: 9am–5pm, Monday–Friday)
Website: http://www.migraine.org.uk

Aims to bridge the gap between the migraine sufferer and the medical world by providing information on all aspects of the condition and its management.

The Migraine Trust
45 Great Ormond Street, London WC1N 3HZ

020 7831 4818
Website: http://www.migrainetrust.org

Neurological Alliance
The Neurological Alliance, PO Box 36731, London SW9 6WY

Tel: 020 7793 5907, Fax: 020 7793 5939
email: info@neurologicalalliance.org.uk
Website: http://www.neurologicalalliance.org.uk

The Organization for Understanding Cluster Headaches (OUCH) UK
Norham House, Mountenoy Road, Moorgate, Rotherham S60 2AJ

24-hour infoline/answer phone: 0161 272 1702 (recording and messages only)
Website: http://www.clusterheadaches.org.uk

Stroke Association
Stroke House, 240 City Road, London EC1V 2PR

Office: 020 7566 0300
Helpline: 0845 303 3100
Email: stroke@stroke.org.uk; website: http://www.stroke.org.uk

Provides a comprehensive series of information leaflets, including *Stroke — questions and answers*, *Sex after stroke*, *Cognitive problems after stroke*, *Stroke: a carers guide*.

Different strokes
Email: info@differentstrokes.co.uk; website: http://www.differentstrokes.co.uk

Provides free services to younger stroke survivors throughout the UK.

Parents and children

Advisory Centre for Education
18 Aberdeen Studios, 22–24 Highbury Grove, London N5 2DQ

General advice line: 0808 800 5793
Website: http://www.ace-ed.org.uk

Independent advice centre for parents, offering free advice on many topics including exclusion from school, bullying, special educational needs and school admission appeals.

Fathers Direct
Website: http://www.fathersdirect.com

Home-Start UK
2 Salisbury Road, Leicester LE1 7QR

0800 068 6368 (8.30am–8pm Monday–Friday, 9am–Midday Saturday)
Website: http://www.home-start.org.uk

Volunteers offer support, friendship and practical support to young families with at least one child under five, who are experiencing difficulties and stress.

The Incredible Years
Website: http://www.incredibleyears.com

A website of programmes for reducing children's aggression and behaviour problems and increasing social competence at home and school.

National Family and Parenting Institute
430 Highgate Studios, 53–79 Highgate Road, London NW5 1TL

020 7424 3460
Email info@nfpi.org; website: http://www.nfpi.org

NEWPIN (Northern Ireland) (local groups)
Development Office, 8 Windsor Avenue, Lurgan, County Armagh BT67 9BG

01762 324 843
Website: http://www.newpin.org.uk

Befriending and support groups for parents of young children who are under stress. Work focuses on alleviating maternal depression and stress. Provides training in parenting skills and family play programmes.

Parentline (and the National Stepfamily Association)
Endway House, The Endway, Hadleigh, Essex SS7 2AN

Office: 01702 554 782
Helpline: 0808 800 2222 (9am–9pm, Monday–Friday; 9.30am–5pm, Saturday; 10am–3pm, Sunday)

Information sheets and books about belonging to a stepfamily: 020 7209 2460

Offers help and advice to parents on all aspects of bringing up children and teenagers. Provides support for parents under stress.

Parents Anonymous (local groups)
6–9 Manor Gardens, London N7 6LA

020 7263 8918

Offers friendship and help to parents who are at risk of abusing their children and those who may have done so. Offers telephone counselling and network of local groups.

Young Minds Parents Information Service
102–108 Clerkenwell Road, London EC1M 5SA

Information service: 0800 018 2138
Website: http://www.youngminds.org.uk

Produces books and leaflets about young people's mental health and offers seminars and training.

Personality (behavioural) disorders

Borderline UK
PO Box 42, Cockermouth, Cumbria CA13 0WB

Email: info@borderlineuk.co.uk; website: http://www.borderlineuk.co.uk

A national user-led network of people within the UK who have been diagnosed with borderline personality disorder.

Borderline
Website: http://www.bpdcentral.com

Mainly for families of people with borderline personality disorder.

Postnatal depression

Association for Postnatal Illness
020 7386 0868

145 Dawes Road, London SW6 7EB
Email: info@apni.org; website: http://www.apni.org

Information on postnatal depression, and will put affected mothers in touch with others who have had similar experiences.

Meet-a-Mum Association (MAMA) (local groups)
376 Bideford Green, Linslade, Leighton Buzzard, Beds LU7 2TY

01525 217 064
Email: meet-a-mum.assoc@blueyonder.co.uk; website: http://www.MAMA.org.uk

Local self-help groups for pregnant women and those with young children.

National Childbirth Trust (local groups)
Alexandra House, Oldham Terrace, London W3 1BE

0870 444 8707
Website: http://www.nctpregnancyandbabycare.com

Information and support on all aspects of pregnancy and childbirth with local groups around the country.

Relationship and sexual problems

BASRT (British Association for Sexual and Relationship Therapy)
020 8543 2707
Email: info@basrt.org.uk; website: http://www.basrt.org.uk

Registered therapists are multidisciplinary and work in the NHS as well as privately.

Brook Advisory Centres
421 Highgate Studios, 53–79 Highgate Road, London NW5 1TL

Helpline: 020 7617 8000 (24-hour)
Ask Brook: 020 7284 6060
Email: admin@brookcentres.org.uk; website: http://www.brook.org.uk

Free counselling and confidential advice on contraception and sexual matters for young people (under 25).

Care for the Family
PO Box 488, Cardiff CF15 7YY

029 2081 1733
Website: http://www.care-for-the-family.org.uk/

Provides help for those experiencing distress from family problems.

The Impotence Association
PO Box 10296, London SW17 9WH

Helpline: 020 8767 7791
Email: theia@btinternet.com; website: http://www.impotence.org.uk

Relate
Herbert Gray College, Little Church Street, Rugby, Warwickshire CV21 3AP

01788 573 241
Helpline: 08451 304 010/0800 456 1310
Website: http://www.relate.org.uk

Counselling for adults with relationship difficulties, whether married or not.

Schizophrenia

Hearing Voices Network (local groups)
91 Oldham Street, Manchester M4 1LW

0161 834 5763
Email: hearingvoices@care4free.net; website: http://www.hearing-voices.org.uk

Self-help groups to allow people to explore their voice-hearing experiences.

Rethink (formerly the National Schizophrenia Fellowship) (local groups)
28 Castle Street, Kingston-upon-Thames, Surrey KT1 1SS

Advice line: 020 8974 6814 (10am–3pm, Monday–Friday)
Email: advice@rethink.org; website: http://www.rethink.org

Scotland
Claremont House, 130 East Claremont Street, Edinburgh EHT 4LB

0131 557 8969

Northern Ireland
'Wyndhurst', Knockbracken Health Care Park, Saintfield Rd, Belfast BT8 8BH

02890 402 323

Monthly social groups for clients with schizophrenia living in the community and support for relatives.

Schizophrenia Association of Great Britain
'Bryn Hyfryd', The Crescent, Bangor, Gwynedd LL57 2AG.

01248 354 048
Email: info@sagb.co.uk; website: http://www.sagb.co.uk

Offers information and support to sufferers, relatives, friends, carers and medical workers.

The UK NHS Portal for Schizophrenia
Website: http://www.nhs.uk/schizophrenia

Web-based information resource for people with schizophrenia and their carers. The site contains a number of user-friendly sections. These include the following: Evidence-based treatment summaries; What is schizophrenia? How is schizophrenia diagnosed? Managing schizophrenia; Living with schizophrenia; Support for carers; and Legal issues.

Self-care for professionals

British Medical Association Stress Counselling Service
0645 200 169

24-hour, free, confidential counselling service available to doctors, their families and medical students, to discuss personal, emotional and work-related problems.

Medical Council on Alcohol
020 7487 4445

National Counselling Service for Sick Doctors
0870 241 0535

Confidential advisory service. Deals with concerns about health issues that might be affecting ability to treat patients safely.

Royal College of Nursing
0345 726 100 (24-hour service for information and advice)
Website: http://www.rcn.org.uk

Self-harm and suicidal feelings

Basement Project
PO Box 5, Abergavenny, Gwent NP7 5XW

01873 856 524

Publications on self-harm, run groups and workshops and work with people (mainly women) who have been abused.

239

Bristol Crisis Service for Women
PO Box 654, Bristol BS99 1XH

Helpline: 0117 925 1119 (9pm–12.30am, Friday and Saturday)
Email: bcsw@womens-crisis-service.freeserve.co.uk

Telephone counselling and information service relating to self-harm. Bi-monthly newsletter *Shout* on self-harm.

National Self-Harm Network
PO Box 16190, London NW1 3WW

Provides information sheets and training.

The Samaritans
46 Marshall Street, London W1V 1LR

Helpline: 08457 909090 (24-hour, daily)
Email: jo@samaritans.org; website: http://www.samaritans.org.uk

Offers confidential emotional support to any person who is despairing or suicidal.

Self Harm Alliance
PO Box 61, Cheltenham, Gloucestershire GL51 8YB

Helpline: 01242 578 820 (6–7pm, Tuesday and Sunday; 11am–1pm, Thursday)
Email: selharmalliance@aol.com; website: http://www.selfharmalliance.org

Helpline, produces monthly newsletters, provides postal and email support, and offers an advocacy service.

Self-Injury and Related Issues (SIARI)
Email: jan@siari.uk; website: http://www.siari.co.uk

Forum for self-harmers.

Sleep problems

British Sleep Society
PO Box 247, Colne, Huntington PE28 3UZ.

Email: enquiries@sleeping.org.uk; website: http://www.sleeping.org.uk

British Snoring and Sleep Apnoea Association
0800 0851 097

Email: info@britishsnoring.co.uk; website: http://www.britishsnoring.com

UKAN (Narcolepsy Association UK)
020 7721 8904
Email: info@narcolepsy.org.uk; website: http://www.narcolepsy.org.uk

Provides help for those suffering from narcolepsy.

Smoking cessation

NHS Smoking Helpline
0800 169 0169 (7am–11pm, daily)

Website: http://www.givingupsmoking.co.uk

NHS Pregnancy Smoking Helpline
0800 169 9169 (12 noon–9pm, daily)

Quit Line Smoking Helpline
0800 00 22 00 (9am–9pm, daily)

Trauma

CombatStress
Tyrwhitt House, Oaklawn Road, Leatherhead, Surrey KT22 0BX

01372 841600
Email: contactus@combatstress.org.uk; website: http://www.combatstress.com

Supports men and women discharged from the armed services and merchant navy who suffer from mental health problems, including post-traumatic stress disorder. It has a regional network of welfare officers who visit people at home or in hospital.

The Medical Foundation for the Care of Victims of Torture
96–98 Grafton Rd, Kentish Town, London NW5 3EJ (open 9am–6pm, Monday–Friday, by appointment)

Clinical department: 020 7813 7777
Website: http://www.torturecare.org.uk

Provides survivors of torture with medical treatment, social assistance and psychotherapeutic support.

Rape Crisis Federation
0115 900 3560 (9am–5pm, Monday–Friday)

Email: info@rapecrisis.co.uk; website: http://www.rapecrisis.co.uk

Victim Support
PO Box 11431, London SW9 6ZH

Supportline: 0845 3030 900 (9am–9pm, Monday–Friday; 9am–7pm, Saturday/Sunday; 9am–5pm bank holidays)
Email: contact@victimsupport.org.uk; website: http://www.victimsupport.com

Provides emotional support and practical information for anyone who has suffered the effects of crime, regardless of whether the crime has been reported.

Women against Rape
020 7482 2496

Email: war@womenagainstrape.net; website: http://www.womenagainstrape.net

Welfare and advice for practical problems

Benefits Enquiry Line
0800 882 2200

Textphone 0800 243 355

For information about Disability Living Allowance, Invalid Care Allowance and other benefits.

Citizens Advice Bureau (See local telephone directory for the number of your nearest bureau)

Main website: http://www.citizensadvice.org.uk (gives directory of all offices and advice by email); Advice guide website: http://www.adviceguide.org.uk

Provides a wide range of free and confidential advice and help. Subjects include social security benefits, housing, family and personal matters, money advice and consumer complaints.

Shelter Helpline

Helpline: 0808 800 4444 (24-hour)

Website: http://www.shelter.org.uk

General advice and help on housing problems.

Mental health in your practice: what does your practice offer?

You may like to consider the following:

Practice organization:

1. A practice policy for what receptionists should do when faced with a patient who is very agitated or describing intentions of harm to self or others.
2. The practice discrimination policy should include a statement that people with mental health problems should not be discriminated against.
3. Some longer slots booked in surgeries to allow for people with emotional problems.
4. Routine follow-up appointments for people prescribed antidepressants, with a doctor or another member of the team, eg chronic disease management systems.
5. Encouraging patients with chronic mental disorders to see the same team member at each visit (shared care).
6. A list of Read codes used by the practice including those with severe or chronic mental illness to ensure regular follow-up and monitoring, including physical health checks. Regular audits of lithium monitoring, benzodiazepine and atypical antipsychotic medication prescribing. Ideally this would be co-ordinated by the practice mental health team lead.
7. Reviewing the 'mental health workload' of each partner. If it falls disproportionately on one or a small number of partners, consider ways of relieving the pressure; alternatively consider acknowledging and supporting the partners' specialization as part of the way the team operates.
8. Practice policy for people who misuse drugs/alcohol.

Information and support for patients:

9. Information leaflets or audiotapes for people suffering mental ill health, including a carers' leaflet, readily available to all team members.
10. Information readily available to patients and all members of the practice team about community or voluntary groups who can help patients suffering mental ill health.

Skills within the primary-care team:

11. Encourage mental health to be part of all clinicians' personal development plan. This includes anti-stigma and stress management training for all staff.
12. Reviewing the skills of all members of the team: doctors, health visitor, practice nurse, counsellor, district nurse, school nurse. What kind of problems/patients is each competent to deal with? Are all members of the team aware of the skills already available within the team?
13. Checking the training and support needs of practice nurses or others who are involved in activities, such as giving depot injections or monitoring of lithium.
14. Developing further primary mental health skills within the team. Consider:

    - structured problem-solving
    - activity planning — depression
    - teaching controlled breathing — anxiety
    - teaching relaxation — anxiety
    - motivational interviewing — alcohol and drug misuse
    - supporting graded exposure to feared situations — anxiety, particularly phobias
    - encouraging more appropriate thinking (cognitive skills) — depression and anxiety

- re-attribution of symptoms from physical to emotional causes
- asking about suicidal intentions
- managing self-harming behaviours.

15. Clinical supervision, peer or external, for team members who take on a significant counselling or mental health workload.

Liaison with community mental health and substance abuse services:

16. Regular, face-to-face meetings with the relevant person from the community mental health team(s) that serve your practice.
17. Arrangements to 'share' people with a severe mental illness and those with substance abuse.
18. Displaying the contact details of the key worker for each person with a severe mental illness prominently on the patient notes.

Psychological therapies:

19. Reviewing the access, via secondary care or non-statutory agencies, to cognitive, behavioural, family or other psychological therapies.

Stress management for the primary-care team:

20. Meeting with members of the practice team to consider how you might provide support for each other to minimize your own stress.
21. Liaison with the primary-care organization to consider some form of regular psychological support system for health professionals.

Suggested issues for practice and PCT audit

You may find the following ideas useful when auditing your practice performance in relation to mental health, in order to improve patient outcomes.

Primary-care process indicators
- Establishment of a register for people with severe mental illness.
- Check that people with severe mental illness are not missing out on routine targets set for the rest of the population (eg immunization, vaccination, prescribing of statins, blood pressure control, cervical smears, and breast screening).
- Arrangement to make a longer than average appointment for people with a mental health problem.
- Access to non-drug treatments within the practice, eg practice counsellor or practice nurse.
- Appropriate prescribing rate for atypical antipsychotics.
- Appropriate prescribing rate for antidepressants.
- Appropriate prescribing rate for methylphenidate (eg implementation of NICE guidance).
- Reduction in benzodiazepine prescribing.
- Number of referrals to specialist services.
- Number of admissions to specialist services.
- Number of referrals to other community services (eg those run by voluntary organisations), and self-help groups.
- Link with the NIMHE (National Institute of Mental Health for England) primary care mental health programme.

Indicators of arrangements between primary and specialist care
- Level of 24-hour services provided to ensure that people managed on the Care Programme Approach (CPA) can, when necessary, see a mental health professional at any time, 24 hours a day, 365 days a year.
- Protocol with which everyone is familiar for urgent referrals to specialist services, where patient can be seen without delay, even if he/she is not yet on the CPA.
- Establishment of referral protocols between primary and specialist care for range of conditions and for range of therapies, including psychological treatments.
- Average time of untreated psychosis in young people experiencing first signs of a psychotic illness (dependent on identification, onward referral and presence of an early intervention team within specialized services).
- Number of channels (one, two, three or more) for making links with specialized services (including specialized staff on site, gateway worker, link worker, routine joint reviews of patients with severe mental illness).
- Frequency with which patients on enhanced CPA have a risk assessment.
- Proportion of patients with a current or recent history of severe mental illness and/or self-harm, who have been detained under the Mental Health Act because of a high risk of suicide, followed up with a face-to-face contact with a mental health professional within 7–14 days of discharge.
- Proportion of people seen in Accident & Emergency after an episode of self-harm, who are seen by their GP within the next three days.
- Shared system for suicide audit.

Acceptability to patients
- Opinion of service users and carers.
- Information provided to patients.

- Receptionists are sympathetic to needs of mental health patients.
- Routine audits of services that include opinions of service-users and carers.

Morbidity outcome indicators

- Routine measurement of mental health outcomes (eg HoNOS — the Health of the Nation Outcome Scales or specific depression and anxiety scores).

Mortality outcome indicators

- The system to address these should be at PCT level, rather than practice level, because of the issue of low frequency.
- Reduction in suicides:
  - Primary-care trusts should track suicides, and check that the right systems are in place to investigate the circumstances, in a manner that promotes effective leaving and change.
  - Promote good-quality risk management (eg action for people who self-harm, checks to ensure those with severe mental illness know whom to contact in an emergency, and automatic triggers in records for rapid follow-up after discharge from hospital).
- Reduction in premature mortality of people with severe mental illness from physical disorders.

Psychological therapies: what are they?

Behavioural therapy

Behavioural therapy is based on the belief that many of our actions are the result of things that we have learned. The focus of behavioural interventions is on definable behaviours that can be readily monitored and addressed in therapeutic interventions. It is a very directive therapy, which sets objectives (in collaboration with the patient) for the patient to attain. Patients are given homework assignments. It is particularly good for treating phobias, obsessional and compulsive behaviour and can also be helpful in dealing with some sexual problems. Anxiety management and exposure therapy are particular types of behavioural therapy.

Anxiety management

This approach involves a varying mixture of behavioural strategies, often taught in a group setting to people with anxiety problems. The strategies commonly include education about the nature of anxiety (eg fight-or-flight response), recognizing hyperventilation, the slow-breathing technique, relaxation training and graded exposure. Stress management, assertiveness training and structured problem solving may also be included, depending on the training and background of the therapist and the needs of the clients.

Graded exposure

Patients who avoid particular places or people because of anxiety (ie those suffering from phobias, Obsessive-compulsive disorder or panic) are encouraged gradually to face the things they fear, starting with easy situations and building up slowly to harder things. Breathing and relaxation techniques are used to help the patient remain in the feared situation until the anxiety diminishes and the patient learns that they can cope with the situation. The clinician supports the client but does not need to accompany them in their assignments.

Cognitive therapy

Cognitive therapy is based on the idea that how you think largely determines the way you feel. Cognitive therapy teaches the individual to recognize and challenge upsetting thoughts. Learning to challenge negative or fear-inducing thoughts helps people think more realistically and feel better. Patients are given homework assignments. Cognitive therapy is more complex than positive thinking. It is usually given in 50-minute sessions over 10–15 weeks.

Cognitive behavioural therapy (CBT)

This is a structured treatment combining elements of cognitive and behavioural therapy approaches, used to change a patient's thought processes and behaviour, in order to bring about relief of symptoms or other practical objectives agreed by the patient. The range of techniques used includes challenging irrational beliefs, replacing the irrational beliefs with alternative ones, thought stopping, exposure, assertiveness and social skills training. Patients are given homework assignments.

Compliance therapy

This is a form of counselling, usually used for people with severe mental illness who are reluctant to take medication. It encourages patients to take an active role in monitoring their illness and negotiating treatment decisions. The patient's views about medication are elicited, ambivalence explored and options considered, in an atmosphere of support and empathy, avoiding blaming. This interactive approach has proved more successful than a simple didactic approach.

Counselling

The term 'counselling' covers a wide range of skills and techniques. Counsellors may, for example, use cognitive or behavioural techniques. In the main, however, it provides a supportive and non-judgemental atmosphere for people to talk over their problems and explore more satisfactory ways of living. Counselling generally deals with specific life situations and is shorter term than analytical psychotherapies — in primary care, usually 6–12 sessions. It is generally used for less severe problems. Counselling is often focused, with counsellors or agencies specializing in particular problems, eg relationship problems, rape or bereavement.

Family interventions for people with schizophrenia

A form of 'psycho-social intervention', this comprises giving information to the patient's family about the illness, and helping them to improve their ability and confidence in tackling problems effectively. The approach is broadly behavioural and the family is encouraged to set realistic goals. This means that the family is able to avoid making unrealistic demands on the patient and to make the environment of the person who is ill less stressful. Relapse rates are reduced.

Interpersonal therapy

Interpersonal psychotherapy uses the connection between the onset of symptoms and current interpersonal problems as a treatment focus. It deals with current, rather than past, relationships, and maintains a clear focus on the patient's social context and dysfunction, rather than their personality. Treatment is carried out by experienced therapists over 10–15 sessions.

Problem solving

Structured problem solving can help patients sort out and deal with stresses that contribute to worry and depression. It involves encouraging the patient to identify specific problems, to order them in terms of importance and then to focus on one problem at a time, writing down potential solutions and identifying specific steps that they might take to implement the solutions. A main aim is to assist people to incorporate the principles of efficient problem solving and goal achievement into their everyday lives. The aim is not for the clinician to solve the patient's problems for them but to give them skills so that they can effectively overcome problems and achieve goals for themselves. Self-management is a key goal, with the clinician adopting the role of teacher or guide.

Psychodynamic therapy (analytical psychotherapies)

These are usually offered by psychotherapy departments after assessment by a psychotherapist. They are based on psychoanalytical ways of understanding human development (Freud and his successors). The therapy concentrates on unconscious conflicts and explores the person's inner world, as well as their external situations. Analytical therapies may be offered on an individual, couple, family or group basis. Individual sessions are usually for 50 minutes over several months. Group sessions usually last an hour a week for a year or more. Couple and family sessions are usually more widespread, with homework tasks set between sessions.

Complementary and alternative treatment

Complementary and alternative medicine (CAM) is a growing provider of healthcare and mental healthcare in the UK. Many people with mental health problems and frank mental illness use both orthodox care and CAM. Irrespective of whether CAM is effective, good practice suggests that primary-care teams and mental health teams should be familiar with the generic issues around CAM, and with the specific complementary interventions used by their patients and the possibility for interaction with orthodox treatments.[1-3] Patients should be asked if they are using any complementary therapies.

There is growing evidence that some complementary interventions may be helpful.[4,5] There is a need for much more research on widely used but still untested interventions and for more research on tightly defined client groups. The Department of Health has recently started a £3.5 million programme to stimulate research capacity in this area.

References

1 Ernst E. Risks associated with complementary therapies. In: Dukes MNG, Aronson JK (eds.) *Meyler's Side Effects of Drugs*, 14th edn. Amsterdam: Elsevier, 2000: 1649–1681.

2 Izzo AA, Ernst E. Interactions between herbal medicines and prescribed drugs: a systematic review. *Drugs* 2001; 15: 2163–2175.

3 Fugh-Berman A, Ernst E. Herb–drug interactions: review and assessment of report reliability. *Br J Clin Pharmacol* 2001; 52: 587–595.

4 Ernst E, Pittler MH, Stevenson C, White AR. *The Desktop Guide to Complementary and Alternative Medicine*. Edinburgh: Mosby, 2001.

5 Holford P. *Optimum Nutrition for the Mind*. London: Piatkus Books, 2003.

Training for primary-care teams in mental health skills

This is a template for a chart for information on local and regional sources of training and support. You might like to compare this with the review of the training needs of your practice team or primary-care organization/local health group. Below we have listed some national resources that may be drawn upon to help fill identified local gaps. The list of national resources is not exhaustive.

Topic	Multidisciplinary training	GPs	Nurses	Receptionists/ non-professionals	Counsellors
Mental health awareness					
Promoting mental health and preventing mental illness					
Communication skills					
Counselling skills					
Problem solving					
Cognitive strategies					
Motivational interviewing					
Depression					
Postnatal depression					
Anxiety					
Schizophrenia					
Dementia					
Re-attribution — somatization					
Suicide and self-harm					
Child and adolescent mental health					
Alcohol misuse					
Drug misuse					

The following providers of courses or training packs are all national organizations. You may wish to adapt this list to include details of your local or regional providers of training.

Training courses

Training courses may be organized locally via educational consortia, university departments of general practice or nursing, health authorities or primary-care groups, often utilizing locally available skills. The following provide courses or training packs on a national or regional basis.

Section of Primary Care Mental Health, Institute of Psychiatry is led by Professor André Tylee and also has a full-time training fellow funded by the Charlie Waller Memorial Trust. The Section provides lectures, seminars and mental health skills masterclasses in collaboration with the Royal College of General Practitioners (RCGP). Masterclasses for GPs have been run at the RCGP on topics such as counselling, cognitive behaviour therapy, dementia, heartsink patients, chronic fatigue, somatization disorder, and a new series is to start. The main teaching activity over the past five years has been the pioneering and development of the 'Teach the Teachers' course, now known as 'Trailblazers'. This course is for pairs of local leaders (one from primary care and one from mental health services) and runs over three two-day modules over six months. The local pairs are helped to prioritize their learning needs and that of their organizations (usually primary-care trusts). They are then helped to plan and deliver a teaching programme for local use or a service improvement. Over 350 participants to date have achieved a great deal at local level with this help. The course began in London as a pilot for the south and west regions and rapidly developed through Yorkshire (Dr Tim Thornton and Mrs Heather Raistrick), West Midlands (Dr David Shiers, Dr Helen Lester and colleagues) and the North East (Dr Dave Tomson and Dr MaryAnne Freer). It is beginning in South London and the eastern region, and it is hoped it will develop soon in East Midlands and the southeast region. Contact details and information can be provided by Professor André Tylee or the Waller Fellow, Institute of Psychiatry, De Crespigny Park, Denmark Hill, London SE5 8AF. Tel: 020 7848 0150; Email: Julie.smith@iop.kcl.ac.uk.

The National Institute for Mental Health in England (NIHME) has several programmes, including a Primary-care Programme. This is chaired by Professor André Tylee from the Section of Primary Care Mental Health at the Institute of Psychiatry and is jointly managed by the London Regional Development Centre (RDC) and the West Midlands RDC. The programme has five key areas: staff development, commissioning, integrating care and services for those with severe and enduring mental illness (SEMI), primary-care users, and research and development. Staff development includes core training for primary-care professionals, leadership development in primary care mental health, multiprofessional learning and training for new workers (eg primary care mental health workers from September 2003). Commissioning involves improving the knowledge and evidence base around commissioning and developing effective partnerships. Regarding the care of those with SEMI, it is essential to have good communication at the interface of primary, mental and social care, to meet the physical, mental and social needs of this group and provide good chronic disease management, as is now customary for asthma and diabetes. Users who only attend primary care will be encouraged to take part in designing and delivering good care together with the relevant user and carer groups. Research and development ideas will emerge and it will be important to prioritize them and stimulate innovative research and service development. The programme has a Board that includes all RDCs, who will be encouraged to lead on each of the five areas. Also on the Board are NATPACT (National Primary and Care Trust), the Primary-care Collaborative, The National Champion, a representative of the Users Programme, and the lead in primary care for the Department of Health. There is a Reference group, which includes all relevant stakeholders, and this will advise and lobby the programme, which has a full-time project manager (Mary Sheppard). Contact Professor André Tylee, Institute of Psychiatry, De Crespigny Park, Denmark Hill, London SE5 8AF. Tel: 020 7848 0150; Email: Julie.smith@iop.kcl.ac.uk.

PRiMHE (Primary Care Mental Health Education) is the UK charity devoted to the provision of mental health support, services and education to primary-care professionals. PRiMHE produces a resource pack for mental health promotion, nurturing social inclusion and managing mental health problems in primary care. The CEO is Dr Chris Manning. The *Resource Pack for Promoting Mental Health, Nurturing*

Social Inclusion and Managing Mental Health Problems in Primary Care in the UK was launched in June 2003. For information about the *PRiMHE* and *Child and Adolescent Mental Health in Primary Care* journals, network, Clarion (website discussion forum), educational meetings, training materials programmes, supportership and subscriptions, contact PRiMHE, The Old Stables, 2A Laurel Avenue, Twickenham TW1 4JA. Tel: 020 8891 6593; Email: info@primhe.org; Website: http://www.primhe.org.

The Sainsbury Centre for Mental Health (SCMH) is an independent mental health charity that can provide bespoke training courses for primary-care teams and primary healthcare teams. It also provides a training course that equips primary-care clinicians for the GMS2 contract, and has published a number of guides and manuals for primary-care clinicians and trusts. Contact Claire Groom, PCAU Project Co-ordinator; tel: 020 7403 8790; Email: claire.groom@scmh.org.uk. Further details of the other services that SCMH provide may be found at http://www.scmh.org.uk.

National Primary Care Research and Development Centre runs a course in psychiatry for GP Registrars and other courses on a needs basis. Contact Dr Linda Gask, School of Primary Care, Rusholme Health Centre, Walmer Street, Manchester M14 5NP. Tel: 0161 256 3015 x220.

Counselling in Primary Care Trust offers consultancy in primary care mental health development, training and psychotherapy research. Contact Dr Graham Curtis-Jenkins, Counselling in Primary Care Trust, 38 Richmond Road, Staines TW18 2AB. Tel: 01784 441 782.

The Counselling and Psychotherapy Training Forum in Healthcare comprises the lead professional organizations and has set standards for training and employment of primary-care counsellors. Contact through Counsellors and Psychotherapists in Primary Care, Queensway House, Queensway, Bognor Regis, West Sussex, PO21 1QT. Tel: 01243 870 701.

Resources for use by trainers

Training packages, including videos, for use in skills-based training (watching the skills demonstrated on the video followed by practising them in role play) are available on the following topics:

- Managing somatic presentation of emotional distress (re-attribution, 2nd edition)
- Helping people at risk of suicide or self-harm
- Problem-based interviewing in general practice
- Depression and suicidal behaviour in adolescents
- Counselling depression in primary care
- Depression in primary care. Part 1: Recognition in general practice
- Depression in primary care. Part 2: How to plan and assess treatment
- Relaxation.

Videos cost £58.75 (including postage). Contact Nick Jordan, Video Producer, University of Manchester, School of Psychiatry and Behavioural Sciences, Wythenshaw Hospital, Manchester M23 9LT. Tel: 0161 291 5926; Email: Nick.Jordan@man.ac.uk. Online catalogue: http://www.man.ac.uk/psych.

Other topics available include the following:

- Anxiety (non-pharmacological approaches)
- Dementia
- Chronic fatigue
- Schizophrenia.

All available from Professor André Tylee, Section of Primary Care Mental Health, Institute of Psychiatry, De Crespigny Park, Denmark Hill, London SE5 8AF. Tel: 020 7848 0150; Email: Julie.smith@iop.kcl.ac.uk.

- Problem solving
  available from Dr Laurence Mynors-Wallis, Consultant Psychiatrist, Alderney Hospital, Ringwood Road, Parkstone, Poole, Dorset BH12 4NB. Tel 01202 305 080; price £10.
- Alcohol misuse (including motivational interviewing)
  available from Dr Barry Lewis, Department of Post-Graduate Medicine, Gateway House, Piccadilly South, Manchester M60 7LP. Tel: 0161 237 2109.
- Child and adolescent mental health
  available from Professor Elena Garralda, Academic Unit of Child and Adolescent Psychiatry, Saint Mary's Hospital, Praed Street, Paddington, London W2 1NY. Tel: 020 7886 1145.
- Triadic consultations with children/adolescents and their parents/carers (CD-ROM-based teaching package including video disc of typical consultations and practice exercises) available from Dr Barry Lewis, Department of Post-Graduate Medicine, Gateway House, Piccadilly South, Manchester M60 7LP. Tel: 0161 237 2109.

Audio tapes on depression and anxiety, stress management and health promotion (relaxation, depression, anxiety, sleep problems) for primary-care professionals are available from Talking Life, 1A Grosvenor Rd, Hoylake, Wirral CH47 2BS. Tel: 0151 632 0662; website: http://www.talkinglife.co.uk.

An interactive CD-ROM teaching/revising basic clinical skills for primary-care clinicians is produced by the Clinical Research Unit for Anxiety Disorders (CRUFAD) in Australia, which is a WHO Collaborating Centre for Mental Health and Substance Abuse. The CD-ROM covers interviewing skills, prescribing skills, patient education, structured problem solving and control of hyperventilation. It costs A$70. Details of this and many other resources, usually based on cognitive behavioural methods, including treatment manuals (suitable for use by counsellors or others with appropriate training) on Obsessive-compulsive disorder, panic, generalized anxiety and phobias can be found on CRUFAD's website (http://www.crufad.unsw.edu.au), or by contacting Professor Gavin Andrews, University of New South Wales Clinical Research Unit for Anxiety Disorders, 299 Forbes Street, Darlinghurst, NSW 2010, Australia. Fax: +61 (612) 9332 4316; Email: gavina@gecko.crufad.unsw.edu.au

CALIPSO, developed at the University of Leeds School of Medicine, provides interactive CD-ROM self-led learning resources for use by GPs, trainee psychiatrists and mental health professionals in clinical identification, treatment and management of mood disorders, depression, anxiety, schizophrenia/paranoid disorders, and dementia. It is also available as a multimedia training package on delivery of Cognitive behavioural therapy in structured groups. For prices and other details, contact University of Leeds Media Innovations Ltd, 3 Gemini Business Park, Sheepscar Way, Leeds LS7 3SB. Tel: 0113 262 1600; Email: s.taylor-parker@media-innovations.ltd.uk; website: http://www.calipso.co.uk.

A learning resource pack for use by health professionals and others on *Understanding Depression in People with Learning Disabilities* is available from Pavilion Publishing Ltd, 8 St. Georges Place, Brighton BN1 4ZZ. Tel: 01273 623222. Price: £125 plus VAT and p&p.

A variety of other resources for trainers are available from MIND, the Mental Health Foundation and the Samaritans. For example, MIND provides inhouse training on mental health awareness and other mental health issues. These training resources are generally aimed at a broad audience, including clinicians, but are not specifically produced for primary care. For catalogues, contact MIND Conference and Training Unit, Granta House, 15–19 Broadway, London E15 4BQ. Tel: 020 8519 2122, and The Mental Health Foundation, 83 Victoria Street, London SW1. Tel: 020 7802 0300.

References

1 World Health Organization. *Schizophrenia: An International Follow-up Study*. Chichester: John Wiley & Sons, 1979. (AIV)

Large outcome study with two-year follow-up, showed that only 10–15% of patients did not recover from their illness in that two-year period. Another shorter-term follow-up study (Lieberman J, Jody D, Geisler S *et al*. Time course and biologic correlates of treatment response in first episode schizophrenia. *Arch Gen Psychiatry* 1993, 50: 369–376) showed that 83% of first-episode psychotic patients treated with antipsychotic medication remitted by one year post-inpatient admission.

2 Kavanagh DJ. Recent developments in expressed emotion and schizophrenia. *Br J Psychiatry* 1992, 160: 601–620. (AIII)

Family support and education, which promotes a more supportive family environment, can reduce relapse rates substantially.

3 Driver and Vehicle Licensing Agency. *At a Glance Guide to Medical Aspects of Fitness to Drive*. URL http://www.dvla.gov.uk.

Further information is available from The Senior Medical Adviser, DVLA, Driver Medical Unit, Longview Road, Morriston, Swansea SA99 ITU, Wales.

4 Atypical antipsychotics appear to be better tolerated, with fewer extrapyramidal side-effects, than typical drugs at therapeutic doses. Even at low doses, extrapyramidal side-effects are commonly experienced with typical drugs. Whether or not atypicals improve the long-term outcome has yet to be established. Risperidone, amisulpride and possibly olanzapine have a dose-related effect. Selected references:

4a American Psychiatric Association. Practice guidelines: schizophrenia. *Am J Psychiatry* 1997, 154(Suppl 4): 1–49. (BII)

This reports 60% of patients receiving acute treatment with typical antipsychotic medication, develop significant extrapyramidal side-effects.

4b Mir S, Taylor D. Issues in schizophrenia. *Pharmaceut J* 1998, 261: 55–58. (CV)

This work reviews evidence on efficacy, safety and patient tolerability of atypical antipsychotics.

4c Duggan L, Fenton M, Dardennes RM *et al*. Olanzapine for schizophrenia (Cochrane Review). In: *The Cochrane Library*. Oxford: Update Software, 1999. (CI)

Twenty-one studies were analysed. Olanzapine was found to be an effective antipsychotic that produced fewer movement side-effects. It did tend to cause more weight gain than the older drugs, however.

4d Hunter RH, Joy CB, Kennedy E *et al*. Risperidone versus typical antipsychotic medication for schizophrenia (Cochrane Review). In: *The Cochrane Library*, Issue 2, 2003. Oxford: Update Software (C1)

Twenty-three studies were analysed. Risperidone might be equally clinically effective as relatively high doses of haloperidol. It causes fewer adverse effects than the side-effect-prone haloperidol.

5 National Institute for Clinical Excellence. *Schizophrenia: Core Interventions in the Treatment and Management of Schizophrenia in Primary and Secondary Care*. Clinical Guideline 1. December 2002. URL http://www.nice.org.uk. (AI)

6 Bollini P, Pampallona S, Orza MJ. Antipsychotic drugs: is more worse? A meta-analysis of the published randomized control trials. *Psychol Med* 1994, 24: 307–316. (AI)

For most patients, higher than moderate doses of antipsychotic drugs bring increased side-effects but no additional therapeutic gains.

7 Dixon LB, Lehman AF, Levine J. Conventional antipsychotic medications for schizophrenia. *Schizophrenia Bull* 1995, 21(4): 567–577. (AI)

This paper produces overwhelming evidence that continuing maintenance therapy reduces risk of relapse. The authors conclude that it is appropriate to taper or discontinue medication within six months to a year for first-episode patients who experience a full remission of symptoms.

8 Taylor D, McConnell D, McConnel H, Kerwin R. *The Bethlem and Maudsley NHS Trust Prescribing Guidelines 2001*. London: Martin Dunitz Ltd, 2000.

9 United Kingdom Psychiatric Pharmacy Group (UKPPG). URL http://www.UKPPG.co.uk.

10a Mental Health Commission. *Early Intervention in Psychosis: Guidance Note*. Wellington, New Zealand, 1999.

b Falloon I, Coverdale J, Laidlaw T *et al*. Family management in the prevention of morbidity of schizophrenia: social outcome of a 2-year longitudinal study. *Psychol Med* 1997, 17: 59–66. (AII)

Involvement of the family is vital. Education is important for engaging individuals and families in treatment and promoting recovery. Psychological therapies may be helpful.

11 Department of Health. *National Service Framework for Mental Health*. London: HMSO, 1999.

12 Consensus (BV). As people reacting to stresses such as unemployment or divorce are at high risk of developing a mental disorder, studies on prevention in high-risk groups may be relevant. These support the offering of social support and problem-solving. [NHS Centre for Reviews and Dissemination. Mental health promotion in high-risk groups. *Effect Health Care Bull* 1997, 3(3): 1–10.]

13 Catalan J, Gath D, Edmonds G, Ennis J. The effects of not prescribing anxiolytics in general practice. *Br J Psychiatry* 1984, 144: 593–602. (BII)

GP advice and reassurance is as effective as administration of benzodiazepines. The mean time spent by the GP for giving advice and reassurance was 12 minutes, compared with 10.5 minutes for giving a prescription.

14a Roth AD, Fonagy P. *What Works For Whom? A Critical Review of Psychotherapy Research*. New York: Guilford Press, 1996. (CII)

The efficacy of counselling in primary-care settings is difficult to assess because of the methodological problems of available research. It seems more appropriate for milder presentations of disorders, however, than for more severe presentations, and evidence is better for counselling focused on a particular client group (eg relationship or bereavement counselling).

14b Bower P, Rowland N, Mellor Clark J *et al*. Effectiveness and cost-effectiveness of counselling in primary care (Cochrane Review). In: *The Cochrane Library*, Issue 2, 2003. Oxford: Update Software. (B1)

Seven studies were analysed. Results showed that counselling is significantly more effective than 'usual care' in the short- but not the long-term. Satisfaction with counselling was high. Patients had a mix of 'emotional disorders'.

15 Rosenberg H. Prediction of controlled drinking by alcoholics and problem drinkers. *Psychol Bull* 1993, 113: 129–139. (BII)

This is a qualitative review of the literature. Successful achievement of controlled drinking is associated with less severe dependence and a belief that controlled drinking is possible.

16 NHS Centre for Reviews and Dissemination. Brief interventions and alcohol use. *Effect Health Care Bull* 1993, 1: 1–12. (AI)

Brief interventions, including assessing drinking and related problems, motivational feedback and advice, are effective. They are most successful for less severely affected patients.

17 Slattery J, Chick J, Cochrane M *et al*. *Prevention of Relapse in Alcohol Dependence*. Health Technology Assessment Report 3. Glasgow: Health Technology Board for Scotland, 2003. URL http://www.htbs.co.uk. (A1)

This study looked at treatments for individuals with alcohol dependence. Psychological treatments are effective but brief psychological treatments have no effect. Acamprosate and naltrexone showed significant beneficial effects.

18 Miller WR, Wilbourne PL. Mesa Grande: a methodological analysis of clinical trials of treatments for alcohol use disorders. *Addiction* 2002, 97(3): 265–277. (A1)

Three hundred and sixty-one studies were analysed. There is strong evidence for the use of psychological treatments and the drugs acamprosate and naltrexone in treatment of alcohol use disorders.

19 McCrady B, Irvine S. Self-help groups. In: Hester R, Miller W (eds.) *Handbook of Alcoholism Treatment Approaches: Effective Alternatives*. 2nd edition. New York: Allyn and Bacon, 2003. (AIV)

This chapter discusses the characteristics of patients who are good candidates for Alcoholics Anonymous (AA). Several studies show AA to be an important support in remaining alcohol-free to patients who are willing to attend.

20 American Psychiatric Association. *Practice Guidelines: Substance Use Disorders*, 1996. (BIV)

Where patients have mild to moderate withdrawal symptoms, general support, reassurance and frequent monitoring is sufficient treatment for two thirds of them, without pharmacological treatment.

21 Collins MN, Burns T, Van den Berk PA, Tubman GF. A structured programme for out-patient alcohol detoxification. *Br J Psychiatry* 1990, 156: 871–874. (BIV)

22 Srisurapanont M, Jarusuraisin N. Opioid antagonists for alcohol dependence (Cochrane Review). In: *The Cochrane Library*, Issue 1, 2003. Oxford: Update Software. (B1)

Nineteen studies were analysed. Naltrexone may decrease alcohol consumption in people with alcohol dependency but their compliance with treatment appears problematic. It should be given with psychological intervention.

23 Duncan D, Taylor D. Chlormethiazole or chlordiazepoxide in alcohol detoxification. *Psychiatr Bull* 1996, 20: 599–601. (AIV)

This paper describes randomized controlled trials that show chlordiazepoxide and chlomethiazole to be of equal efficacy; however, chlordiazepoxide is a safer alternative (there is a risk of fatal respiratory depression with alcohol and chlomethiazole) and chlomethiazole is no longer recommended for outpatient use.

24 Cook CC, Hallwood PM, Thomson AD. B vitamin deficiency and neuropsychiatric syndromes in alcohol misuse. *Alcohol Alcoholism* 1998, 33(4): 317–336.

25 Kranzler H, Burleson J, Del Boca F *et al*. Buspirone treatment of anxious alcoholics: a placebo-controlled trial. *Arch Gen Psychiatry* 1994, 51: 720–731. (BII)

26 Hughes JC, Cook CC. The efficacy of disulfiram: a review of outcome studies Addiction 1997, 92(4): 381–395. (C1)

Thirty-eight studies were analysed. Support for the general use of oral disulfiram is equivocal, mostly leading to reduced quantity of alcohol consumed and a reduced number of drinking days.

27 Alcohol Concern. *Brief Interventions Guidelines*. London, 1997.

Available from Alcohol Concern, Waterbridge House, 32–36 Loman Street, London SE1 OEE, UK. Tel: +44 20 7928 7377. URL http://www.alcoholconcern.org.uk.

28 Holder H, Longabaugh R, Miller W, Rubonis A. The cost effectiveness of treatment for alcoholism: a first approximation. *J Stud Alcohol* 1991, 52: 517–540. (AI)

Treatments aim to improve self-control and social skills — for example, relationship skills, assertiveness and drink refusal.

29 Hunt G, Axrin N. A community reinforcement approach to alcoholism. *Behav Res Ther* 1973, 11: 91–104. (AI)

This approach uses behavioural principles and includes training in job finding, support in developing alcohol-free social and recreational activities, and an alcohol-free social club.

30 Raphael B. Preventive intervention with the recently bereaved. *Arch Gen Psychiatry* 1997, 34: 1450–1454. (BIII)

This work demonstrates that 'high-risk' bereaved people who receive counselling have fewer symptoms of lasting anxiety and tension than those who do not.

31 Kato PM, Mann T. A synthesis of psychological interventions for the bereaved. *Clin Psychol Rev* 1999, 19(3): 275–296. (C1)

Fourteen studies were analysed. A slight improvement is seen for individual therapies.

32 Manic Depression Fellowship. *Inside Out: A Guide to Self-Management of Manic Depression*. London, 1995.

Available from the Manic Depression Fellowship, 8–10 High Street, Kingston-upon-Thames, London KT1 1EY, UK. This advice is based on self-management training, 7–12 sessions of which have been shown to increase time between manic episodes. See Perry A, Tarrier N, Morris R *et al*. Randomised control trial of efficacy of teaching patients with bipolar disorder to identify early symptoms of relapse and obtain treatment. *Br Med J* 1999, 318: 149–152. (BII) Teaching patients to recognise early symptoms of manic relapse and seek early treatment is associated with important clinical improvements in time to first manic relapse, social functioning, and employment.

33 Chou JC-Y. Recent advances in treatment of acute mania. *J Clin Psychopharm* 1991, 11: 3–21. (BII)

Antipsychotics are effective in mania, and they appear to have a more rapid effect than lithium.

34 Rifkin A, Doddi S, Karajgi B *et al*. Dosage of haloperidol for mania. *Br J Psychiatry* 1994, 165: 113–116. (BII)

Doses of haloperidol over 10 mg a day in management of mania confer no benefit.

35 American Psychiatric Association. *Practice Guidelines: Bipolar Disorder*. Washington, DC, 1996. (AII)

Four randomized control trials show that benzodiazepines are effective, in place of, or in conjunction with, a neuroleptic in sedating acutely agitated, manic patients.

36a Cookson J. Lithium: balancing risks and benefits. *Br J Psychiatry* 1997, 171: 113–119. (BIII)

36b Dali I. Mania. *Lancet* 1997, 349: 1157–1160.

36c Bowden C, Brugger A, Swann A *et al*. Efficacy of divolproex versus lithium and placebo in the treatment of mania. The Depakote Mania Study Group. *JAMA* 1994, 271: 918–924. (CII)

This is a randomized controlled trial. Lithium is as effective as valproate and more effective than placebo.

36d A Cochrane Review will soon be available: Bhagwagar Z, Goodwin G, Geddes J. Lithium for acute mania (Protocol for a Cochrane Review). In: *The Cochrane Library*, Issue 2, 2003. Oxford: Update Software.

37a Zornberg G, Pope H Jr. Treatment of depression in bipolar disorder: new directions for research. *J Clin Psychopharmacol* 1993, 13: 397–408. (BIII)

A review of nine controlled studies shows a high response rate to lithium for acute bipolar depression. Response may take six to eight weeks to become evident, however.

37b A Cochrane Review will soon be available. Gijsman HJ, Rendell J, Geddes J, Nolen WA, Goodwin GM. Antidepressants for bipolar depression (Protocol for a Cochrane Review). In: *The Cochrane Library*, Issue 2, 2003. Oxford: Update Software.

37c A Cochrane Review will soon be available. Bhagwagar Z, Goodwin G and Geddes J. Lithium for bipolar depression (Protocol for a Cochrane Review). In: *The Cochrane Library*, Issue 2, 2003. Oxford: Update Software.

38a Goodwin G. Lithium revisited: a re-examination of the placebo-controlled trials of lithium prophylaxis in manic-depressive disorder. *Br J Psychiatry* 1995, 167: 573–574. (BIII)

Trials show prophylactic use of lithium to be effective, although most trials have had methodological flaws.

38b Berghofer A, Kossmann B, Muller-Oerlinghausen B. Course of illness and pattern of recurrence in patients with affective disorders during long-term lithium prophylaxis: a retrospective analysis over 15 years. *Acta Psychiatr Scand* 1996, 93: 349–354.

The prophylactic effect of lithium can be maintained over at least 10 years.

39 Burgess S, Geddes J, Hawton K, Townsend E, Jamieson K, Goodwin G. Lithium or maintenance treatment of mood disorders (Cochrane Review). In: *The Cochrane Library*, Issue 1, 2003. Oxford: Update Software. (A1)

Nine studies were analysed. Lithium was more effective than placebo in preventing relapse in bipolar disorder. Caution should be exercised in abruptly stopping lithium therapy in patients who have been taking it successfully for some time, because of the high risk of relapse.

40 Macritchie K, Geddes J, Scott J *et al*. Valproate for acute mood episodes in bipolar disorder (Cochrane Review). In: *The Cochrane Library*, Issue I. Oxford: Update Software, 2003. (A1)

Ten studies were analysed. No significant difference in efficacy was seen between valproate and lithium or between valproate and carbamazepine. Valproate might be less effective in reducing manic symptoms than olanzapine but it could cause less sedation and weight gain.

41 Schou M. Effects of long-term lithium treatment on kidney function: an overview. *J Psychiatry* Res 1988, 22: 287–296.

This is a qualitative literature review.

42 Goodwin GM. Recurrence of mania after lithium withdrawal. Implications for the use of lithium in the treatment of bipolar affective disorder. *Br J Psychiatry* 1994, 164(2): 149–152. (BIII)

Fourteen studies were analysed. More than 50% of new episodes of illness occurred within three months of treatment cessation. Lithium should not be introduced for the prophylactic treatment of bipolar illness unless or until the doctor and patient understand that it must be used for a minimum of two years. If after two years there is no worthwhile benefit, it is more likely that harm, in the form of premature recurrence of mania, will be done.

43 An Independent Working Group. *Working Party on CFS/ME to the Chief Medical Officer for England and Wales*. London: Department of Health, 2002.

44 Fukuda K, Strauss SE, Hickie I, Sharp M *et al*. and the International Chronic Fatigue Study Group. The Chronic Fatigue Syndrome: a comprehensive approach to its definition and study. *Ann Intern Med* 1994, 121: 953–959.

45 Abbey S, Garfinkel P. Chronic fatigue syndrome and depression: cause, effect or covariate. *Rev Infect Dis* 1991, 13(suppl 1): S73–S83.

46 Prins J, Bleijenberg G, Rouweler E *et al*. Doctor–patient relationship in primary care of chronic fatigue syndrome: Perspectives of the doctor and the patient. *J Chronic Fatigue Syndrome* 2001, 7: 3–15.

47 Butler C, Rollnick S. Missing the meaning and provoking resistance: a case of myalgic encephalomyelitis. *Family Pract* 1996, 13: 106–109.

48 Whiting P, Bagnall A, Sowden A *et al*. Interventions for the treatment and management of chronic fatigue syndrome: a systematic review. *JAMA* 2001, 286: 1360–1368. (AI)

Forty-four studies were analysed. Interventions that have shown promising results include cognitive behavioural therapy and graded exercise therapy.

49 Fulcher K, White P. Randomised controlled trial of graded exercises in patients with chronic fatigue syndrome. *Br Med J* 1997, 314: 1647–1652. (AII)

Fatigue, functional capacity and fitness were significantly better after exercise than after flexibility treatment in patients with chronic fatigue syndrome.

50 Powell P, Bentall R, Nye F, Edwards R. Randomised controlled trial of patient education to encourage graded exercise in chronic fatigue syndrome. *Br Med J* 2001, 322: 387–390. (AII)

Treatment of patients with Chronic fatigue syndrome incorporating evidence-based physiological explanations for symptoms was effective in encouraging self-managed graded exercise. This resulted in substantial improvement compared with standardized medical care.

51 Price JR, Couper J. Cognitive behaviour therapy for chronic fatigue syndrome in adults (Cochrane Review). In: *The Cochrane Library*, Issue 4, 1998. Oxford: Update Software. (AI)

Three studies were analysed. Cognitive behaviour therapy appears to be an effective and acceptable treatment for adult outpatients with chronic fatigue syndrome.

52 Essame C, Phelan S, Aggett P, White P. Pilot study of a multidisciplinary inpatient rehabilitation of severely incapacitated patients with chronic fatigue syndrome. *J Chronic Fatigue Syndrome* 1998, 4: 51–60. (CIV)

This is a descriptive outcome study of multidisciplinary inpatient rehabilitation. Intervention might be effective, but the studies carried out have not been well controlled.

53 Cox, Findley L. Severe and very severe patients with chronic fatigue syndrome: perceived outcome following an inpatient programme. *J Chronic Fatigue Syndrome* 2000, 7: 33–47. (CIV)

This is a descriptive outcome study of an inpatient unit. There is a tentative trend towards positive outcomes.

54 Consensus, plus some — usually small — trials. For example, Donnan P, Hutchinson A, Paxton R *et al*. Self-help materials for anxiety: a randomized controlled trial in general practice. *Br J Gen Pract* 1990, 40: 498–501. (BV)

An audiotape and booklet were given to patients with chronic anxiety. Intervention led to reduced scores for depression, as well as for anxiety.

55 Lima M, Moncrieff J. Drugs versus placebo for the treatment of dysthymia (Cochrane Review). In: *The Cochrane Library*, Issue 2, 2003. Oxford: Update Software. (AI)

Fifteen studies were analysed. There is some evidence of efficacy of most antidepressants in dysthymia (chronic, mild depressive syndrome) that has been present for at least two years.

56 McLean J, Pietroni P. Self care — who does best? *Soc Sci Med* 1990, 30(5): 591–596. (BIII)

This describes a controlled trial of a general-practice-based class teaching self-care skills, relaxation, stress management, medication, nutrition and exercise. Significant improvements were seen and maintained after one year.

57 Catalan J, Gath DH, Anastasiades P *et al*. Evaluation of a brief psychological treatment for emotional disorders in primary care. *Psychol Med* 1991, 21: 1013–1018. (BII)

This paper describes a small randomized control trial. Patients — selected for high symptom scores — did significantly better with problem-solving therapy than with routine care. Other patients — with lower symptom scores —who were not treated showed similar improvement to the treated group.

58a Roth AD, Fonagy P. *What Works For Whom? A Critical Review of Psychotherapy Research*. New York: Guilford Press, 1996. (CII)

This work concludes that the efficacy of counselling in primary-care settings is difficult to assess because of the methodological problems of available research. Counselling seems more appropriate for milder than for more severe disorders, and evidence seems better for counselling focused on a particular client group (eg relationship or bereavement counselling).

58b See reference 14b.

59 Adams CE, Eisenbruch M. Depot fluphenazine for schizophrenia (Cochrane Review). In: *The Cochrane Library*, Issue 2, 2003. Oxford: Update Software. (CI)

The use of depot fluphenazine continues to be based on clinical judgement rather than on evidence from methodical evaluation within trials.

60 Kendrick T, Millar E, Burns T, Ross F. Practice nurse involvement in giving depot neuroleptic injections: development of a patient assessment and monitoring checklist. *Prim Care Psychiatry* 1998, 4(3): 149–154 (AIV)

Of the 25% of people with schizophrenia who have no specialist contact, many have a practice nurse as their only regular professional contact. Levels of knowledge of schizophrenia and its treatment of those nurses was often no better than a lay person's.

61 Kemp R, Kirov G, Everitt B, David A. A randomised controlled trial of compliance therapy: 18-month follow-up. *Br J Psychiatry* 1998, 172: 413–419. (AII)

Patients who received specific counselling regarding their attitudes towards their illness and drug treatment were five times more likely to take medication without prompting compared with controls.

62 Pharoah FM, Mari JJ, Streiner D. Family intervention for schizophrenia (Cochrane Review). In: *The Cochrane Library*, Issue 2, 2003. Oxford: Update Software. (AI)

Thirteen studies were analysed. Families receiving this intervention, which promotes a more supportive family environment, can expect the family member with schizophrenia to relapse less and to be in hospital less.

63 Cormac I, Jones C, Campbell C, Silveira da Mota Neto J. Cognitive behaviour therapy for schizophrenia (Cochrane Review). In: *The Cochrane Library*, Issue 2, 2003. Oxford: Update Software. (AI)

Thirteen studies were analysed. Four small trials show that cognitive behaviour therapy is associated with substantially reduced risk of relapse.

64 Rabins PV. Psychosocial and management aspects of delirium. *Int Psychoger* 1991, 3(2): 319–324. (BV)

This is a review of 21 papers, concluding that the evidence base is very thin.

65a Inouye SK, Bogardus ST Jr, Charpentier PA *et al.* A multicomponent intervention to prevent delirium in hospitalized older patients. *N Engl J Med* 1999, 340: 669–676. (CIII)

Intervention was associated with significant improvement in the degree of cognitive impairment among patients with cognitive impairment at admission, and with a reduction in the rate of use of sleep medication among all patients.

65b A Cochrane Review will soon be available. Britton A, Russell R. Multidisciplinary team interventions for delirium in patients with chronic cognitive impairment (Cochrane Review). In: *The Cochrane Library*, Issue 2, 2003. Oxford: Update Software Issue 4, 2003.

66 Rummans TA, Evans JM, Krahn LE, Fleming KC. Delirium in elderly patients: evaluation and management. *Mayo Clinic Proc* 1995, 70(10): 989–998. (BV).

This reviews 55 papers, concluding that the evidence base is thin.

67 Ballard C, Grace J, McKeith I *et al.* Neuroleptic sensitivity in dementia with Lewy bodies and Alzheimer's disease. *Lancet* 1998, 351: 1032–1033. (CV)

This is a case-register study. Other interventions should be explored before the use of neuroleptics in patients with dementia, particularly in those with dementia with Lewy bodies.

68 Eccles M, Clark J, Livingstone M *et al.* North of England evidence-based guidelines development project: guidelines for the primary-care management of dementia. *Br Med J* 1998, 317: 802–808.

69 National Institute for Clinical Excellence. *Guidance on the Use of Donepezil, Rivastigmine and Galantamine for the Treatment of Alzheimer's Disease* (Technology appraisal guidance 19). London: NICE, 2001. URL http://www.nice.org.uk. (AI)

70 Areosa Sastre A, Sherriff F. Memantine for dementia (Cochrane Review). In: *The Cochrane Library*, Issue 1, 2003. Oxford: Update Software. (BI)

Seven studies were analysed. Results are awaited from two large trials, but those to date suggest a small beneficial effect from 20 or 30 mg/day of memantine on cognitive function measured at 6 and 28 weeks and on global function in patients with mild to moderately severe Alzheimer's disease, vascular and mixed dementia.

71 Reisberg B, Doody R, Stoffler A *et al.* Memantine in moderate-to-severe Alzheimer's disease. *N Engl J Med* 2003, 348(14): 1333–1341. (BII)

Memantine reduced clinical deterioration in moderate to severe Alzheimer's disease, a phase associated with distress for patients and burden on caregivers, for which other treatments are not available. It was not associated with a significant frequency of adverse events.

72 NICE will publish a guideline on the management of depression in February 2004.

73 Lawlor DA, Hopker SW. The effectiveness of exercise as an intervention in the management of depression: systematic review and meta-regression analysis of randomised controlled trials. *Br Med J* 2001, 322: 763–767. (BI)

Fourteen studies were analysed. The effectiveness of exercise in reducing symptoms of depression cannot be determined because of a lack of good-quality research on clinical populations with adequate follow-up.

74 Greden JF. Anxiety or caffeinism: a diagnosis dilemma. *Am J Psychiatry* 1974, 131: 1089–1092. (AV)

75 Schuckit M. Alcohol and major depressive disorder: a clinical perspective. *Acta Psychiatrica Scand* 1994, 377: 28–32. (AIV)

76 Wallin M, Rissanen A. Food and mood: relationship between food, serotonin and affective disorders. *Acta Psychiatr Scand* 1994, 377(Suppl): 36–40. (CV)

Quoted in *Guidelines for the Treatment and Management of Depression by Primary Health Care Professionals.* National Health Committee of New Zealand, 1996.

77 Schulberg H, Katon W, Simon G, Rush AJ. Best clinical practice: guidelines for managing major depression in primary care. *J Clin Psychiatry* 1999, 60(Suppl 7): 19–24. (BII)

The authors conclude that recovery rates for an acute episode of major depression in primary care are similar for guideline-driven pharmacotherapy and depression-specific psychotherapies, such as interpersonal therapy and problem-solving treatments. Medication takes four to six weeks to show effect and psychotherapies six to eight weeks. Another conclusion from this paper is that recent randomized controlled trials conducted in primary care show a 50–60% response rate to all classes of antidepressants in primary-care patients.

78 Lave J, Frank R, Schulberg H, Kamlet M. Cost-effectiveness of treatments for major depression in primary-care practice. *Arch Gen Psychiatry* 1998, 55(7): 645–51. (BII)

The authors describe a high-quality randomized control trial comparing standardized treatment by nortriptyline, interpersonal psychotherapy and primary physician's usual care (*n* >90 for each group) for major depression in primary care. Both standardized therapies were better than usual care, and more expensive. Those taking drugs did slightly better with respect to both quality of life and economic outcomes.

79 Paykel E, Hollyman J, Freeling P, Sedgwick P. Prediction of therapeutic benefit from amitriptyline in mild depression: a general practice, placebo-controlled trial. *J Affective Disord* 1988, 14: 83–95. (BIII)

Antidepressants do not show efficacy in mild, acute depression.

80 NHS Centre for Reviews and Dissemination, University of York. The treatment of depression in primary care. *Effect Health Care* 1993, March(5): 1–12. (AII)

Effective strategies to improve the detection and appropriateness of treatment of depression in primary care are available.

81a Prien R, Kupfer D. Continuation drug therapy for major depressive episodes: how long should it be maintained? *Am J Psychiatry* 1986, 143: 18–23. (BII)

The authors conclude that patients treated for a first episode of uncomplicated depression, who respond well to an antidepressant, should receive a full therapeutic dose for at least 16–20 weeks after achieving full remission.

81b A Cochrane Review will soon be available. Carney S, Geddes JR, Furukawa T *et al.* Duration of treatment with antidepressants in depressive disorder (Protocol for a Cochrane Review). In: *The Cochrane Library*, Issue 2, 2003. Oxford: Update Software Issue 4, 2003.

82a Reimherr F, Amsterdam J, Quitkin F *et al.* Optimal length of continuation therapy in depression: a prospective assessment during long-term fluoxetine treatment. *Am J Psychiatry* 1998, 155: 1247–1253. (BIII)

82b A Cochrane Review will soon be available. Cipriani A, Brambilla P, Barbui C, Hotopf M. Fluoxetine versus other types of pharmacotherapy for depression (Protocol for a Cochrane Review). In: *The Cochrane Library*, Issue 2, 2003. Oxford: Update Software Issue 4, 2003.

83 Kupfer D, Frank E, Perel J *et al.* Five-year outcomes for maintenance therapy: possible mechanisms and treatments. *J Clin Psychiatry* 1998, 59: 279–288.

This is a study carried out by psychiatric patients. There are no comparable clinical trials of the efficacy of maintenance treatment in reducing recurrence of depression in primary care.

84 Donoghue J. Sub-optimal use of tricyclic antidepressants in primary care: Editorial. *Acta Psychiatrica Scand* 1998, 98(6): 429–431. (CV)

85 Furukawa TA, McGuire H, Barbui C. Meta-analysis of effects and side-effects of low dosage tricyclic antidepressants in depression: systematic review. *Br Med J* 2002, 325: 991–995. (AI)

Treatment of depression in adults with low dose tricyclics is justified.

85b A Cochrane Review will soon be available. Furukawa T, McGuire H, Barbui C. Low dosage tricyclic antidepressants for depression (Cochrane Review). In: *The Cochrane Library*, Issue 4, 2003. Oxford: Update Software.

86 Linde K, Mulrow CD. St John's wort for depression (Cochrane Review). In: *The Cochrane Library*, Issue 2, 2003. Oxford: Update Software. (AI)

Twenty-seven studies were analysed. St John's Wort demonstrated beneficial effects in mild and moderate depressive disorders. St John's Wort extracts have fewer short-term side-effects than older antidepressants; however, the preparations available on the market could vary considerably in their pharmaceutical quality.

87 Thiede HM, Walper A. Inhibition of MAO and CoMT by *Hypericum* extracts and hypericin. *J Geriat Psychiatr Neurol* 1994, 7(Suppl 1): S54–S56.

88 Interactions with tyramine-containing foods (eg beans, some cheeses, yeast, bovril, bananas, pickled herrings), are theoretically possible. However, there is, to date, an absence of spontaneous reports of these problems occurring.

89 Izzo AA, Ernst E. Interactions between herbal medicines and prescribed drugs: a systematic review. *Drugs* 2001, 15: 2163–75. (BIII)

Interactions between herbal medicines and synthetic drugs exist and can have serious clinical consequences. Healthcare professionals should ask their patients about the use of herbal products and consider the possibility of herb–drug interactions.

90a DeRubeis RJ, Crits-Cristoph P. Empirically supported individual and group psychological treatments for adult mental disorders. *J Consulting Clin Psychol* 1998, 66(1): 37–52. (BI)

This work supports cognitive behaviour therapy, behaviour therapy and structured problem-solving. Studies reviewed are based in secondary care.

90b Churchill R, Hunot V, Corney R *et al*. A systematic review of controlled trials of the effectiveness and cost-effectiveness of brief psychological treatments for depression. *Health Technol Assess* 2001, 5(35): 1–173. (AI)

Brief psychological treatments, particularly those derived from cognitive/behavioural models, are beneficial in the treatment of people with depression managed outside the hospital setting.

90c Mynors-Wallis LM, Gath DH, Lloyd-Thomas AR, Tomlinson D. Randomised controlled trial comparing problem-solving treatment with amitriptyline and placebo for major depression in primary care. *Br Med J* 1995, 310: 441–445. (AII)

Where the therapies have been compared with each other, none appears clearly superior to the others. More variance in outcomes may be due to the strength of the therapeutic relationship, rather than to the treatment method used. Problem-solving is the easiest therapy to learn and can be provided by GPs and primary-care nurses. Brief cognitive behaviour therapy is difficult to deliver, even using trained therapists (Scott J. Editorial: Psychological treatments for depression — an update. *Br J Psychiatry* 1995, 167: 289–292). Evidence for the effectiveness of therapies in depression in primary care tends to be weaker than in major depressive disorder in secondary care.

91a Thase M, Greenhouse J, Frank E *et al*. Treatment of major depression with psychotherapy or psychotherapy–pharmacotherapy combinations. *Arch Gen Psychiatry* 1997, 54: 1009–1015. (CIV)

Combined therapy was not significantly more effective than psychotherapy alone in patients with milder depression; a highly significant advantage was observed in more severe recurrent depressions. Poorer outcomes were also observed in women and older patients.

91b A Cochrane Review will soon be available. Churchill R, Wessely S, Lewis G. Combinations of pharmacotherapy and psychotherapy for depression (Cochrane Review). In: *The Cochrane Library*, Issue 4, 2003. Oxford: Update Software.

92a Evans M, Hollon S, De Rubeis R *et al*. Differential relapse following cognitive therapy and pharmacotherapy of depression. *Arch Gen Psychiatry* 1992, 49: 802–808. (BII)

It appears that providing cognitive therapy during acute treatment prevents relapse.

92b A Cochrane Review will soon be available. Churchill R, Wessely S, Lewis G. Antidepressants alone versus psychotherapy alone for depression (Protocol for a Cochrane Review). In: *The Cochrane Library*, Issue 4, 2003. Oxford: Update Software.

93 Ostler KJ, Thompson C, Kinmonth ALK *et al*. Influence of socio-economic deprivation on the prevalence and outcome of depression in primary care: the Hampshire Depression Project. *Br J Psychiatry* 2001, 178(1): 12–17.

The authors show a strong link between high indices of deprivation and poor prognosis for depression in primary care.

94 Golding JM. Intimate partner violence as a risk factor for mental disorders: a meta-analysis. *J Family Violence* 1999, 14: 99–132. (CIV)

This is a literature review of 38 studies. Existing research is consistent with the hypothesis that intimate partner violence increases the risk for mental health problems such as depression, suicidality, Post-traumatic stress disorder and drug abuse.

95 Home Office. *Domestic Violence: Finding from a New British Crime Survey Self-Completion Questionnaire*. London: Home Office Research Studies, 1999.

96 Richardson J, Coid J, Petruckevitch A *et al*. Identifying domestic violence: cross-sectional study in primary care. *Br Med J* 2002, 324: 274–277 (CIV)

This is a survey and review of medical records. Health professions should be aware of domestic violence, but the case for screening has not been made. One in six subjects surveyed objected to screening.

97 Ramsay J, Richardson J, Carter YH *et al*. Should health professionals screen women for domestic violence? Systematic review. *Br Med J* 2002, 325: 314 (CIV)

Twenty studies in surveys and interventions studies were reviewed. Most subject were in favour of screening. None of the studies measured quality of life, mental health outcomes or potential harm from screening programmes.

98 Burton S, Regan L, Kelly L. *Supporting Women and Challenging Men: Lessons From the Domestic Violence Intervention Project*. Bristol: Policy Press, 1998 (CIV)

Women benefit from the combination of forms of support, with support groups being the most effective in combating shame, self-blame and the destruction of self-belief, which can strongly inhibit a woman's attempts to end violence. Although two in three men dropped out of the programme, there was a substantial impact on attitudes and behaviour for most men who did complete it.

99 Abel E. Psychosocial treatments for battered women: a review of the empirical research. *Res Social Work Practice* 2000, 10: 55–77.

100 Kaltenbach K, Finnegan L. Children of maternal substance misusers. *Curr Opin Psychiatry* 1997, 10: 220–224.

Most harm to children is indirect, for example via ill health of the mother, poor antenatal care or cigarette smoking. There is a smaller risk of direct harm caused by heroin — growth retardation — and cocaine and amphetamines.

101 Miller W, Rollnick S. *Motivational Interviewing: Preparing People to Change Addictive Behaviour*. New York: Guilford Press, 1991. (AV)

102a Gossop M, Stewart D, Marsden J. *NTORS at One Year: The National Treatment Outcome Research Study. Change in Substance Use, Health and Criminal Behaviour One Year After Intake*. London: Department of Health, 1998. (A1)

102b Ward J, Mattick R, Hall W. *Maintenance Treatment and Other Opioid Replacement Therapies*. London: Harwood Academic Press, 1997.

102c Jeffries V, Gabbay M, Carnwath T. *Treatments for Opiate Users in Primary Care*. Monograph for Enhancing Shared Care Project, Chapel Road, Sale, Manchester M33 7FD, UK.

103 Lader M, Russell J. Guidelines for the prevention and treatment of benzodiazepine dependence: summary of a report from the Mental Health Foundation. *Addiction* 1993, 88(12): 1707–1708.

104 Royal College of Psychiatrists. *Benzodiazepines: Risks, Benefits and Dependence — A Re-Evaluation*. London: The Royal College of Psychiatrists, UK. URL http://www.rcpsych.ac.uk/publications/cr/cr59.htm.

105 The Task Force to Review Services for Drug Misusers. *Report of an Independent Review of Drug Treatment Services in England*. London: DoH, 1995.

106 American Psychiatric Association. *Practice Guidelines: Substance Use Disorders*. Washington DC, 1996. (BII)

This publication reports a large randomized controlled trial replicated in a controlled trial comparing drug counselling, drug counselling plus supportive psychotherapy, and drug counselling plus cognitive behaviour therapy for methadone maintenance patients. Those with moderate to high depression or other psychiatric symptoms did better with either therapy in addition to drug counselling. For patients with low levels of psychiatric symptoms, all three treatments were equally effective.

107 Khantzian E. The primary-care therapist and patient needs in substance abuse treatment. *Am J Drug Alcohol Abuse* 1988, 14: 159–167.

The authors review studies of relapse prevention through, for example, encouraging improved social and other relationships and activities.

108 Department of Health, The Scottish Office, The Welsh Office and DHSS Northern Ireland. *Drug Misuse and Dependence: Guidelines on Clinical Management*, 1999.

109 Amato L, Davoli M, Ferri M, Ali R. Methadone at tapered doses for the management of opioid withdrawal (Cochrane Review). In: *The Cochrane Library*, Issue 2, 2003. Oxford: Update Software. (AI)

Tapered methadone seems to be useful and causes fewer side-effects than other medicated detoxification methods. Moreover, the rate of completion is higher. However, relapse rates are high.

110 Marsch LC. The efficacy of methadone maintenance interventions in reducing illicit opiate use, HIV risk behaviour and criminality: a meta-analysis. *Addiction* 1998, 93: 515–532. (A1)

This is a systematic review of 11 studies. Results demonstrate a consistent, statistically significant relationship between methadone maintenance treatment and the reduction of illicit opiate use, HIV risk behaviours and drug- and property-related criminal behaviour.

111 Mattick RP, Kimber J, Breen C, Davoli M. Buprenorphine maintenance versus placebo or methadone maintenance for opioid dependence (Cochrane Review). In: *The Cochrane Library*, Issue 2, 2003. Oxford: Update Software. (BI)

Buprenorphine is an effective intervention for use in the maintenance treatment of heroin dependence, but it is not more effective than methadone at adequate doses.

112 Gowing L, Farrell M, Ali R, White J. Alpha2 adrenergic agonists for the management of opioid withdrawal (Cochrane Review). In: *The Cochrane Library*, Issue 2, 2003. Oxford: Update Software. (BI)

Ten studies compared a treatment regimen based on an alpha2-adrenergic agonist, with one based on reducing doses of methadone. Participants stay in treatment longer with methadone regimens, which may provide greater opportunity for psychosocial intervention. Methadone regimes may be preferable for withdrawal in outpatient settings where the risk of relapse to heroin use is high. Methadone might also facilitate transfer to maintenance treatment, should completion of withdrawal become unlikely. For those who are well prepared for withdrawal and seeking earlier resolution of withdrawal symptoms, alpha2-adrenergic agonist treatment may be preferred. Clonidine and lofexidine appear equally effective for inpatient settings, but the lower incidence of hypotension makes lofexidine more suited to use in outpatient settings.

113 Brown AS, Fleming PM. A naturalistic study of home detoxification from opiates using lofexidine. *J Psychopharmacol* 1998, 12: 93–96.

114 McLellan AT, Arndt IO, Metzger DS. The effects of psychosocial services in substance abuse treatment. *JAMA* 1993, 269: 1953–1959. (BII)

Patients who received employment help, psychiatric care and family therapy had better outcomes than those who received counselling, who in turn had better outcomes than those who received methadone only.

115 NICE will publish a guideline on the management of eating disorders in January 2004.

116 Fairburn CG, Harrison PJ. Eating disorders. *Lancet* 2003, 361: 407–416. (AI)

This is an up-to-date evidence-based review of all aspects of eating disorders including their management. A specific form of cognitive behaviour therapy is the most effective treatment for patients with eating disorders, although few patients seem to receive it in practice. Treatment of anorexia nervosa and atypical eating disorders has received remarkably little research attention.

117 A Cochrane review will soon be available. Schmidt U, Perkins S, Winn S *et al*. Self-help and guided self-help for eating disorders (Protocol for a Cochrane Review). In: *The Cochrane Library*, Issue 4, 2003. Oxford: Update Software.

118 Bacaltchuk J, Hay P. Antidepressants versus placebo for people with bulimia nervosa (Cochrane Review). In: *The Cochrane Library*, Issue 2, 2003. Oxford: Update Software. (AI)

Sixteen studies were analysed. The use of a single antidepressant agent was clinically effective for the treatment of bulimia nervosa compared with placebo, with an overall greater remission rate but a higher dropout rate. No differential effect regarding efficacy and tolerability among the various classes of antidepressants could be demonstrated.

119 Treasure J, Schmidt U. Anorexia nervosa. *Clinical Evidence* 2002, 8: 903–913. (AI)

No evidence was found of beneficial effects for tricyclic antidepressants or SSRIs.

120 Russell GFM, Szmukler GI, Dare C, Eisler I. An evaluation of family therapy in anorexia nervosa and bulimia nervosa. *Arch Gen Psychiatr* 1987, 44: 1047–1056. (CIII)

Patients with anorexia nervosa with onset at or before age 18 and of less than three year's duration did better with family therapy than individual therapy. Moreover, older patients did better with individual therapy. However, a major UK review, while supporting these recommendations, states that there are currently no high-quality reviews of psychological treatments for anorexia nervosa (Gloaguen V, Cottraux J, Cucherat M *et al.* A meta-analysis of the effects on cognitive therapy in depressed patients. *J Affect Disord* 1998, 49: 59–72).

121 A Cochrane review will soon be available. Hay P, Bacaltchuk J, Claudino A, Ben-Tovim D. Individual psychotherapy in the outpatient treatment of adults with anorexia nervosa (Cochrane Review). In: The Cochrane Library, Issue 4, 2003. Oxford: Update Software.

122a Bacaltchuk J, Hay P, Trefiglio R. Antidepressants versus psychological treatments and their combination for bulimia nervosa (Cochrane Review). In: *The Cochrane Library*, Issue 2, 2003. Oxford: Update Software (AI)

Seventeen studies were looked at. Using a more conservative statistical approach, combination treatments were superior to single psychotherapy. Psychotherapy appeared to be more acceptable to subjects. When antidepressants were combined with psychological treatments, acceptability of the latter was significantly reduced.

122b Hay PJ, Bacaltchuk J. Psychotherapy for bulimia nervosa and binging (Cochrane Review). In: *The Cochrane Library*, Issue 2, 2003. Oxford: Update Software. (AI)

Thirty-four studies were analysed. There is small body of evidence supporting the efficacy of cognitive-behaviour therapy in bulimia nervosa and similar syndromes.

123 Eating Disorders Special Interest Group, Royal College of Psychiatry. Primary Care Protocol for the Management of Adults with Eating Disorders. URL http://www.rcpsych.ac.uk/college/sig/eatdis.htm.

124 Smith D, Defalla BA, Chadwick DW. The misdiagnosis of epilepsy and the management of refractory epilepsy in a specialist clinic. *Q J Med* 1999, 92: 15–23.

125 Crawford PM, Appleton R, Betts T, Duncan J, Guthrie E, Morrow J. Best practice guidelines for the management of women with epilepsy. *Seizure* 1998, 8: 201–217.

126 NICE are due to publish a guideline on the management of Epilepsy in June 2004.

127 Marson A, Ramaratnam S. Epilepsy. *Clinical Evidence* 2002, 8: 1313–28. (AI)

Reviews in people with drug-resistant partial epilepsy have found that adding gabapentin, levetiracetam, lamotrigine, oxcarbazepine, tiagabine, topiramate, vigabatrin or zonisamide to their usual treatment significantly reduces seizure frequency (compared with adding placebo). Adding second-line drugs compared with adding placebo increases the frequency of adverse effects. Randomized controlled trials have found that immediate treatment of single seizures with antiepileptic drugs (compared with no treatment) reduces seizure frequency over a two-year follow-up period. No evidence was found that treatment alters long-term prognosis. Long-term antiepileptic drug treatment is potentially harmful.

128 Berg AT, Shinnar S. The risk of seizure recurrence following a first unprovoked seizure: a quantitative review. *Neurology* 1991, 41: 965–972.

129 Marson AG, Williamson PR, Hutton JL *et al.*; on behalf of the epilepsy monotherapy trialists. Carbamazepine versus valproate monotherapy for epilepsy (Cochrane Review). In: *The Cochrane Library*, Issue 2, 2003. Oxford: Update Software. (AI)

Eight studies were analysed. There was some evidence to support the policy of using carbamazepine as the first treatment of choice in partial epilepsies, but no evidence to support the choice of valproate in generalized epilepsies. Confidence intervals were too wide to confirm equivalence, however.

130 Sirven JI, Sperling M, Wingerchuk DM. Early versus late antiepileptic drug withdrawal for people with epilepsy in remission (Cochrane Review). In: *The Cochrane Library*, Issue 2, 2003. Oxford: Update Software. (BI)

Seven studies were examined. There is evidence to support waiting for at least two or more seizure-free years before discontinuing anti-epileptic drugs (AEDs) in children, particularly if patients have an abnormal EEG and partial seizures. There is insufficient evidence to establish when to withdraw AEDs in paediatric patients with generalized seizures. There is no evidence to guide the timing of withdrawal of AEDs in adult seizure-free patients.

131 Shear K, Schulberg H. Anxiety disorders in primary care. *Bull Menninger Clinic* 1995, 59(2; Suppl A): 73–82. (BI)

Studies of psychoeducation and minimal intervention in primary care show much promise as first-line interventions for anxiety disorders in primary care. More severely ill patients require more specialist intervention.

132 NICE will publish a guideline on Anxiety (generalized) in June 2004. (AI)

133 Hawton K, Kirk J. Problem-solving. In: Hawton K, Salkovskis PM, Kirk J, Clark DM (eds.) *Cognitive Therapy for Psychiatric Problems: A Practical Guide*. Oxford: Oxford University Press, 1989: 406–426. (AII)

134 See reference 13.

135a Gould RA, Otto MW, Pollack MH, Yap L. Cognitive behavioural and pharmacological treatment of generalised anxiety disorder: a preliminary meta-analysis. *Behaviour Ther* 1997, 28(2): 285–305. (BI)

This paper discusses the effectiveness of different treatments for anxiety. Buspirone had a much lower effect size than either benzodiazepines or antidepressants, and its onset is slow (up to four weeks). However, problems with dependence and withdrawal are minimal compared with benzodiazepines. Cognitive behaviour therapy (CBT) and anxiety management were the most efficacious psychological treatments; each was equally efficacious in the short term. Gains of CBT and anxiety management were maintained at six months.

135b Lader MH, Bond AJ. Interaction of pharmacological and psychological treatments of anxiety. *Br J Psychiatry* 1998, 173(Suppl 34): 165–8.

Firm conclusions are not possible. Observations suggest using benzodiazepines for treating anxiety initially, as these produce rapid symptomatic improvement; then psychological treatments can take over.

135c A Cochrane review will soon be available. Gale C, Kapczinski F, Busnello JV *et al.* Benzodiazepines for generalized anxiety (Protocol for a Cochrane Review). In: *The Cochrane Library*, Issue 4, 2003. Oxford: Update Software.

136a Kapczinski F, Lima MS, Souza, JS, Schmitt, R. Antidepressants for generalized anxiety disorder (Cochrane Review). In: *The Cochrane Library*, Issue 2, 2003. Oxford: Update Software (AI)

Fifteen studies were examined. Antidepressants are superior to placebo in treating general anxiety disorder (GAD) and are tolerated by GAD patients.

136b A Cochrane review will soon be available. Kapczinski F, Ribeiro L, Quevedo J *et al.* 5HT-1 agonists for generalized anxiety (Protocol for a Cochrane Review). In: *The Cochrane Library*, Issue 4, 2003. Oxford: Update Software.

137 Tyrer P. Use of beta-blocking drugs in psychiatry and neurology. *Drugs* 1980, 20: 300–308.

138 Kupshik G, Fisher C. Assisted bibliotherapy: effective, efficient treatment for moderate anxiety problems. *Br J Gen Pract* 1999, 49: 47–8. (BIII)

Learning self-help skills through reading, supported by contact with a clinician, significantly improved symptoms. More patients improved with more clinician contact, especially if less educated.

139 Bower P, Richards D, Lovell, K. The clinical and cost-effectiveness of self-help treatments for anxiety and depressive disorders in primary care: a systematic review. *Br J Gen Pract* 2001, 51: 838–845. (AI)

Self-help treatments may have the potential to improve the overall cost-effectiveness of mental health service provision.

140. Steiner TJ, Scher AI, Stewart WF *et al.* The prevalence and disability burden of adult migraine in England and their relationships to age, gender and ethnicity. *Cephalalgia* 2003; **23**: 519–527.

141. Rasmussen BJ, Jensen R, Schroll M, Olesen J. Epidemiology of headache in a general population – a prevalence study. *J Clin Epidemiol* 1991; **44**: 1147–1157.

142. Schwartz BS, Stewart WF, Simon D, Lipton RB. Epidemiology of tension-type headache. *JAMA* 1998; **279**: 381–383.

143. British Association for the Study of Headache. *Guidelines for all doctors in the diagnosis and management of migraine and tension-type headache, 2nd edition (revised)*. BASH 2003 at www.bash.org.uk.

144. Srikiatkhachorn A, Phanthurachinda K. Prevalence and clinical features of chronic daily headache in a headache clinic. *Headache* 1997; **37**: 277–280.

145. Limmroth V, Katsarava Z, Fritsche G *et al.* Features of medication overuse headache following overuse of different acute headache drugs. *Neurology* 2002; **59**: 1011–1014.

146. International Headache Society Classification Subcommittee. International classification of headache disorders, 2nd edition. *Cephalalgia* 2004; **24 (suppl 1)**:1–160.

147. Steiner TJ. Headache burdens and bearers. *Funct Neurol* 2000; **15 (suppl 3)**: 219–223.

148. Lipton RB, Bigal ME, Kolodner K *et al.* The family impact of migraine: population-based studies in the USA and UK. *Cephalalgia* 2003; **23**: 429–440.

149. Rasmussen BK, Olesen J. Migraine with aura and migraine without aura: an epidemiological study. *Cephalalgia* 1992; **12**: 221–228.

150. MacGregor EA. Menstruation, sex hormones and headache. *Neurol Clin* 1997; **15**: 125—141.

151. MacGregor EA, Guillebaud J (on behalf of the Clinical and Scientific Committee of the Faculty of Family Planning and Reproductive Health Care of the Royal College of Obstetricians and Gynaecologists). Recommendations for clinical practice: Combined oral contraceptives, migraine and stroke. *Br J Fam Planning* 1998; **24**: 53–60.

152. World Health Organization. *Improving access to quality care in family planning. Medical eligibility criteria for contraceptive use* (2nd edition). Geneva: WHO 2000.

153. Ferrari MD, Roon KI, Lipton RB, Goadsby PJ. Oral triptans (serotonin 5-HT$_{1B/1D}$ agonists) in acute migraine treatment: a meta-analysis of 53 trials. *Lancet* 2001; **358**: 1668–1675.

154. Ramadan NM, Schultz LL, Gilkey SJ. Migraine prophylactic drugs: proof of efficacy, utilization and cost. *Cephalalgia* 1997; **17**: 73–80.

155. Hopkinson HE. Treatment of cardiovascular diseases. In Rubin P (ed), *Prescribing in pregnancy*. London: BMJ Publishing Group 1995, p. 98.

156. Rothrock JF. Clinical studies of valproate for migraine prophylaxis. *Cephalalgia* 1997; **17**: 81–83.

157. Steiner TJ, Lange R, Voelker M. Aspirin in episodic tension-type headache: placebo-controlled dose-ranging comparison with paracetamol. *Cephalalgia* 2003; **23**: 59–66.

158. Kudrow L. Treatment of cluster headache. *Headache Quart* 1993; **4**: 42–47.

159. Gabai IJ, Spierings ELH. Prophylactic treatment of cluster headache with verapamil. *Headache* 1989; **29**: 167–168.

160. Schnider P, Aull S, Baumgartner C *et al.* Long-term outcome of patients with headache and drug abuse after inpatient withdrawal: five-year follow-up. *Cephalalgia* 1996; 16: 481–485.

161. Hering R, Steiner TJ. Abrupt outpatient withdrawal of medication in analgesic-abusing migraineurs. *Lancet* 1991; **337**: 1442–1443.

162. World Federation of Neurology Research Group on Neuromuscular Diseases. El Escorial World federation of Neurology criteria for the diagnosis of amyotrophic lateral sclerosis. *J Neurol Sci* 1994; **124S**: 96–107.

163. Brockington A, Shaw PJ. Developments in the treatment of motor neurone disease. *Advances in Clinical Neuroscience and Rehabilitation* 2003 (In press).

164. Miller RG, Rosenberg JA, Gelinas DF *et al.* Practice parameter: the care of the patient with amyotrophic lateral sclerosis (an evidence-based review): report of the quality standards subcommittee of the American Academy of neurology. ALS Practice Parameters Task Force. *Neurology* 1999; **52**: 1311–1323.

165. Langmore SE, Kasarskis EJ, Manca ML, Olney R. Enteral feeding for amyotrophic lateral sclerosis: *Protocol for a Cochrane review* 2003.

166. Lannacone S, Ferini-Strambi L. Pharmacological treatment of emotional lability. *Clinical Neuropharmacol* 1996; **19**: 532–535.

167. Bourke SC, Bullock RE, Williams TL *et al*. Non-invasive ventilation in ALS: indications and effect on quality of life. *Neurology* 2003; **61**: 171–177.

168. Miller RG, Mitchell JD, Lyon M, Moore DH. Riluzole for amyotrophic lateral sclerosis (ALS)/motor neurone disease (MND). *Cochrane Database Systematic Review* 2002; **CD001447**.

169. National Institute of Clinical Excellence. Guidance on the use of riluzole (rilutek) for the treatment of motor neurone disease. *National Institute of Clinical Excellence* 2001.

170. Compston A, Coles A. Multiple Sclerosis. *Lancet* 2002; 359: 1221–1231.

171. McDonald WI, Compston A, Edan G *et al*. Recommended diagnostic criteria for Multiple Sclerosis: Guidelines from the international panel on the diagnosis of Multiple Sclerosis. *Ann Neurol* 2001; 50: 121–127.

172. Rice GA, Incorvara B, Munan L *et al*. Interferon in relapsing-remitting Multiple Sclerosis. In: *The Cochrane Library*, Issue 2, 2002.

173. Burgess M. MS symptoms and their treatment. In: *Multiple Sclerosis: Theory & Practice for Nurses*. London: Whurr 2002, pp. 72–100.

174 NICE will publish a guideline on the management of Obsessive-compulsive disorder in February 2005.

175 Greist JH, Marks IM, Baer L *et al*. Behaviour therapy for obsessive compulsive disorder guided by a computer or by a clinician compared with relaxation as a control. *J Clin Psychiatry* 2002, 63: 138–145 (CII)

This is a randomized controlled trial. Computer-guided behaviour therapy was effective for patients with Obsessive compulsive disorder, although clinician-guided behaviour therapy was even more effective. Systematic relaxation was ineffective.

176 Freeston MH, Ladouceur R. The cognitive-behavioural treatment of obsessions. In: Caballo VE (ed) *International Handbook of Cognitive and Behavioural Treatment of Psychological Disorders*. Oxford: Pergamon, 1998: 127–160.

177 Salkovskis PM, Kirk J. Obsessional disorders. In: Hawton K, Salkovskis PM, Kirk J, Clark M (eds.) *Cognitive Behaviour Therapy for Psychiatric Disorders*. Oxford: Oxford University Press, 1988: 129–168.

178 Stern R, Drummond L. *The Practice of Behavioural and Cognitive Psychotherapy*. Cambridge: Cambridge University Press, 1991

179 Marks IM. *Fears, Phobias and Rituals*. New York: Oxford University Press, 1987.

180 Soomro GM. Obsessive compulsive disorder. *Clinical Evidence* 2002, 8: 991–1002. (AI)

This is a review. Selective serotonin reuptake inhibitors, behaviour therapy, cognitive therapy and combined treatment (fluvoxamine and behaviour therapy) are beneficial in Obsessive-compulsive disorder.

181 Cottraux J, Note I, Yao SN *et al*. A randomized controlled trial of cognitive therapy versus intensive behavior therapy in Obsessive-compulsive disorder. *Psychother Psychosom* 2001, 70(6): 288–297. (BII)

This is a randomized controlled trial. Cognitive therapy and behaviour therapy were equally effective for patients with Obsessive-compulsive disorder.

182 de Haan E, Hodgduin KA, Buitecaar JK *et al*. Behavior therapy versus clomipramine for the treatment of obsessive-compulsive disorder in children and adolescents. *J Am Acad Child Adolesc Psychiatry* 1998, 37(10): 1022–1029. (CII)

This is a randomized controlled trial. Behaviour therapy is shown to be a good alternative to drug treatment.

183 Swinson RP, Soulios C, Cox BJ, Kuch K. Brief treatment of emergency-room patients with panic attacks. *Am J Psychiatry* 1992, 149: 944–946. (BIII)

People presenting to Accident and Emergency with panic who went on to have psychoeducation and exposure instructions improved significantly more at follow-up compared with controls.

184 Kumar S, Oakley-Browne. Panic disorder. *Clinical Evidence* 2002, 8: 1003–1009. (AI)

Selective-serotonin reuptake inhibitors and tricyclic antidepressants are effective in Panic disorder.

185a American Psychiatric Association. Practice guideline for the treatment of patients with panic disorder. *Am J Psychiatry* 1998, 155(Suppl): 1–26. (AII)

Tricyclic antidepressants (TCAs), selective serotonin re-uptake inhibitors, monoamine oxidase inhibitors and benzodiazepines had roughly comparable short-term efficacy in patients with panic disorder. Benzodiazepines help in the very short term if very rapid control of symptoms is critical. TCA side-effects might be problematic. Discontinuation of medication commonly leads to relapse, so longer-term use is recommended — 2–18 months —after which period, the relapse rate is unknown.

185b A Cochrane review will be available soon. Mendes HA, Lima MS, Hotopf MH. Serotonin reuptake inhibitors and new generation antidepressants for panic disorder (Protocol for a Cochrane Review). In: *The Cochrane Library*, Issue 4, 2003. Oxford: Update Software.

186 Barlow DH, Gorman JM, Shear KM *et al*. Cognitive behavioural therapy, imipramine or their combination for panic disorder: a RCT. *JAMA* 2000, 283: 2529–2536. (BII)

Combining imipramine and cognitive behaviour therapy (CBT) appears to confer limited advantage acutely but more substantial advantage by the end of maintenance. Each treatment worked well immediately following treatment and during maintenance; CBT appeared durable in follow-up.

187 Haug TT, Blomhoff S, Hellstrom K *et al*. Exposure therapy and sertraline in social phobia: 1-year follow-up of a randomised controlled trial. *Br J Psychiatry* 2003, 101: 312–318. (BII)

Exposure therapy alone yielded a further improvement during follow-up, whereas exposure therapy combined with sertraline and sertraline alone showed a tendency towards deterioration after the completion of treatment.

188 Marks I, Swinson P, Basoglu M *et al*. Alprazolam and exposure alone and combined in panic disorder with agoraphobia. A controlled study in London and Toronto. *Br J Psychiatry* 1993, 162: 776–787. (BII)

Where agoraphobic fear and avoidance is present, with panic, exposure — a behavioural treatment — proved to be twice as effective as alprazolam.

189. Hughes AJ, Daniel SE, Kilford L, Lees AJ. Accuracy of clinical diagnosis of idiopathic Parkinson's disease: a clinico-pathological study of 100 cases. *J Neurol Neurosurg Psychiatry* 1992; **55**: 181–184.

190. Hughes AJ, Ben-Shlomo Y, Daniel S, Lees AJ. What features improve the accuracy of clinical diagnosis in Parkinson's disease. *Neurology* 1992; **42**: 1142–1146.

This large series of post-mortem-proven Parkinson's disease studied the reliability of the clinical diagnosis of idiopathic PD, and the frequency of a particular symptom and its reliability in making a diagnosis of PD.

191. Gelb DJ, Oliver E, Gilman S. Diagnostic criteria for Parkinson's disease. *Arch Neurol* 1999; **56**: 33–39.

A clinical diagnostic classification based on a thorough review of the literature concerning the sensitivity and specificity of the clinical features of PD.

192. Ben-Shlomo Y. How far are we in understanding the cause of Parkinson's disease? *J Neurol Neurosurg Psychiatry* 1996; **61**: 4–16.

Thorough review of current understanding of the evidence about the epidemiology of PD.

193. Betchen SA, Kaplitt M. Future and current surgical therapies in Parkinson's disease. *Curr Opin Neurol* 2003; **16**: 487–493.

194. Fung VS, Morris JG, Pell MF. Surgical treatment for Parkinson's disease. *Med J Australia* 2002; **177**: 1130–1142.

195 UK Department of Health guidelines on personality disorder. *Personality Disorder: No Longer a Diagnosis of Exclusion. Policy Implementation Guidance for the Development of Services for People with Personality Disorder.* URL http://www.doh.gov.uk/mentalhealth/personalitydisorder.htm.

196 Benzodiazepines are effective in many cases in suppressing panic in the short term. They are not effective for chronic panics or phobias — there is no evidence that any gains continue when drugs are withdrawn, and there is some evidence that they do not. Where patients are doing exposure therapy by gradually facing the fear, there is some evidence that benzodiazepines actually interfere with maintenance of longer-term gains. Selected references (BII):

196a See references 185a and 188.

196b A Cochrane review will be available soon. van der Linden GJH, van Balkom JLM, Zung-dirwayi N, Stein DJ. Pharmacotherapy for social phobia (Protocol for a Cochrane Review). In: *The Cochrane Library*, Issue 4, 2003. Oxford: Update Software.

197 NICE will publish a guideline on the management of Post-traumatic stress disorder in January 2005.

198 Rose S, Bisson J, Wessley S. Psychological debriefing for preventing post traumatic stress disorder (Cochrane Review). In: *The Cochrane Library*, Issue 1, 2003. Oxford: Update Software. (AI)

The routine use of single-session debriefing given to non-selected trauma victims cannot be recommended at present.

199 Bisson JI.Early interventions following traumatic events. *Psychiatric Ann* 2003, 33: 37–44. (BI)

The authors review randomized controlled trials and conclude that the evidence base does not support routine early intervention but that multiple session cognitive behavioural early interventions might help.

200a Foa EB, Keane TM, Friedman MJ (eds.) *Effective Treatments for PTSD.* New York: Guildford Press, 2000.

This work summarizes evidence for a wide variety of treatment approaches for Post-traumatic stress disorder. Cognitive therapy and exposure therapy emerge as the psychological treatments with the best evidence for efficacy.

200b Bisson JI., Andrew M. Psychological treatment of Post-traumatic stress disorder (PTSD) (Protocol for a Cochrane Review). In: *The Cochrane Library*, Issue 2, 2003. Oxford: Update Software.

201 Marks I, Lovell K, Noshirvani H *et al.* Treatment of Post-traumatic stress disorder by exposure and/or cognitive restructuring: a controlled study. *Arch Gen Psychiatry* 1998, 55: 317–25. (BII)

This randomized control trial shows that exposure, cognitive restructuring, or both combined, were equally effective in Post-traumatic stress disorder and better than relaxation without exposure.

202 Shepherd J, Stein K, Milne R. Eye movement desensitization and reprocessing in the treatment of Post-traumatic stress disorder: a review of an emerging therapy. *Psychol Med* 2000, 30(4): 863–871. (AI)

This is a systematic review of 16 studies. Eye movement desensitization and reprocessing might be as effective as imaginal exposure therapy and more effective than relaxation techniques in Post-traumatic stress disorder but it is unclear if it is the technique or the imaginal exposure component that is effective.

203 Stein DJ, Zungu-Dirwayi N, Van der Linden GJ, Seedat S. Pharmacotherapy for post-traumatic stress disorder (Cochrane Review). In: *The Cochrane Library*, Issue 2, 2003. Oxford: Update Software. (AI)

Fifteen studies were examined. The research base is limited but there is increasing evidence that drugs can help in Post-traumatic stress disorder. Sertraline and paroxetine have been the most researched and have been shown to be effective. There is good evidence for the efficacy of fluoxetine and some evidence for tricyclic antidepressants and monoamine oxidase inhibitors.

204 Ray KL, Hodnett ED. Caregiver support for postpartum depression (Cochrane Review). In: *The Cochrane Library*, Issue 2, 2003. Oxford: Update Software. (CI)

Women with postpartum (postnatal) depression who are supported by caregivers are less likely to remain depressed, although the most effective support from caregivers remains unknown.

205 Harris B, Huckle P, Thomas R *et al.* The use of rating scales to identify postnatal depression. *Br J Psychiatry* 1989, 154: 813–817

206 Appleby L, Warner R, Whitton A, Faragher B. A controlled study of fluoxetine and cognitive behavioural therapy in the treatment of postnatal depression. *Br Med J* 1997, 314: 932. (BII)

Both fluoxetine and cognitive-behavioural counselling given as a course of therapy are effective treatments for non-psychotic depression in postnatal women. After an initial session of counselling, additional benefit results from either fluoxetine or further counselling

207 Holden JM, Sagovsky R, Cox JL. Counselling in a general practice setting: a controlled study of health visitor intervention in treatment of postnatal depression. *Br Med J* 1989, 298: 223–6. (BII)

Counselling by health visitors is valuable in managing non-psychotic postnatal depression.

208 O'Hara M, Stuart S, Gorman L, Wenzel A. Efficacy of interpersonal psychotherapy for postnatal depression. *Arch Gen Psychiatry* 2000, 57: 1039–1045. (BII)

Interpersonal psychotherapy is an efficacious treatment for postpartum depression. It reduced depressive symptoms and improved social adjustment, and represents an alternative to pharmacotherapy, particularly for women who are breastfeeding.

209 Hoffbrand S, Howard L, Crawley H. Antidepressant treatment for post-natal depression (Cochrane Review). In: *The Cochrane Library*, Issue 2, 2003. Oxford: Update Software Ltd (CI)

One study was examined. Women with postnatal depression can be treated effectively with fluoxetine, which is as effective as a course of cognitive-behavioural counselling in the short-term.

210 Altshuler LL, Cohen L, Szuba MP *et al.* Pharmaceutical management of psychiatric illness during pregnancy. *Am J Psychiatry* 1996, 153: 592–606. (BI)

This is a review. The use of psychotropic medications during pregnancy is appropriate in many clinical situations and should include thoughtful weighing of risk of prenatal exposure with risk of relapse following drug discontinuation.

211 NICE will publish a guideline on the management of self-harm in March 2004.

212 Hawton K, Townsend E, Arensman E *et al*. Psychosocial and pharmacological treatments for deliberate self-harm (Cochrane Review). In: *The Cochrane Library*, Issue 2, 2003. Oxford: Update Software. (AI)

Twenty-three studies were analysed. Promising results were found for problem-solving therapy, provision of a card to allow emergency contact with services, depot flupenthixol for recurrent repeaters of self-harm and long-term psychological therapy for female patients with borderline personality disorder and recurrent self-harm.

213 Ralph D, McNicholas T; for the Erectile Dysfunction Alliance. UK Management Guidelines for Erectile Dysfunction. *Br Med J* 2000, 321: 499–503.

214a Montorsi F, Salonia A, Deho F *et al*. Pharmacological management of erectile dysfunction. *Br J Urol Int* 2003, 91(5): 446–454. (CI)

214b Vitezic D, Pelcic-Mrsic J. Erectile dysfunction: oral pharmacotherapy options. *Int J Clin Pharmacol Ther* 2002, 40(9): 393–403. (AI)

214c Werneke U, Crowe M. Review of patients with erectile dysfunction attending the Maudsley Psychosexual Clinic in 1999: the impact of sildenafil. *Sex Relation Ther* 2002, 17(4): 171–185. (CIV)

Sildenafil has a very satisfactory efficacy/safety profile in all patient categories.

214d A Cochrane Review will be available soon. Fink H, Wilt T, MacDonald R *et al*. Sildenafil for erectile dysfunction (Protocol for a Cochrane Review). In: *The Cochrane Library*, Issue 4, 2003. Oxford: Update Software.

215a Kuan J, Brock G. Selective phosphodiesterase type 5 inhibition using Tadalafil for the treatment of erectile dysfunction. *Expert Opin Invest Drugs* 2002, 11(11): 1605–1613. (AI)

This is a review. Tadalafil is likely to play an important role in the management of erectile dysfunction across a broad spectrum of aetiologies, once past the ongoing regulatory review process. Side-effects are generally mild to moderate.

215b A Cochrane Review will be available soon. Urciuoli R, Cantisani TA, Carlini M *et al*. Prostaglandin E1 for treatment of erectile dysfunction (Protocol for a Cochrane Review). In: *The Cochrane Library*, Issue 4, 2003. Oxford: Update Software.

216 Padma-Nathan H, Hellstrom WJG, Kaiser RE *et al*. Treatment of men with erectile dysfunction with transurethral alprostadil. *N Engl J Med* 1997, 336: 1–7. (AII)

217 Linet OI, Ogrine FG. Efficacy and safety of intracavernosal alprostadil in men with erectile dysfunction. *N Engl J Med* 1996, 334: 873–877. (AII)

218 Kupfer DJ, Reynolds CF. Management of insomnia. *N Engl J Med* 1997, 336: 341–346.

219 Ancoli-Israel S. Insomnia in the elderly: a review for the primary-care practitioner. *Sleep* 2000, 23(Suppl 1): S23–S30.

220 Edinger JD, Wohlgemuth WK. The significance and management of persistent primary insomnia: the past, present and future of behavioural insomnia therapies. *Sleep Med Rev* 1999, 3: 101–118.

221 Stores G. Dramatic parasomnias. *J R Soc Med* 2001, 94: 173–176.

222 Royal College of Physicians. *Nicotine Addiction in Britain. A Report of the Tobacco Advisory Group of the Royal College of Physicians*. London: Royal College of Physicians, 2000

223 Rigotti NA. Clinical practice. Treatment of tobacco use and dependence. *N Engl J Med* 2002, 346(7): 506–512. (CIV)

224 National Institute for Clinical Excellence. *Guidance on the Use of Nicotine Replacement Therapy and Bupropion for Smoking Cessation*. URL http://www.nice.org.uk. (AI)

Both drugs are effective in smoking cessation.

225 Jackson G, Bobak A, Chorlton I *et al*. Smoking cessation: a consensus statement with special reference to primary care. *ICGP* 2001, 55: 385–392

226 Raw M, McNeill A, West R. Smoking cessation guidelines for health professionals. *Thorax* 1998, 53(Suppl 5,Part 1): S1–S19.

227 West R, McNeill A, Raw M. Smoking cessation guidelines for health professionals: an update. *Thorax* 2000, 55(12), 987–999.

228 Silagy C, Mant D, Fowler G, Lancaster T. Nicotine replacement therapy for smoking cessation. (Cochrane Review). In: *The Cochrane Library*, Issue 2, 1999. Oxford: Update Software. (AI)

One hundred and ten studies were analysed. All forms of nicotine replacement therapy can help people quit smoking, almost doubling long-term success rates.

229 Gubitz G, Sandercock P. Stroke management. *Clin Evidence* 2002; 8: 169–183. (AI)

This systematic review in people with ischaemic stroke found that giving aspirin (compared with placebo) within 48 hours of stroke onset significantly reduces death or dependency at six months and significantly increases the numbers making a complete recovery. Specialist stroke rehabilitation units significantly reduce death or dependency after a median follow-up of one year compared with usual non-specialist care.

230 Clinical Evidence Writers on Stroke Prevention. Stroke prevention. *Clin Evidence* 2002; 8: 184–208. (AI)

Antiplatelet treatment reduces the risk of serious vascular events in people with previous stroke or transient ischaemic attack (TIA) compared with placebo or no antiplatelet treatment. Antihypertensive treatment reduced stroke among people with a previous stroke or TIA, whether they were hypertensive or not. Low-dose aspirin (75–100 mg) daily is as effective as higher doses in the prevention of serious vascular events.

231 PROGRESS Collaborative Group. Randomised trial of a perindopril-based blood-pressure-lowering regimen among 6,105 individuals with previous stroke or transient ischaemic attack. *Lancet* 2001; 358: 1033–1041. (BII)

This blood-pressure-lowering regimen reduced the risk of stroke among both hypertensive and non-hypertensive individuals with a history of stroke or transient ischaemic attack.

232 Sandercock P, Gubitz G, Foley P, Counsell C. Antiplatelet therapy for acute ischaemic stroke (Cochrane Review). In: *The Cochrane Library*, Issue 2, 2003. Oxford: Update Software. (AI)

Nine studies were analysed. Antiplatelet therapy with aspirin at 160–300 mg daily, started within 48 hours of onset of presumed ischaemic stroke, reduces the risk of early recurrent ischaemic stroke without a major risk of early haemorrhagic complications and improves long-term outcome.

233 Antithrombotic Trialists' Collaboration. Collaborative meta-analysis of randomised trials of antiplatelet therapy for prevention of death, myocardial infarction, and stroke in high-risk patients. *Br Med J* 2002; 324: 71–86. (Erratum appears in *Br Med J* 2002; 324: 141.) (AII)

Aspirin (or another oral antiplatelet drug) is protective in most types of patient at increased risk of occlusive vascular events, including those with ischaemic stroke or previous stroke. Low-dose aspirin (75–100 mg) is an effective antiplatelet regimen for long-term use, but in acute settings an initial loading dose of at least 150 mg may be required. Adding a second antiplatelet drug to aspirin may produce additional benefits in some clinical circumstances, but more research into this strategy is needed.

234 Hankey GJ, Sudlow CLM, Dunbabin DW. Thienopyridine derivatives (ticlopidine, clopidogrel) versus aspirin for preventing stroke and other serious vascular events in high vascular risk patients (Cochrane Review). In: *The Cochrane Library*, Issue 2, 2003. Oxford: Update Software. (AI)

Four studies were analysed. Thienopyridine derivatives are modestly but significantly more effective than aspirin in preventing serious vascular events in patients at high risk (and specifically in transient ischaemic attack/ischaemic stroke patients), but there is uncertainty about the size of the additional benefit.

235 Heart Protection Study Collaborative Group. MRC/BHF Heart Protection Study of cholesterol lowering with simvastatin in 20,536 high-risk individuals: a randomised placebo-controlled trial. *Lancet* 2002, 360: 7–22. (CII)

Among the high-risk individuals studied, these antioxidant vitamins appeared to be safe. Although this regimen increased blood vitamin concentrations substantially, however, it did not produce any significant reductions in the five-year mortality from, or incidence of, any type of vascular disease, cancer or other major outcome.

236 Mayou R, Farmer A. ABC of psychological medicine. Functional somatic symptoms and syndromes. *Br Med J* 2002; 325: 265–268

237 Goldberg R, Dennis H, Novack M, Gask L. The recognition and management of somatization: what is needed in primary care training. *Psychosomatics* 1992, 33(1): 55–61. (BV)

238 Smith GR, Rost K, Kashner M. A trial of the effect of a standardised psychiatric consultation on health outcomes and costs in somatising patients. *Arch Gen Psych* 1995, 52(3): 238–243. (BII)

239 Fishbain DA, Cutler RB, Rosomoff HL, Rosomoff HL. Do antidepressants have an analgesic effect in psychogenic pain and somatoform pain disorder? A meta-analysis. *Psychosom Med* 1998, 60(4): 503–509.

240 Speckens A, Van Hemert A, Spinhoven P *et al*. Cognitive behavioural therapy for medically unexplained physical symptoms: a randomized controlled trial. *Br Med J* 1995, 311: 1328–1332. (BII)

Six to 16 sessions of cognitive behaviour therapy were conducted in medical outpatients. Intervention was found to be effective and acceptable to patients, and gains were maintained at 12-month follow-up.

241 Kashner TM, Rost K, Cohen B *et al*. Enhancing the health of somatization disorder patients: effectiveness of short-term group therapy. *Psychosomatics* 1995, 36: 924–932. (BII)

Randomized controlled trial of 70 patients in primary care offered eight sessions of group therapy. Improvement, both physical and emotional, were maintained.

242 Guthrie E. Emotional disorder in chronic illness: psychotherapeutic interventions. *Br Med J* 1996, 168(30): 265–273.

243 Hill P, Taylor E. An auditable protocol for treating attention deficit/hyperactivity disorder. *Arch Dis Child* 2001, 84: 404–409.

The authors suggest a good-practice protocol with a checklist.

244 Jensen PS, Hinshaw SP, Swanson JM *et al*. Findings from the NIMH Multimodal Treatment Study of ADHD (MTA): implications and applications for primary care providers. *J Dev Behav Pediatrics* 2001, 22(1): 60–73. (AII)

This is a randomized controlled trial. Results indicated that medication (usually methylphenidate) and combination interventions were substantially superior to behavioural and community care interventions for attention-deficit hyperactivity disorder symptoms. High-quality medication treatment characterized by careful, yet adequate, dosing, three-times-daily methylphenidate administration, monthly follow-up visits and communication with schools conveyed substantial benefits to those children that received it.

245 A Cochrane Review will be available soon. Zwi M, Pindoria S, Joughin C. Parent training interventions in attention-deficit/hyperactivity disorder (Protocol for a Cochrane Review). In: *The Cochrane Library*, Issue 4, 2003. Oxford: Update Software.

246 National Institute for Clinical Excellence. *Guidance on the Use of Methylphenidate (Ritalin, Equasym) for Attention-Deficit/Hyperactivity Disorder in Childhood*. Technology appraisal guidance No.13, 2000; URL http://www.nice.org.uk. (AI)

Services specializing in attention-deficit/hyperactivity disorder (ADHD) should ensure that methylphenidate is used as part of a comprehensive treatment programme for children with a diagnosis of severe ADHD.

247 Ramchandani P, Joughin C, Zwi M. Attention deficit hyperactivity disorder in children. *Clinical Evidence* 2002, 8: 280–290. (AI)

Methylphendate alone or combined with behavioural treatments and dexamphetamine are beneficial for ADHD.

248 Diggle T, McConachie HR, Randle VRL. Parent-mediated early intervention for young children with autism spectrum disorder (Cochrane Review). In: *The Cochrane Library*, Issue 2, 2003. Oxford: Update Software.

Two studies were analysed. There is some evidence that parent training might provide benefits to both children and parents. However, large-scale randomized controlled trials are needed, to involve both short- and long-term outcome information, to evaluate for which children parent-mediated early intervention might be most beneficial, and to include economic evaluations.

249 Black D. Bereavement. In: Rutter M, Taylor E (eds.) *Child and Adolescent Psychiatry*, 4th edn. Oxford: Blackwell Science, 2002: pp. 299–308.

This is a review of treatments and interventions.

250 Harris-Hendriks J, Black D, Kaplan T. *When Father Kills Mother — Guiding Children Through Trauma and Grief*, 2nd edn. London: Routledge, 2000.

This is a comprehensive review of the effects of traumatic bereavement on children and details of treatments.

251 Sharp S. How much does bullying hurt? The effects of bullying on the personal well being and educational progress of secondary aged students. *Education Child Psychol* 1995, 12(2): 81–88.

252 Hawker D, Boulton M. Twenty years' research on peer victimisation and psychosocial maladjustment: a meta-analytic review of cross-sectional studies. *J Child Psychol Psychiatry* 2000, 42(4): 441–455. (CI)

This is a meta-analysis of cross-sectional studies. Results suggest that victimization is most strongly related to depression, and least strongly to anxiety. There was no evidence that victimization is more strongly related.

253 Deater-Decker K. Recent research examining the role of peer relations in the development of psychopathology. *J Child Psychol Psychiatry* 2001, 42(5): 565–580.

254 Dawkins J. Bullying in schools: Doctors' responsibilities. *Br Med J* 1995, 310: 274–275.

255 Kaltiala-Heino R, Rimpela M, Marttunen M, Rimpela A, Rantanen P. Bullying, depression and suicidal ideation in Finnish adolescents. *Br Med J* 1999, 319: 348–51. (CV)

Adolescents who are being bullied and those who are bullies are at an increased risk of depression and suicide. The need for psychiatric intervention should be considered not only for victims of bullying but also for bullies.

256 Bannon MJ, Carter YH. *The Role of Primary Care in the Protection of Children from Abuse and Neglect*. A joint position paper with the Royal College of Paediatrics and Child Health and endorsed by the NSPCC. London: RCGP Publications, 2003.

257 Home Office/CPS/Department of Health Practice. *Guidance Provision of Therapy for Child Witnesses Prior to a Criminal Trial*. URL http://www.doh.gov.uk/scg/therapy/therapybooklet.htm

258 Kazdin A. Psychosocial treatments for conduct disorder in children. *J Child Psychol Psychiatry* 1997, 38: 161–178. (CII)

This is a literature review. Promising treatments include problem-solving skills training, parent management training, functional family therapy and multisystemic therapy.

259 Scott S, Spender Q, Doolan M *et al*. Multicentre controlled trial of parenting groups for child antisocial behaviour in clinical practice. *Br Med J* 2001, 323: 194–197. (CIII)

Parenting groups effectively reduce serious antisocial behaviour in children in real-life conditions. Follow-up is needed to see if the children's poor prognosis is improved and criminality prevented.

260 Woolfenden SR, Williams K, Peat J. Family and parenting interventions in children and adolescents with conduct disorder and delinquency aged 10–17 (Cochrane Review). In: *The Cochrane Library*, Issue 2, 2003. Oxford: Update Software. (AI)

Eight trials were analysed. Current evidence suggests that family and parenting interventions for juvenile delinquents and their families have beneficial effects on reducing time spent in institutions. This has an obvious benefit to the participant and their family, and may result in a cost saving for society.

261 NICE will publish a guideline on the management of depression in children and adolescents in March 2005.

262 Robin A, Gilroy M, Dennis AB. Treatment of eating disorders in children and adolescents. *Clin Psychol* 1998, 18(4): 421–446. (CIV)

263 Eisler I, Le Grange D, Asen E. Family interventions. In: Treasure J, Schmidt U, van Furth E (eds.) *Handbook of Eating Disorders*. Chichester: John Wiley and Sons, 2003.

264 *Action for Health*, DoH publication about Health Action Plans, available from the Department of Health, PO Box 777, London SE1 6XH, UK.

Acknowledgements

The primary-care guide to mental and neurological disorders would not have been possible without the advice, support and collaboration of primary-care workers, researchers, WHO Collaborating Centres and other agencies. The WHOCC wishes to express its particular thanks to the following for their valuable collaboration.

SECOND EDITION

UK version
Expert input on particular topics was generously provided by the following people.

Adult guidelines
Ms Liz Armstrong, Former Director, National Depression Care Training Centre; Dr Christopher Bass, Consultant in Liaison Psychiatry, Department of Psychological Medicine, The John Radcliffe Hospital, Oxford; Dr Jonathan Bisson, Consultant Liaison Psychiatrist, Department of Liaison Psychiatry, Cardiff and Vale NHS Trust; Dr Mike Boggild, Consultant Neurologist, The Walton Centre for Neurology and Neurosurgery NHS Trust, Liverpool; Lynn Bracewell, National Clinical Classifications Service Manager, NHS Information Authority, Winchester; Dr Tom Brown, Consultant Liaison Psychiatrist, Glasgow Liaison Psychiatry Services, Stobhill Hospital, Glasgow; Professor Terry Brugha, Professor of Psychiatry, Section of Social and Epidemiological Psychiatry, University of Leicester; Dr Josie Butcher, General Practitioner, Director Psychosexual Counselling Service Cheshire and Wirral Partnership Trust, Course Leader and Clinical Director MSc/PGDip Psychosexual Therapy Unit, Central Lancashire; Dr Alan Cohen, Director of Primary Care, Sainsbury Centre for mental health; Cheryl Cowley, Programme Lead Director, HIP for CHD, Nottingham; Dr Mike Crawford, Senior Lecturer in Psychiatry, Imperial College London; Dr Martin Deahl, Consultant Psychiatrist, Shelton Hospital; Gareth Dear, Data Quality and Classification Advisor, National Clinical Classification Services, NHS Information Authority, Winchester; Dr Michael Farrell, Senior Lecturer and Consultant Psychiatrist, National Addiction Centre, Institute of Psychiatry and South London and Maudsley Trust; Professor Gene Feder, Professor of Primary Care Research and Development, Institute of Community Health Sciences, Barts and The London, Queen Mary's School of Medicine and Dentistry; Professor Leslie Findley, Consultant Neurologist, National ME Centre, Disablement Services Centre, Harold Wood Hospital; Professor Peter Goadsby, Wellcome Senior Research Fellow, The Headache Group, Institute of Neurology, National Hospital for Neurology and Neurosurgery, London; Dr Alain Gregoire, Honorary Senior Lecturer and Director, Rural Mental Health Research, Department of Psychiatry, University of Southampton; Dr Andrew Hodgkiss, Consultant Liaison Psychiatrist, Department of Liaison Psychiatry, St Thomas' Hospital, London; Professor Tony Kendrick, Professor of Primary Medical Care, Director of Community Clinical Sciences Division, University of Southampton Medical School; Professor Mike Kerr, Professor of Learning Disability Psychiatry, Honorary Consultant in Neuropsychiatry, University of Wales College of Medicine, Cardiff; Ms Gundi Kiemle, Consultant Clinical Psychologist (Sexual Health), Bolton Hospitals NHS Trust; Professor Malcolm Lader, Emeritus Professor of Clinical Psychopharmacology, Institute of Psychiatry, King's College London; Professor Glyn Lewis, Professor of Psychiatric Epidemiology, University of Bristol; Dr Anne Lingford-Hughes, Senior Lecturer, Division of Psychiatry, University of Bristol; Dr Nicholas Losseff, Institute of Neurology, National Hospital for Neurology and Neurosurgery, London; Dr Heather Major, Senior Medical Advisor, DVLA, Swansea; Professor Isaac Marks, Emeritus Professor of Experimental Psychopathology, Institute of Psychiatry, King's College London; Dr Paul Moran,

Senior Research Fellow, Health Services Research Department, Institute of Psychiatry, King's College London; Professor Greg O'Brien, Professor of Developmental Psychiatry, Northgate Hospital, Morpeth; Ruth Page, Business Analyst/Data Modeller, Data and Information Standards Programme, NHS Information Authority, Winchester; Ms Carol Paton, Chief Pharmacist, Oxleas NHS Trust; Professor Robert Peveler, Professor of Psychiatry, University of Southampton; Professor Tony Pinching, Associate Dean for Cornwall, Peninsula Medical School, Royal Cornwall Hospital; Dr Louise Robinson, Clinical Senior Lecturer in Mental Health for Older People, Centre for Health Services Research, University of Newcastle upon Tyne; Dr Suzanna Rose, Project Leader, Berkshire Traumatic Stress Service; Dr Ulrike Schmidt, Senior Lecturer in Psychiatry, Eating Disorders Research Unit, Institute of Psychiatry, King's College London; Dr Isobel Scriven, Assistant Psychologist, Berkshire Traumatic Stress Service; Professor Tom Sensky, Professor of Psychological Medicine, Imperial College London, Honorary Consultant Psychiatrist, West London Mental Health NHS Trust; Professor Pamela Shaw, Consultant in Neurology, Royal Hallamshire Hospital, Sheffield; Dr David Smart, General Practitioner, Leicester Terrace Health Centre, Northampton; Dr G Mustafa Soomro, Honorary Research Fellow, Community Psychiatry, St George's Hospital, London; Dr George Stein, Consultant Psychiatrist, Farnborough Hospital; Professor Gregory Stores, Professor of Developmental Neuropsychiatry, Department of Psychiatry, University of Oxford; Dr Malcolm Steiger, Consultant Neurologist, The Walton Centre for Neurology and Neurosurgery NHS Trust, Liverpool; Dr Tim Steiner, Reader in Clinical Physiology, Imperial College London, Director and Trustee of World Headache Society and European Headache Federation; Dr Geraldine Strathdee; Consultant Psychiatrist and Clinical Director, Bromley Directorate, Oxleas NHS Trust; Dr Graham Venables, Consultant Neurologist and Clinical Director, Neuroscience, Sheffield Teaching Hospital; Professor Charles Warlow, Professor of Medical Neurology, Clinical Neuroscience, Western General Hospital, Edinburgh; Professor Simon Wessely, Professor of Epidemiological and Liaison Psychiatry, Institute of Psychiatry; Dr Richard Woof, Clinical Lecturer, University of Birmingham, General Practitioner, Corbett Medical Practice, Associate Specialist, St Richard's Hospice, Worcester; Professor AH Young, School of Neurology, Neurobiology and Psychiatry, The Royal Victoria Infirmary, Newcastle-upon-Tyne.

Child and adolescent guidelines
Professor Anthony Bailey, Cheryl and Reece Scott Professor of Psychiatry, University Section of Child and Adolescent Psychiatry, Park Hospital, Oxford; Dr Michael Bannon, Consultant Paediatrician, Northwick Park Hospital, Associate Dean in Postgraduate Medicine, London Deanery; Dr Dora Black, Honorary Consultant Child and Adolescent Psychiatrist, Traumatic Stress Clinic, London; Professor Yvonne Carter, Head of Division of Community Sciences, Barts & The London; Dr Sam Cartwright-Hatton, NHS Executive Research Fellow, University of Manchester Department of Child and Adolescent Psychiatry, Professor Ilana Crome, Academic Director of Psychiatry and Professor of Addiction Psychiatry, Keele University Medical School; Dr Mina Fazel, Warneford Hospital, Oxford; Dr Gillian Forrest, Senior Research Fellow, Section of Child and Adolescent Psychiatry, Oxford University; Professor Elena Garralda, Professor in Child and Adolescent Psychiatry, Imperial College School of Medicine, London; Dr Danya Glaser, Consultant in Child and Adolescent Psychiatry, Great Ormond Street Hospital, London; Professor Ian Goodyer, Professor of Child and Adolescent Psychiatry, Section of Developmental Psychiatry, University of Cambridge; Professor Richard Harrington, Professor of Child and Adolescent Psychiatry, Royal Manchester Children's Hospital; Professor Peter Hill, Department of Psychological Medicine, Great Ormond Street Hospital; Professor Chris Hollis, Head of Division of Psychiatry, University of Nottingham; Dr Lionel Jacobson, Honorary Lecturer, Department of General Practice, University of Wales College of Medicine; Ms Claire Norton, Senior Pharmacist, Birmingham Children's Hospital; Dr Paul Ramchandani, MRC Training Fellow in Health Services Research, University of Oxford Department of

Psychiatry; Dr Gill Salmon, Consultant Child and Adolescent Psychiatrist, Trehafod Child and Adolescent Clinic; Dr Stephen Scott, Reader in Child Health and Behaviour, King's College London, Consultant Child and Adolescent Psychiatrist, Maudsley Hospital; Dr Mima Simic, Child and Adolescent Eating Disorders Team, Institute of Psychiatry, King's College London; Dr TI Williams, Consultant Clinical Psychologist, Berkshire Healthcare NHS Trust, Visiting Research Fellow, School of Psychology, University of Reading

UK National Editorial Team

Professor Edzard Ernst, Professor of Complementary Medicine, Institute of Health and Social Care Research, Peninsula Medical School, Exeter; Professor Rachel Jenkins, Director, WHO Collaborating Centre for Research and Training for Mental Health, Institute of Psychiatry; Dr Barry Lewis, Associate Director Postgraduate GP Education, University of Manchester, General Practitioner, Castleton Health Centre, Rochdale; Dr Albert Persaud, Director of Black and Ethnic Minority R&D Group, Department of Health, London; Professor Debbie Sharp, Professor of Primary Health Care, University of Bristol; Professor Eric Taylor, Professor of Child and Adolescent Psychiatry, Department of Child and Adolescent Psychiatry, Institute of Psychiatry; Jim Thompson, Director, Depression Alliance; Professor André Tylee, Professor of Primary Care Mental Health, Institute of Psychiatry, Chair of the Primary Care Board, NIMHE, Editor, *Primary Care Mental Health*; Professor Charles Warlow, Professor of Medical Neurology, Clinical Neurosciences, Western General Hospital, Edinburgh.

UK National Consensus Groups

Adult guidelines

Ms Melanie Atkinson, Primary Care Mental Health Worker, West Sussex Health & Social Care Trust; Professor Terry Brugha, Professor of Psychiatry, Section of Social and Epidemiological Psychiatry, University of Leicester; Dr Eleanor Cole, Consultant Psychiatrist, South London & Maudsley NHS Trust; Dr Michael Farrell, Senior Lecturer and Consultant Psychiatrist, National Addiction Centre, Institute of Psychiatry and South London & Maudsley NHS Trust; Dr Mark Gabbay, Senior Lecturer in General Practice, University of Liverpool; Professor Rachel Jenkins, Director, WHO Collaborating Centre for Research and Training for Mental Health, Institute of Psychiatry; Professor Tony Kendrick, Professor of Primary Care, Department of Primary Medical Care, University of Southampton; Dr Sue Lamerton, Specialist Registrar in Treatment of Addictions, Gloucester Partnership Trust; Dr Helen Lester, Senior Lecturer in Primary Care, Department of Primary Care, University of Birmingham; Dr Barry Lewis, Associate Director Postgraduate GP Education, University of Manchester, General Practitioner, Castleton Health Centre, Rochdale; Professor Glyn Lewis, Professor of Psychiatric Epidemiology, University of Bristol; Professor Isaac Marks, Emeritus Professor of Experimental Psychopathology, King's College London; Dr Dele Olajide, Consultant Psychiatrist, Maudsley Hospital and Honorary Senior Lecturer, Institute of Psychiatry; Dr Sue Plummer, MRC Fellow in Health Services Research, Institute of Psychiatry, King's College London; Professor Tom Sensky, Professor of Psychological Medicine, Imperial College London, Honorary Consultant Psychiatrist, West London Mental Health NHS Trust; Professor Debbie Sharp, Professor of Primary Health Care, University of Bristol; Dr David Shiers, Primary Care Lead, NIMHE, West Midlands, General Practitioner, North Staffordshire; Jim Thompson, Director, Depression Alliance; Professor Nigel Wellman, Professor of Health and Human Sciences, Thames Valley University & Consultant Nurse, Berkshire Healthcare NHS Trust; Professor Simon Wessely, Professor of Epidemiological and Liaison Psychiatry, Institute of Psychiatry; Dr Richard Woof, Clinical Lecturer, University of Birmingham, General Practitioner, Corbett Medical Practice, Associate Specialist, St Richard's Hospice, Worcester

Child and adolescent guidelines

Professor Elena Garralda, Professor in Child and Adolescent Psychiatry, Imperial College School of Medicine, London; Professor Richard Harrington, Department of Child Health and Adolescent Psychiatry, Royal Manchester Children's Hospital; Dr Danya Glaser, Consultant Child and Adolescent Psychiatrist, Great Ormond Street Hospital; Professor Robert Goodman, Professor of Brain and Behavioural Medicine, Institute of Psychiatry; Dr John James, Consultant to the Institute for Health Sector Development, London; Dr Barry Lewis, Associate Director Postgraduate GP Education, University of Manchester, General Practitioner, Castleton Health Centre, Rochdale; Dr Quentin Spender, Consultant and Senior Lecturer in Child and Adolescent Psychiatry, West Sussex Health and Social Care NHS Trust and St George's Hospital Medical School, London; Professor Eric Taylor, Professor of Child and Adolescent Psychiatry, Department of Child and Adolescent Psychiatry, Institute of Psychiatry; Mr Mervyn Townley, Consultant Nurse, CAMHS, Gwent NHS Trust

Commentators

Adult guidelines

Professor Johan A. Aarli, Professor of Neurology, Chairman, Department of Clinical Neurosciences, University of Bergen, Liaison Officer to FRO and to WHO; Dr Shakeel Ahmad, Consultant General, Adult and Neuropsychiatry; Mary Baker, President of Parkinson's Disease Association, President of the European Federation of Neurological Associations, Vice President of the European Brain Council; Dr Anthony Bateman, Consultant Psychiatrist in Psychotherapy/Honorary Senior Lecturer, Royal Free and University College Medical School, London; Professor Dinesh Bhugra, Professor of Mental Health and Cultural Diversity, Institute of Psychiatry; Dr MF Boyle, General Practitioner, The Health Centre, Linlithgow; Professor Julian Bogousslavsky, Chairman, Department of Neurology, Lausanne, President-Elect, International Stroke Society; Professor Alistair Burns, Professor of Mental Health in the Elderly, Withington Hospital; Professor Chris Butler, Professor of Primary Care Medicine, Department of General Practice, University of Wales College of Medicine; Dr Richard Byng, Honorary Lecturer in General Practice and Primary Care, GKT, King's College, London; Professor David Clark, Professor of Psychology and Head of Department, Department of Psychology, Institute of Psychiatry; Dr Alan Cohen, Director of Primary Care, Sainsbury Centre, Chair of the London Regional Development Centre; Professor Arthur Crisp, Emeritus Professor of Psychological Medicine, University of London at St George's Hospital Medical School; Professor Anke Ehlers, Wellcome Principal Research Fellow, Department of Psychology, Institute of Psychiatry; Professor Chris Fairburn, Wellcome Principal Research Fellow and Professor of Psychiatry, Department of Psychiatry, University of Oxford; Dr Andrew Farmer, Department of Primary Health Care, University of Oxford; Professor Anne Farmer, Professor of Psychiatric Nosology, Institute of Psychiatry; Professor Mark Freeston, Director of Research and Training, Newcastle Cognitive and Behaviour Centre; Dr Mark Gabbay, Senior Lecturer in General Practice, University of Liverpool; Dr Clare Gerada, Director of Primary Care NHS Clinical Governance Support Team, RCGP Director of Drugs Training Unit, General Practitioner; Professor Else Guthrie, Professor of Psychological Medicine and Medical Psychotherapy, Department of Psychiatry, Manchester Royal Infirmary; Dr Willie Hamilton, Research Fellow, University of Bristol; Dr Margaret Hannah, Consultant in Public Health, Fife NHS Board; Dr Madelyn Hicks, Consultant Psychiatrist, South London & Maudsley NHS Trust, Lecturer, Department of Social Medicine, Harvard Medical School, Honorary Research Worker, Department of Health Services Research, Institute of Psychiatry; Chris Holley, Consultant Nurse, Sexual Abuse and Women's Issues, South Staffordshire Healthcare NHS Trust; Professor Sheila Hollins, Professor of Psychiatry of Learning Disability, Department of Mental Health, St George's Hospital Medical School, London; Professor Amanda Howe,

Professor of Primary Care, School of Medicine, Health Policy & Practice, University of East Anglia; Dr Steve Iliffe, Department of Primary Health Care, Royal Free and University College Medical School, London; Dr Navneet Kapur, Senior Lecturer in Psychiatry, Centre for Suicide Prevention, University of Manchester; Professor Tony Kendrick, Professor of Primary Care, University of Southampton; Dr David Kessler, Senior Clinical Research Fellow, Division of Primary Health Care, Bristol University; Professor Mike King, Professor of Psychiatry, Royal Free and University College Medical School, London; Professor Shon Lewis, Professor of Adult Psychiatry, School of Psychiatry and Behavioural Sciences, University of Manchester; Dr Anne Lingford-Hughes, Senior Lecturer, Division of Psychiatry, University of Bristol; Professor Alistair MacDonald, Professor of Psychiatry of Old Age, Lewisham and Guy's Mental Health Trust, London; Dr Viv Mak, Consultant in Psychiatry of the Elderly; Professor Anthony Mann, Professor of Epidemiological Psychiatry, King's College London; Professor Isaac Marks, Emeritus Professor of Experimental Psychopathology, King's College London; Dr Robert Mayer, GP Principal, Highgate Group Practice, London; Dr Colin Murray Parkes, Consultant Psychiatrist, St Christopher's Hospice, Syndenham and St Joseph's Hospice, Hackney, Life President of Cruse Bereavement Care, Editor *Bereavement Care*; Professor Sheila Payne; Dr Jack Piachaud, Consultant in Learning Disability, St Mary's Hospital, London; Dr Sue Plummer, MRC Fellow in Health Services Research, Institute of Psychiatry; Dr Nikki Rizvi, General Practitioner, London; Dr Suzanna Rose, Project Leader, Berkshire Traumatic Stress Service; Dr Chiara Samele, Non-Clinical Lecturer and Senior Researcher, Institute of Psychiatry, King's College Hospital; Professor Debbie Sharp, Professor of Primary Health Care, University of Bristol; Dr David Shiers, Primary Care Lead, NIMHE, West Midlands, General Practitioner, North Staffordshire; Dr Tim Steiner, Reader in Clinical Physiology, Imperial College London, Director and Trustee of World Headache Society and European Headache Federation; Dr Tim Stokes, Senior Lecturer in General Practice, Clinical Governance Research & Development Unit, University of Leicester; Professor Graham Thornicroft, Section of Community Psychiatry, Institute of Psychiatry; Professor André Tylee, Professor of Primary Care Mental Health, Institute of Psychiatry, Chair of the Primary Care Board, NIMHE, Editor, *Primary Care Mental Health*; Dr Graham Venables, Consultant Neurologist and Clinical Director, Neurosciences, Sheffield Teaching Hospital.

Child and adolescent guidelines
Professor Yvonne Carter, Head of Division of Community Sciences, Barts & The London; Dr Tim Chambers, Consultant Physician and Nephrologist, Bristol Royal Hospital for Sick Children; Dr Myra Cooper, Isis Education Centre, Warneford Hospital, Oxford; Dr Judith Dawkins, Consultant Child and Adolescent Psychiatrist, Surrey; Dr Sharon Davies, Institute of Psychiatry, London; Dr Mary Eminson, Consultant Child and Adolescent Psychiatrist, CAMHS, Royal Bolton Hospital; Dr Isobel Heyman, Consultant Child Psychiatrist, Department of Child Psychiatry, Institute of Psychiatry, London; Dr Gillian Forrest, Senior Research Fellow, Section of Child and Adolescent Psychiatry, Oxford University; Dr Willie Hamilton, Research Fellow, University of Bristol; Dr Bob Jezzard, Department of Health, London; Professor Joe Kai, Professor of Primary Care, University of Nottingham; Dr Daphne Keen, Consultant Developmental Paediatrician, Community Child Health, St George's Hospital, London; Dr Barry Lewis, Associate Director Postgraduate GP Education, University of Manchester, General Practitioner, Castleton Health Centre, Rochdale; Dr Aidan Macfarlane, Independent International Consultant in the Strategic Planning of Child and Adolescent Services; Dr Robert Mayer, GP Principal, Highgate Group Practice, London; Dr Julian Morrell, Consultant Child and Adolescent Psychiatrist, Winnicott Research Unit, Department of Psychology, Reading University; Dr George Smerdon, General Practitioner, St Ives, Huntingdon; Dr Quentin Spender, Consultant and Senior Lecturer in Child and Adolescent Psychiatry, West Sussex Health and Social Care NHS Trust and St George's Hospital Medical School, London; Dr Jennifer Tyrrell, Consultant Paediatrician, Royal United Hospital, Bath; Dr Avril Washington,

Consultant Paediatrician, Homerton University Hospital, London; Professor Bill Yule, Professor of Applied Child Psychology, Institute of Psychiatry, London.

References: Rachel Churchill and Hugh McGuire of The Cochrane Collaboration Depression, Anxiety & Neurosis group (CCDAN), Institute of Psychiatry, graded and provided comment on the references and provided the Cochrane reviews. *Codes*: Dr Alan Cohen of the Sainsbury Centre for Mental Health, Cheryl Cowley, Health Information and Nurse Practitioner, The National Programme for IT (NPfIT) — Primary Care Team, Lynn Bracewell, National Clinical Classifications Service Manager NHS Information Authority, Winchester and Gareth Dear, Data Quality and Classification Advisor, National Clinical Classification Service, NHS Information Authority, Winchester supplied the equivalent clinical terms for the ICD-10 codes. *Resources*: Ruth Jenkins, Mike Morgan and Lynette Timms checked the contact details for the resources section. *Project Management*: Overall project management was initiated by Dr Sue Collinson and completed by Lucy Gardner, under the direction of Rachel Jenkins.

FIRST EDITION

Expert input on particular topics was generously provided by the following people.

Dr Sube Banerjee, Dr Tom Carnwath, Professor Anna Cooper, Dr Michael Crowe, Dr Katy Drummond, Dr Jim Dyer, Dr Mike Farrell, Dr Mark Gabbay, Dr Clare Garrada, Dr Linda Gask, Professor Sir David Goldberg, Professor Sheila Hollins, Dr Gundi Kiemle, Professor Tony Kendrick, Professor Malcolm Lader, Professor Alistair MacDonald, Professor Isaac Marks, Mr John Park, Mr Stephen Popplestone, Ms Sue Plummer, Professor Jan Scott, Dr Ulrike Schmidt, Dr James Strachan, Mr David Taylor, Dr André Tylee, Dr John Turvill, Professor Simon Wessely. Jo Paton researched the evidence base and compiled the references and notes section and adapted the patient leaflets. Lynette Timms checked all the contact details for the Community Resources.

UK National Editorial Team
David Goldberg, Linda Gask, Rachel Jenkins, Barry Lewis, Jo Paton, Debbie Sharp, André Tylee. Overall management and co-ordination of the project was carried out by Jo Paton, under the direction of Rachel Jenkins.

UK National Consensus Group
Ms Elizabeth Armstrong, Director, National Depression Care Training Centre; Dr Sube Banerjee, Lecturer, Institute of Psychiatry, Dr Mary Burd, Primary Care Psychology and Counselling Service; Dr Richard Byng, Lecturer, Department of General Practice and Primary Care, UMDS; Professor Anna Cooper, Professor of Psychiatry and Learning Disability, Glasgow University; Dr Katie Drummond, Psychiatrist of Disability; Ms Joan Foster, Chair, Counsellors in Primary Care; Dr Mark Gabbay, Senior Lecturer, Department of General Practice, Liverpool University; Dr Clare Garrada, RCGP Mental Health Task Force and Senior Policy Advisor, Department of Health; Dr Linda Gask, Reader in Psychiatry, University of Manchester; Professor Sir David Goldberg, Professor of Psychiatry, Institute of Psychiatry; Professor Glyn Harrison, Professor of Psychiatry, Bristol University; Professor Sheila Hollins, Department of Psychiatry of Disability, St George's Hospital; Professor Rachel Jenkins, Director, WHO Collaborating Centre for Research and Training for Mental Health; Professor Tony Kendrick, Professor of General Practice, University of Southampton; Dr David Kessler, GP, PriMHE; Professor Malcolm Lader, Professor of Clinical Psychopharmacology, Institute of Psychiatry; Dr Chris Manning, GP, co-Chair PriMHE; Dr Richard Maxwell, GP, PriMHE; Ms Sue Plummer, Research Nurse, Department of Psychiatric Nursing, Institute of Psychiatry; Professor Debbie Sharp, Professor of General Practice, University of Bristol; Professor Simon Wessely, Institute of Psychiatry; Dr Ellen Wilkinson, Lecturer, Department of Mental Health, Bristol

University; Dr Alastair Wright, GP, formerly Editor, *British Journal of General Practice*; Ms Jo Paton, Researcher, Institute of Psychiatry.

Commentators

The following people also provided valuable comments: Marion Beeforth, Service User; Nigel Duerdoth, Mental Health Foundation; John Mellor Clark, Psychological Therapies Research Centre; Dr Peter Orton, GP Advisor, Royal Society of Medicine; Dr Salman Rawaf, Public Health Department, MSW Health Authority; Ms Jackie Carnell, General Secretary, Community Practitioners and Health Visitors Association; Ms Jo Hesketh, Director, The Queens Nursing Institute; Ms Karen Gupta, Chair, Practice Nurse Forum, Royal College of Nursing; Mr Ian Moore, Community Mental Health Team Association; Brian Rodgers, Community Psychiatric Nurse Association.

International version

J Banda (Zambia), D Berardi (Italy), A Bertelsen (Denmark), E Busnello (Brazil), A Carla (France), J E Cooper (UK), N Dedeoglu (Turkey), M P Deva (Malaysia), D Goldberg (UK), M Gomel (Australia), O Gureje (Nigeria), C Hunt (Australia), R Jenkins (UK), S Murthy (India), K Ogel (Turkey), C Pull (Luxembourg), D Roy (Canada), G E Simon (USA), P Verta (France), M Von Korff (USA) and N Wig (India).

D Goldberg and G E Simon were chief consultants for the project and compiled the information for each category of disorder.

Overall management and coordination of the project was carried out by Dr T B Ustun.

World Organization of National Colleges and Academies and Academic Associations of General Practitioners/Family Physicians (WONCA)
C Bridges-Webb and H Lamberts.

World Psychiatric Association
N Sartorius and JJ López-Ibor Jr.

National Institute of Mental Health, USA
K Magruder, D Reiger, J Gonzalez and G Norquist.

Bristol version

The editorial team were Catherine Crilly, Jonathan Evans, Glynn Harrison, Gemma McCann, Debbie Sharp, Cameron Smith, Ellen Wilkinson. Brendan Blair assisted with the guide to the Mental Health Act.

Permissions

We are grateful to the following organizations who kindly granted copyright permission for us to reproduce or adapt their work:

Radcliffe Medical Press: The School Refusal guideline was adapted from School refusal. In: Spender Q, Salt N, Dawkins J *et al.* (eds.) *Child Mental Health in Primary Care*. Oxford: Radcliffe Medical Press, 2001.

The World Health Organization Division of Mental Health and Substance Abuse: Material from *Mental Disorders in Primary Care: a WHO Educational Package*: Patient leaflets numbers 3–2, 4, 6, 9 and 10, all the interactive summary cards and the diagnostic checklists.

World Health Organization Collaborating Centres in Mental Health, Sydney and London: Extracts from Andrews G, Jenkins R (eds.) *Management of Mental Disorders*, UK Edition. Sydney: World Health Organization Collaborating Centre for Mental Health and Substance Abuse, 1999 — used in patient leaflets numbers 1, 2, 3, 5, 7–2, 8 and 9 and Social and living skills checklist (11–4).

Mental Health Foundation: Extract from *Managing Anxiety and Depression: a Self-Help Guide*, used in patient leaflet 1–2.

Nottingham Alcohol and Drug Team: Extract from *Problem Drug Use*, used in patient leaflet 7–1.

This Guide has been endorsed by the following groups:

WHO Collaborating Centre for Mental Health Research & Training, Institute of Psychiatry, King's College London

The Royal College of Psychiatrists

The Royal College of General Practitioners

The Royal College of Physicians Joint Specialty Committee for Neurology

The Royal College of Nursing

NIMHE (National Institute for Mental Health in England)

Neurological Alliance

European Federation of Neurological Association

The Patients Association

PriMHE (Primary Care Mental Health Education)

Mental Health Nurses Association

The Association of Counsellors and Psychotherapists in Primary Care

The Queen's Nursing Institute

Community Practitioners' and Health Visitors' Association

www.mentalneurologicalprimarycare.org

Interactive summary cards

The pages that follow contain summaries of information about the six disorders most common in primary care.

These are designed to be used interactively within the consultation, to help the practitioner explain key features of the disorder to the patient and enter into discussion about a possible management plan. They can be printed out and mounted on either side of an A4 card for ease of use.

Mental health in primary care
Alcohol problems

There is one unit of alcohol in:
½ pint of ordinary strength beer, lager or cider
¼ pint of extra strength beer, lager or cider
1 small glass of white (8 or 9% ABV) wine
⅔ small glass of red (11 or 12% ABV) wine
1 single measure of spirits (30 ml)

Common symptoms

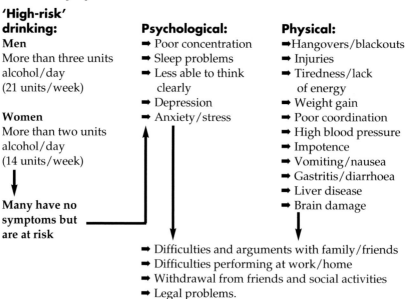

'High-risk' drinking:

Men
More than three units
alcohol/day
(21 units/week)

Women
More than two units
alcohol/day
(14 units/week)

Many have no symptoms but are at risk

Psychological:
➡ Poor concentration
➡ Sleep problems
➡ Less able to think clearly
➡ Depression
➡ Anxiety/stress

Physical:
➡Hangovers/blackouts
➡ Injuries
➡ Tiredness/lack of energy
➡ Weight gain
➡ Poor coordination
➡ High blood pressure
➡ Impotence
➡ Vomiting/nausea
➡ Gastritis/diarrhoea
➡ Liver disease
➡ Brain damage

➡ Difficulties and arguments with family/friends
➡ Difficulties performing at work/home
➡ Withdrawal from friends and social activities
➡ Legal problems.

Alcohol problems are treatable
Alcohol problems *do not* mean weakness
Alcohol problems *do not* mean you are a bad person
Alcohol problems *do* mean that you have a medical problem or a lifestyle problem.

What treatments can help?
Both therapies are most often needed:

Supportive therapy:
➡ to reduce drinking
➡ to stop drinking
➡ for stress
➡ for prevention of life problems
➡ for education of the family members for support.

Medication:
➡ for moderate to severe withdrawal
➡ for physical problems
➡ consider for relapse prevention.

Alcohol problems

Set goals: acceptable levels of drinking

Who?	How many drinks?	How often?
Men	No more than three units	Each day (only for five days/week)
Women	No more than two units	Each day (only for five days/week)

Have two non-alcohol drinking days/week.

Keep in mind: the less the person drinks, the better it is.

➡ Pregnancy
➡ Physical alcohol dependence
➡ Physical problems made worse by drinking
➡ Driving, biking
➡ Operating machinery
➡ Exercising (swimming, jogging, etc.)

➡ Recommendation is not to drink

Determine action: how to reach target levels

➡ Keep track of your alcohol consumption
➡ Turn to family and/or friends for support
➡ Have one or more non-alcoholic drinks before each drink
➡ Delay the time of day that you drink
➡ Take smaller sips

➡ Engage in alternative activities at times that you would normally drink (eg when you are feeling bored or stressed)
➡ Switch to low-alcoholic drinks
➡ Decide on non-drinking days (two days or more per week)

➡ Eat before starting to drink
➡ Join a support group
➡ Quench your thirst with non-alcoholic drinks
➡ Avoid or reduce time spent with heavy-drinking friends
➡ Avoid bars, cafés or former drinking places.

Review progress: are you keeping on track?

Questions to ask:
➡ Am I keeping to my goals?
➡ What are the difficult times?
➡ Am I losing motivation?
➡ Do I need more help?

Progress tips:
➡ Every week, record how much you drink over the week
➡ Avoid these difficult situations or plan activities to help you cope with them
➡ Think back to your original reasons for cutting down or stopping
➡ Come back for help, talk to family and friends.

Mental health in primary care
Anxiety

Common symptoms
Psychological:
- Tension
- Worry
- Panic
- Feelings of unreality
- Fear of going crazy
- Fear of dying
- Fear of losing control

Physical:
- Trembling
- Sweating
- Heart pounding
- Light headedness
- Dizziness
- Muscle tension
- Nausea
- Breathlessness
- Numbness
- Stomach pains
- Tingling sensation

Disruptive to work, social or family life

Anxiety disorders are common and treatable
Anxiety *does not* mean weakness
Anxiety *does not* mean losing the mind
Anxiety *does not* mean personality problems
Severe anxiety *does* mean a disorder which requires treatment.

Common forms of anxiety

Generalized anxiety disorder:
- Persistent/ excessive worry
- Physical symptoms.

Panic disorder:
- Sudden intense fear
- Physical symptoms
- Psychological symptoms.

Social phobia:
- Fear/avoidance social situations
- Fear of being criticized
- Physical symptoms
- Psychological symptoms.

Agoraphobia:
- Fear/avoidance of situations where escape is difficult
- Leaving familiar places alone
- Physical symptoms
- Psychological symptoms.

What treatments can help?
Both therapies are most often needed:
Supportive therapy for:
- slow breathing/relaxation
- exposure to feared situations
- realistic/positive thinking
- problem solving.

Medication:
- for severe anxiety
- for panic attacks.

Anxiety

About medication

Short term
➡ use for severe anxiety
➡ can be addictive and ineffective when used in the long term

Side-effects
➡ are important to report

Counselling
➡ (emotional support and problem-solving) is always recommended with medication

Ongoing review
➡ of medication use is recommended.

Slow breathing to reduce physical symptoms of anxiety

➡ Breath in for three seconds and out for three seconds, and pause for three seconds before breathing in again.
➡ Practise 10 minutes morning or night (five minutes is better than nothing).
➡ Use before and during situations that make you anxious.
➡ Regularly check and slow down breathing throughout the day.

Change attitudes and ways of thinking

'My chest is hurting and I can't breathe, I must be having a heart attack.'

Instead:

'I am having a panic attack, I should slow my breathing down and I will feel better.'

'I hope they don't ask me a question, I won't know what to say.'

Instead:

'Whatever I say will be OK, I am not being judged. Others are not being judged, why should I be?'

'My partner has not called as planned. Something terrible must have happened.'

Instead:

'They might not have been able to get to a phone. It is very unlikely that something terrible has happened.'

Exposure to overcome anxiety and avoidance

Easy stage ⟶ **Moderate stage** ⟶ **Hard stage**
(eg walking on own) (eg lunch with a friend) (eg shopping with a friend)

➡ Use slow breathing to control anxiety
➡ Do not move to the next stage until anxiety decreases to an acceptable level.

Mental health in primary care
Chronic tiredness

Common symptoms

Compared with previous level of energy, and compared with people known to you:

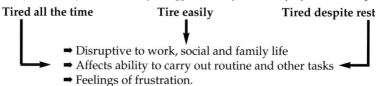

Tired all the time   **Tire easily**   **Tired despite rest**

➡ Disruptive to work, social and family life
➡ Affects ability to carry out routine and other tasks
➡ Feelings of frustration.

Chronic fatigue syndrome is a much rarer condition, diagnosed when substantial physical and mental fatigue lasts longer than six months and there are no significant findings on physical or laboratory investigation.

Common triggers

Psychological triggers:
➡ Depression
➡ Stress
➡ Worry
➡ Anxiety.
➡ Doing too much activity
➡ Doing too little activity.

Physical triggers:
➡ Anaemia
➡ Bronchitis
➡ Asthma
➡ Diabetes
➡ Arthritis.
➡ Thyroid disorder
➡ Influenza
➡ Alcohol/ drug use
➡ Bacterial, viral and other infections.

Medication:
➡ Steroids
➡ Antihistamines.

What treatments can help?
Both therapies are most often needed:

Supportive therapy for:
➡ depression
➡ worry/anxiety
➡ stress/life problems
➡ lifestyle change
➡ level of physical activity.

Medication:
➡ for other mental or physical disorders
➡ anti-depressants are sometimes useful
➡ there are no effective medications specific to fatigue and the main treatment follows psychological lines.

Chronic tiredness

Behavioural strategies

➡ Examine how well you are sleeping.

➡ Have a brief rest period of about two weeks, in which there are no extensive activities.

➡ After the period of brief rest, gradually return to your usual activities.

➡ Plan pleasant/enjoyable activities into your week.

➡ Gradually build up a regular exercise routine.

➡ Do not push yourself too hard; remember to build up all activities gradually and steadily.

➡ Try to have regular meals during the day.

➡ Try to keep to a healthy diet.

➡ Use relaxation techniques, for example, slow breathing.

Slow breathing for relaxation

➡ Breath in for three seconds

➡ Breath out for three seconds

➡ Pause for three seconds before breathing in again

➡ Practise for 10 minutes at night (five minutes is better than nothing).

Increase level of physical activity

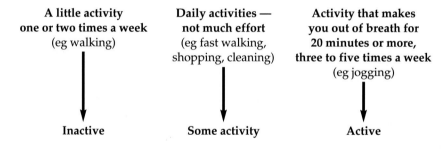

A little activity one or two times a week (eg walking)	Daily activities — not much effort (eg fast walking, shopping, cleaning)	Activity that makes you out of breath for 20 minutes or more, three to five times a week (eg jogging)
↓	↓	↓
Inactive	**Some activity**	**Active**

Mental health in primary care
Depression

Common symptoms

Mood and motivation:
- ➡ Continuous low mood
- ➡ Loss of interest or pleasure
- ➡ Hopelessness
- ➡ Helplessness
- ➡ Worthlessness

Psychological:
- ➡ Guilt/negative attitude to self
- ➡ Poor concentration/ memory
- ➡ Thoughts of death or suicide
- ➡ Tearfulness

Physical:
- ➡ Slowing down or agitation
- ➡ Tiredness/lack of energy
- ➡ Sleep problems
- ➡ Disturbed appetite (weight loss/increase)

- ➡ Difficulties carrying out routine activities
- ➡ Difficulties performing at work
- ➡ Difficulties with home life
- ➡ Withdrawal from friends and social activities.

Depression is common and treatable

- ➡ Depression *does not* mean weakness
- ➡ Depression *does not* mean laziness
- ➡ Depression *does mean* that you have a medical disorder which requires treatment.

Common triggers

Psychological:
Major life events, eg
- ➡ Recent bereavement
- ➡ Relationship problems
- ➡ Unemployment
- ➡ Moving house
- ➡ Stress at work
- ➡ Financial problems.

Other:
- ➡ Family history of depression
- ➡ Childbirth
- ➡ Menopause
- ➡ Seasonal changes
- ➡ Chronic medical conditions
- ➡ Alcohol and substance use disorders.

Illness:
- ➡ Infectious diseases
- ➡ Influenza
- ➡ Hepatitis.

Medication:
- ➡ Antihypertensives
- ➡ H2 blockers
- ➡ Oral contraceptives
- ➡ Corticosteroids.

What treatments can help?

Both therapies are most often needed:

Supportive therapy for:
- ➡ stress/life problems
- ➡ patterns of negative thinking
- ➡ prevention of further episode.

Medication:
- ➡ for depressed mood or loss of interest/ pleasure for two or more weeks and at least four of the symptoms mentioned earlier
- ➡ for little response to supportive therapy (counselling)
- ➡ for recurrent depression
- ➡ for a family history of depression.

About medication

Effective
Usually works faster than other methods.
Treatment plan
must be strictly adhered to.
Drugs
➡ are not addictive
➡ interact in a harmful way with alcohol
➡ improvement takes time, generally three weeks for a response
➡ do not take in combination with St John's wort.

Side-effects
must be reported, but generally start improving within 7–10 days.
Progress
➡ same medication should continue unless a different decision is taken by the doctor
➡ medication should not be discontinued without doctor's knowledge in case a drug is not effective, another drug may be tried.

Time period
Medication to be continued at least four to six months after initial improvement.
Ongoing review
is necessary over the next few months.

Increase time spent on enjoyable activities

➡ Set small achievable, daily goals for doing pleasant activities
➡ Plan time for activities and increase the amount of time spent on these each week

➡ Plan things to look forward to in future
➡ Keep busy even when it is hard to feel motivated
➡ Try to be with other people/family members.

Problem-solving plan

Discuss
problems with partner/family members, trusted friend or counsellor.
Distance
yourself to look at problems as though you were an observer.

Options
Work out possible solutions to solve the problems.
Pros and cons
Examine advantages and disadvantages of each option.

Set a time frame
to examine and resolve problems.
Make an action plan
for working through the problems over a period of time.
Review
progress made in solving problems.

Change attitudes and way of thinking

'I will always feel this way; things will never change.'

Instead:

'These feelings are temporary. With treatment, things will look better in a few weeks.'

'It's all my fault. I do not seem to be able to do anything right.'

Instead:

'These are negative thoughts that are the result of depression. What evidence for this do I really have?'

Mental health in primary care
Sleep problems

Common symptoms

→ Difficulty falling asleep
→ Frequent awakening

→ Early morning awakening
→ Restless or unrefreshing sleep

→ Difficulties at work and in social and family life
→ Makes it difficult to carry out routine or desired tasks.

Common causes

Psychological:	Physical: Medical problems:	Lifestyle:	Environmental:
→ Depression	→ Overweight	→ Too hot or too cold	→ Noise
→ Anxiety	→ Heart failure	→ Tea, coffee and alcohol	→ Pollution
→ Worries	→ Nose, throat and lung disease	→ Heavy meal before sleep	→ Lack of privacy
→ Stress.	→ Sleep apnoea	→ Daytime naps	→ Over-crowding.
	→ Narcolepsy	→ Irregular sleep schedule.	
	→ Pains.		
	Medication:		
	→ Steroids		
	→ Decongestants		
	→ Others.		

What treatments can help?

Supportive therapy is the preferred treatment

Supportive therapy for:
→ stress/life problems
→ depression
→ worry
→ changes in lifestyle and sleep habits.

Medication:
→ for temporary sleep problems
→ for short-term use in chronic problems to break sleep cycle.

Sleep problems

About medication

Short term
→ use for short period of time.

Long term
→ when used in the long term, there may be difficulties stopping, leading to dependence.

Side-effects
→ are important to report.

Harmful
→ when alcohol and other drugs are used.

Ongoing review
→ of medication use is recommended.

Lifestyle change strategies

→ Try to minimize noise in your sleep environment; if necessary consider ear plugs.

→ Try to make sure that the room in which you are sleeping is not too hot or cold.

→ Reduce the amount of alcohol, coffee and tea that you drink, especially in the evenings.

→ Try to avoid eating immediately before going to sleep.

→ Try to have your dinner earlier in the evening, rather than later.

→ Don't lie in bed trying sleep. Get up and do something relaxing until you feel tired.

→ Have regular times for going to bed at night and waking up in the morning.

→ Reduce mental and physical activity during the evenings.

→ Increase your level of physical activity during the day; build up a regular exercise routine.

→ Avoid daytime naps, even if you have not slept the night before.

→ Use relaxation techniques, eg slow breathing.

Slow breathing for relaxation

→ Breath in for three seconds
→ Breath out for three seconds
→ Pause for three seconds before breathing in again
→ Practise for 10 minutes at night (five minutes is better than nothing).

More evaluation may be needed:
→ if someone stops breathing during sleep (sleep apnoea)
→ if there is a daytime sleepiness without possible explanation.

Mental health in primary care
Unexplained somatic complaints

Common, unexplained physical problems

- Headaches
- Chest pains
- Difficulty in breathing
- Difficulty in swallowing

- Nausea
- Vomiting
- Abdominal pain
- Lower back pain

- Skin rashes
- Frequent urination
- Diarrhoea
- Skin and muscle discomfort.

Associated worries and concerns

- Associated symptoms and problems
- Beliefs (about what is causing the symptoms)
- Fear (of what might happen).

Physical symptoms are real

A vicious circle can develop:
- Emotional stress can cause physical symptoms or make them worse.
- Physical symptoms can lead to more emotional stress.
- Emotional stress can make physical symptoms worse.

Headaches
Difficulty in swallowing
Chest pain/difficulty in breathing   →
Abdominal pain/nausea/vomiting
Frequent urination/diarrhoea/impotence
Skin rashes

may all be
caused or made worse
by stress, anxiety
worry, anger, depression

What treatments can help?

Supportive treatment most often needed:

- Effective reassurance, after history and detailed physical examination.
- Management of stress/life problems.
- Treatment of associated depression, anxiety, alcohol problems.
- Learning to relax.
- Avoiding patterns of negative thinking.
- Increasing levels of physical activity.
- Increasing positive/pleasurable activities.

Unexplained somatic complaints

Useful strategies

Reassurance
➡ Stress often produces physical symptoms or makes them worse.
➡ There are no signs of serious illness.
➡ You can benefit from learning strategies to reduce the impact of your symptoms.

Slow breathing to reduce common physical symptoms
(eg muscle tension, hot and cold flushes, headaches, chest tightness)
➡ Breath in for three seconds and out for three seconds and pause for three seconds before breathing in again.
➡ Practise 10 minutes morning or night (five minutes is better than nothing).
➡ Use before and during situations that make you anxious.
➡ Regularly check and slow down breathing throughout the day.

Change attitudes and way of thinking

'I can't understand why the tests are negative. I feel the pain; it is probably something really unusual that I have.'

Instead: 'The pain is real, but I've been checked out physically and I have had all the relevant tests. Many other things, such as worry and stress, can cause these pains.'

'Maybe my doctor has missed something. I should try another doctor or better still a specialist instead.'

Instead: 'It is very unlikely that these doctors have missed something. It is unlikely that a specialist would say anything different. Maybe I should examine whether stress, tension, or my lifestyle is contributing to the pain.'

'Why won't this pain go away. I'm not feeling well; I've probably got cancer.'

Instead: 'This is not the first time that I've thought that there was *something* terribly *wrong* and *in fact* nothing serious developed. I should learn to relax and focus my thoughts on other things to distract myself from the pains.'

Increase level of physical activity

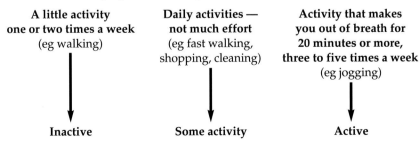

A little activity one or two times a week (eg walking)	Daily activities — not much effort (eg fast walking, shopping, cleaning)	Activity that makes you out of breath for 20 minutes or more, three to five times a week (eg jogging)
Inactive	Some activity	Active

Index